Healing Traditions

University of Pennsylvania Press
Studies in Health, Illness, and Caregiving

Joan E. Lynaugh, General Editor

A complete listing of the books in this series is available from the publisher

Publications of the American Folklore Society
New Series

Elaine Lawless, General Editor

Healing Traditions

Alternative Medicine and the
Health Professions

Bonnie Blair O'Connor

PENN

University of Pennsylvania Press

Philadelphia

10 9 8 7 6 5 4 3 2

Published by
University of Pennsylvania Press
Philadelphia, Pennsylvania 19104-4011

Library of Congress Cataloging-in-Publication Data
O'Connor, Bonnie Blair.
  Healing traditions: alternative medicine and the health
professions / Bonnie Blair O'Connor.
     p.   cm. — (Studies in health, illness, and caregiving)
(Publications of the American Folklore Society. New series)
  Includes bibliographical references and index.
  ISBN 0-8122-3184-8 (cloth). — ISBN 0-8122-1398-X (paper)
  1. Alternative medicine—United States.   2. AIDS (Disease)—
Alternative treatment—United States.   3. Hmong Americans—
Medicine.   I. Title.   II. Series.   III. Series: Publications of the
American Folklore Society. New series.
[DNLM: 1. Alternative Medicine.   2. Health Services
Research—United States.   WB 890 018h 1994]
R733.036   1994
610—dc20
DNLM/DLC
for Library of Congress   94-32190
                                                                      CIP

For Malachi

Contents

Illustrations

Acknowledgments

Suppose a book appears, as this one does, under the name of a single author. This curious selective recognition of one person who happened to put together a number of ideas and write them down in a certain way obscures the efforts and contributions of many others. It conjures images of the lone scholar diligently producing "a work." But, while many aspects of the production of a book are quite solitary, it is fundamentally a social operation, actively involving many people in many processes: providing information, generating and recombining ideas, stimulating thinking, offering critiques, managing the logistics, and providing the degree of exemption from other social obligations that the one who writes requires.

My greatest debt of gratitude is to my husband, Mal O'Connor. My intellectual companion as well as my sweetheart and my friend, he has had an incalculable and sustaining role in this enterprise. He has listened and discussed endlessly, contributing many insights and refinements. An amazing organizer, he often jotted notes as I poured forth confusion; these he crystallized quickly into cogent outlines that furnished me the framework of my arguments and enabled me to write through them. He claims he only gave back what he heard, but what he heard was always honed by his keen analytical abilities on its way to the note page. He has shown amazing grace and patience throughout this project, and often had more fortitude than I. During the three-month "home stretch," while I did nothing but go to work and write, Mal did literally everything else it takes to run a house and keep a life together. I am dearly beholden to him for all of his love, participation, support, and unstinting generosity.

My intellectual debt to Dave Hufford is apparent throughout the book. For years I have benefited from his pioneering approach to this subject matter, his rigorous logic, his careful concern with definition, his astute and constructive criticism, and his warmly collaborative nature. He has shared many of his own papers and manuscripts with me in their formative stages, and has helped me to develop my arguments both by suggestion and by his own extraordinary example. He has been a valued teacher, colleague, and friend who has offered many sound and careful critiques and plenty of moral support. After many years of our ongoing discussion I cannot always separate what I take to be my thoughts from the foundation he has laid and the insights he has inspired. More often than I am able to know it and give it, credit for an idea probably ought to go to Dave.

Much of the content of this work was furnished by my informants and field consultants over the years. Many people have participated, often giving hospitality as well as insights and information. They have been willing to entrust to me their privacy, their experiences of sickness and health, and the explication of some of their most cherished beliefs. Their collective personal knowledge and experience became my data. For this project I am especially indebted to the members of the Hmong and PWA communities of Philadelphia for their immeasurable help. Ironically, it is quite possible that a number of the people who contributed so much of its substance may never see this book. In several instances we met and parted as strangers, with warm and animated hours of conversation in between. Some will have no appetite for an academic description of much that they already know. Some do not read English. Some are no longer living. I hope that I have represented them all well and fairly, for I am to a certain extent their scribe.

Colleagues too have been generous with their time and expertise. Jonathan Lax and Dave Hufford have been true mentors, for whom I am most appreciative. Thanks to Ray Birdwhistell, Bruce Thowpaou Bliatout, Janet Fleetwood, Randi Freedman, Diane Goldstein, Dave Hufford, Kiyoshi Kuromiya, Jonathan Lax, June Lowenberg, Joan Lynaugh, Mal O'Connor, Sally Peterson, Anne Scott, Patricia Smith, Xoua Thao, and Barre Toelken for having read (and sometimes re-read) earlier drafts of various chapters or sections and offered their expert advice and critiques. They have saved me from some egregious errors, but are certainly in nowise responsible for any that remain. Jonathan Lax and Kiyoshi Kuromiya gave expert advice and helped to guide portions of my fieldwork. Christian Fuersich raised the term "research assistant" to new heights of meaning in his thoroughness, insight, persistence, and personal involvement with the outcome; safe to say the manuscript would not have met its deadline without his considerable efforts. Dave Zuckerman provided essential research and production assistance and critical technical backup; Nicole Witoslawski produced the graphics; Monica Lawton handled tedious but critical details; and Thalawyn cheerfully chased down innumerable articles for months on end. All of these people made critical contributions to the book which I could not have provided myself.

Portions of my fieldwork were supported in part by a University of Pennsylvania Research Foundation seed grant and by the Lois Mattox Miller Fellowship in Medical Humanities at the Medical College of Pennsylvania. Warwick Anderson secured the grant that made the HIV clinical practice survey possible, and wrestled skillfully and good-naturedly with its results. Our collaboration and colleagueship have been a pleasure. My colleagues in the Department of Community and Preventive Medicine at the Medical College of Pennsylvania have been extraordinarily accommodating, giving me latitude and taking up my slack on a number of occasions, for which I owe them many thanks.

I am richly blessed with family members who love me, and who are my friends as well as my kin. I am deeply grateful to my parents and in-laws, Pat and Sissy Blair and Mal and Tina O'Connor, for moral and financial support and boundless encouragement, and to the rest of my family—Lisa Blair, Lula Mae Jones, and my brothers- and sisters-in-law—for love and forbearance, and for cheering me on. To many other friends not named, my gratitude for their kindness for keeping me in their attentions and affections during a pretty long stretch of antisocial behavior and precious little reciprocity. I hope they'll all hold me to my promises to act like a regular human again "after the book."

Introduction

In addition to conventional Western medicine, there are a great number and variety of systems of health belief and practice active in the United States today. Far from dying out in the face of advances in scientific medicine, many nonbiomedical health belief systems are growing in popularity. Included among these are both long-standing traditional systems (often referred to as "folk medicine") and newer developments and syncretisms such as the many approaches grouped together under the rubrics of holistic health or New Age healing (sometimes referred to as "popular medicine"). I refer to this entire range of folk and popular healing modalities as vernacular health belief (or healing) systems. Together with conventional medicine, these vernacular health care resources constitute a pluralistic American health culture. Contrary to entrenched stereotypes, use of vernacular health care modalities is not confined to "marginal" groups, and only a small number of such systems are used to the virtual exclusion of conventional medicine.

It is now fairly well established that ordinary people's health care strategies frequently involve the use of *both* conventional medical and nonconventional approaches, in varying combinations. Use of nonconventional modalities may be undertaken on an occasional or event-specific basis, or as a part of routine preventive and therapeutic health behavior. This pattern is found across ethnicities, races, social classes, religious preferences, and educational statuses. The possibilities encompass healing modalities ranging from religious and metaphysical practices, to mental and spiritual contemplation, to physical and manipulative therapies, to dietary regimens and supplements, to botanical medicines; and frames of reference ranging from traditional or revitalized ethnic cultures, to humanistic holism, to patient activism, to New Age self-empowerment and self-improvement philosophies.

This book is a study of vernacular health belief systems, and of some of the ways in which people's experiences, beliefs, and values influence their health care choices. It addresses the issues of how people define health and illness; how and why people believe they become sick; how they decide what to do about it; under whose care they decide to do which things; and what some of the implications of these beliefs and decisions are for health professionals in the conventional Western medical system. The health beliefs and practices examined in this study are representative of the United States in the 1980s and 1990s. The belief systems cited as examples have originated in a wide range of cultural contexts and geographic locations. They have long histories, substantial social support, and reputations for efficacy sustained by experience and observation. Even the most recently developed variations, however innovative or novel their syntheses of philosophies and practices may appear, have deep historical roots in other healing traditions. All of the systems illustrated in this work are in active use here and now. In fact, many are enjoying a renewal of vigor and an expansion of clients and proponents, and this revitalization is also taking place on an international scale.

Purpose and Intent

I intend for this work to be equally useful to social scientists and to health professionals, and to have practical applications as well as theoretical and descriptive interest and value. I mean for the messages to come clear that nonbiomedical health belief systems are alive and well everywhere; that their use is rational and purposeful; and that their use is something that specific cultural heritage groups as well as so-called "mainstream" Americans have in common (Hufford 1988a). I am convinced that it behooves clinicians and health planners to be aware of this phenomenon, and to learn how to respect it and work *with* it, confining their objections only to those aspects that are medically dangerous. This will require considerable rethinking on the part of academic and medical authorities. It raises the larger issues of patients' values and points of view, and of their authoritative agency: patients decide what they are going to do about their health, including whether and when to go to the conventional medical system, and how to respond to medical advice. It raises the matter of why health professionals ought to engage patients as whole and reasonable people who bring with them to the clinical encounter many resources that shape both that encounter and many other aspects of their general health, illness, and care.

I use the term "health belief systems" and several variants thereof. In this category I include conventional, Western, scientific, "official" medicine equally with folk and popular (vernacular) healing, and the usage should be understood in this inclusive sense throughout the work. It is not my intention to evaluate specific health belief systems or their claims, nor to adopt either a partisan or an adversarial position with respect to any system. I cannot speak to efficacy, except to report how users of various healing systems understand and evaluate it. Rather, I hope to demonstrate ways in which health belief systems can be thoroughly investigated and described in their own terms, holding judgments in abeyance until adequate information is available upon which to base them, and until judgment is absolutely necessary. It is important that inspection of these commonly employed health care resources not be made only through the prescriptive lens of the conventional medical system if we are to gain a genuine understanding of what people actually do to take care of their health in addition to (and sometimes instead of) going to the doctor.

In this sense, this work is a plea for academic and professional neutrality and open-mindedness. Through neutral observation (neither advocating nor condemning), it is possible to achieve careful descriptions of the variety of health belief systems active in the United States; to understand how reasonable and intelligent people make use of them; to understand what differing systems hold in common and where they diverge; to appreciate the rational interconnections of their elements; and to identify some likely points of conflict among them. To the extent that any may conflict with conventional biomedicine, only a genuine understanding of the goals and rationales of all parties can facilitate efforts to come to an equitable resolution: one in which the values and mandates of professionals and laypersons alike have received full and fair consideration, and in which the desired degree of participation of the layperson (or patient) in determining the course of his or her own care has been encouraged and respected.

With these goals in mind, I ask readers to consider the ways in which the two broad domains of conventional medicine and vernacular health systems are similar and different. All are rooted in and shaped by particular cultural milieux. They selectively assign importance to a variety of phenomena and interpret them according to culturally derived theories and assumptions. They are alike in their essential structural elements and in the mental processes that are involved in making assessments and arriving at conclusions. Each is dedicated to what is internally defined to be proper treatment of sickness and promotion of health. Neither domain is monolithic, for each encompasses a tremendous variety of values, convictions, mandates, preferences, and practices. Greater than their internecine differences and disagreements, however, are the essential differences between these two broad domains: differences in worldview and content, in the range of concerns they address, in their modes of activity, in their sources of knowledge, in their internal structures for legitimation, and in their relative positions of legitimacy or accreditation in the larger society.

Research Settings and Methods

This work applies ethnographic methods to the study of health beliefs and practices as they are readily discoverable on the American landscape. Participant observation, field interviews, and the personal narratives of informants and field consultants provide the bulk of the primary data for my illustrative examples and for the two detailed studies that comprise the third and fourth chapters. The broad foundation of this work has included twelve years of field interviews and participant observation with clients, healers, and teachers in a wide variety of vernacular health belief systems. These open-ended interviews have been designed to elicit descriptions of specific health beliefs and practices in an ongoing attempt to discover (1) how people form and act upon their beliefs about the nature and causes of health and illness and the goals and means of treatment; and (2) how users of nonconventional health care modalities construct their relationships with conventional medicine. The bulk of this fieldwork has been conducted in the greater Philadelphia and surrounding tri-state area (Pennsylvania, New Jersey, Delaware).

Questions motivating the research have included: How are health belief systems interconnected with the larger cultural systems of which they are a part? How do people learn about, enter into, and evaluate vernacular health belief systems? What is the relationship between specific experiences (of sickness, of recovery, of both conventional and vernacular healing interventions) and a person's health beliefs? How do specific values and experiences shape perceptions of and responses to health, illness, and care? To what extent do personal beliefs and values incongruent with those of biomedicine affect patient modification of conventional therapeutic regimens? Under what circumstances do people decide to alter or augment conventional medical care? How do people come to have the "courage of their convictions" or to rely upon the authority of their own experience in making health care decisions? How and when can accommodations be made between proponents of belief systems that are divergent or even in some respects mutually contradictory?

Group-specific ethnographic fieldwork forms the basis of two descriptive chapters, which make a pair of contrast studies: of a small ethnic minority group and one person's illness, and of a large "mainstream" population and a widespread epidemic. One study describes the course of negotiations between conventional medicine and a young

Hmong man with chronic liver disease, while the other looks at the tremendous range of vernacular responses to HIV/AIDS in the mostly white, middle-class, gay PWA community. Fieldwork consisted of participant observation in a wide variety of settings, cross-cultural mediation, and direct interviewing. These chapters help to illustrate in some detail the differences that are possible between laypersons' points of view and the medical model. Taken together, they also illustrate that use of nonbiomedical healing strategies is found in all kinds of population cross sections.

One case study recounts the interaction of a young Hmong refugee and the American biomedical system. I first met Mr. L. through my husband, who collaborated with him on a Hmong oral history project in 1984 and 1985. We were friends at the time he became ill in 1987, and it was through our friendship that I became involved with his case. During the discovery and occasional acute episodes of his chronic illness over the next couple of years, I acted on many occasions as a mediator between Mr. L. (and members of his family and community) and the physicians and nurses providing both his inpatient and outpatient medical care. In this role, my task was to explain to both the Hmong and the medical cultural groups the health-related ideas, goals, preferences, objections, and restrictions held by the other group, and to facilitate, where possible, a negotiated settlement on treatment and follow-up care. My role was purely explanatory, never advisory. During the course of these years, I spoke at length with Mr. L. and various family and community members, sometimes in formal interviews and often conversationally. Most of my participant observation was carried out at two university-affiliated teaching hospitals, in both inpatient and outpatient units, medical and surgical services. Some took place at family and community events. Few interviews were tape-recorded, owing largely to the circumstances under which they were conducted. Exchanges reported in this chapter are reconstructed from field notes made both during and immediately following clinical encounters and during informal conversations, and are excerpted from verbatim transcripts of those interviews that were recorded.

The second study deals with the alternative therapies movement for HIV/AIDS. I became involved in this work through interest in testing a hypothesis. It seemed likely that wherever there was a serious disease for which conventional medicine had little to offer, there would be alternative therapies: people actively engaged in seeking their own treatments, unwilling to wait for the imprimatur of science and medicine. I joined two or three of the local grass-roots AIDS organizations, got on their mailing lists, and began to go to their meetings. I subscribed to the grass-roots and "underground" newsletters as I found out about them. I could never have anticipated the astonishing extent and sophistication of what I was about to learn. My fieldwork began with participant observation in alternative therapies discussion groups sponsored by the local organizations. Approximately thirty-five people attended the groups that I attended during a period of four months; almost all were gay men. In consideration of the privacy of the participants, no tape recordings were made at these meetings. I soon gained a generous and knowledgeable mentor and a couple of well-informed advisors in the community, who helped to guide my fieldwork and background research and who reviewed my interpretations of data. I became a co-investigator in a clinical practice survey seeking information about uses of alternative therapies, and subsequently began to conduct extensive ethnographic interviews with people who had used alternative therapies. Exchanges reported are reconstructed from field notes of participant observations, cited from correspondence and conversations with members of the community, and drawn from verbatim transcripts of tape-recorded interviews of the later stages of fieldwork (still in progress at the time of this writing).

The HIV/AIDS case study illuminates the development of a vernacular health care treatment, support, and information network under conditions of medical urgency coupled with dissatisfaction with institutional responses. Epidemics provide exceptional conditions for documenting the proliferation and dissemination of therapeutic responses, both conventional and vernacular, and for examining the special strains placed on the socially sanctioned accreditation agencies by the lack of adequate "legitimated" treatments. The use of vernacular therapies for HIV/AIDS is extensive, but it is as yet relatively little documented in the medical or social science literature. On the other hand, abundant information, continually updated, can be found in the gay press, in treatment-specific grass-roots newsletters, and in private print and oral circulation in the PWA (People with AIDS) community.

A Note on Usages

In this book, I refer to or draw examples from a large number of health belief systems. A few are described in considerable detail, while others are summarized very briefly, or referred to almost in passing. Each of these systems is as complex in its workings and underlying theories as is modern biomedicine; several have been the subjects of numerous books. I have had to summarize in many places, as including comprehensive descriptions of every system mentioned would have made this into an encyclopedic work of several volumes. Book-length references for specific systems are given in textual citations and in notes, for those wishing to find more complete information. I ask the understanding of readers who are quite well versed in these systems, for the limitations that a work of this type imposes on thoroughness of representation.

Any description of a belief system is to some extent a composite and an idealization: it reflects the assembly within a single descriptive sweep of as many of the components of a complex repertoire as have come to the writer's notice. It represents only a "freeze-frame" moment in a dynamic and always-changing phenomenon. Several caveats apply. Naturally, there will be things that have been simplified and things that have been missed. Naturally, too, no individual participant in a system represents (or has even *heard of*) all of the aspects of the "big picture." There is as much diversity within a system as there is among systems. To avoid endless tangential disclaimers and digressions, it is necessary to refer to systems and their participants in generalizations much of the time, and to use vague terms like "many" and "most" to discuss trends and prevalent attitudes. Attempts to be too precise would distort the tremendous complexity and infinite variability of the actual picture of vernacular health belief and practice.

Readers are asked to accept these usages as they are intended, and to recall at every mention of any group or belief system that none of us must permit generalizations that are descriptive conveniences to become or to contribute to stereotypes of individuals or of populations. Two other linguistic conveniences also require explanation: (1) "health beliefs" should be taken to imply associated practices or behaviors, even where not expressly mentioned; and (2) "medicine" or "medical" should be taken to refer broadly to the professional health care system, whose branches and subdivisions incorporate the "medical model," and not to refer only to physicians and their practices.

All informants and participants in my fieldwork are identified in the ways in which they have preferred to be named. Some are identified by their own initials, some by pseudonymous initials; some by two initials, and some only by one. Where actual full names of healers, their clients, or field consultants and informants are used, it is with their express permission. While this variation of usage precludes tidy consistency throughout the book, I have found it appropriate and pleasing because it reflects the individual preferences of those who have furnished me with the material to make a book.

Audience

The audience for whom this work is written is intended to be wide and diverse. I hope that it will be useful to health professionals and healers of all sorts, to social scientists and behavioral scientists of various disciplinary affiliations, to educators of many stripes, and to other generally interested parties. I have tried to avoid overuse of disciplinary jargon and have included a glossary to help to translate the indigenous terms of one discipline for readers from other linguistic training grounds, as well as to make clear the specific operational meanings I intend for some common terms. As I am a folklorist, I have written as a folklorist, and my greater familiarity with my own discipline will show. This should not be construed as a suggestion that the knowledge or methods of the discipline of folklore are superior to those of other disciplines or systems, nor that they should replace respected methods in use in other disciplines and venues. I wish to stress not merely the utility and productivity but the absolute necessity of interdisciplinary collaboration in addressing and understanding the subject matter of this work. Equally, I wish to stress the necessity of including in this interdisciplinary enterprise not only the academic or conventional professional bodies of knowledge, but also the vernacular and the nonconventional professional bodies of knowledge.

Synopsis of Contents

The focal point of this study is the meeting of conventional, institutionalized medical values and the great variety of vernacular belief and practice which, taken together, make up the full spectrum of contemporary American health care resources. The book sets out some terms by which studies of nonconventional healing systems can be made, studies that can be used to facilitate interactions between conventional medicine and other health belief systems. Descriptive and theoretical points are illustrated throughout by examples drawn from a variety of vernacular health belief systems that are quite active in the United States at the present time.

Chapter 1 establishes operational definitions for essential terms, identifies the central propositions and theoretical orientation of the book, and introduces a schema for studying belief systems both individually and comparatively. All health belief systems, including conventional medicine, are treated as products of culture, shaped by the cultural contexts in which they arise. My interpretive framework is the cultural construction of knowledge and of descriptions of reality (Berger and Luckmann 1967). Health belief systems are discussed as rational cognitive constructs—a characteristic which can form the basis for negotiation between or among divergent belief systems (such as conventional medicine and any vernacular health belief system). Conformity of basic assumptions or final conclusions with those of the officially accredited, academic canon of knowledge is considered an inaccurate and inappropriate criterion for gauging the rationality of a vernacular belief system.

Chapter 2 briefly summarizes the literature of several fields that have dealt with folk belief and with folk medicine or vernacular health belief systems. The review includes descriptions of the analytical frameworks used by various disciplines, theories of culture and of the production of knowledge, attitudes taken toward the subject of "unofficial" belief and practice, and the relationships of observer to observed which have shaped research and analysis in this complex subject area.

Chapters 3 and 4 provide in-depth descriptions of two vernacular health belief systems and their interactions with conventional medicine: Hmong traditional culture and its views on health, illness, and other related concerns; and the HIV alternative therapies movement.

The fifth and final chapter expands the discussion into broader considerations of cultural influence, cultural diversity, and the importance of the patient's point of view with respect to health, illness, and care. Illustrations focus on provider education, medical ethics, and the issues of patient education and "compliance." I urge a reallocation of authority in relations between patients and health professionals, one which grants genuine recognition to patients as agents of their own health care. Such a move will require (among other things) recognition of the actual prevalence and distribution of vernacular health beliefs and practices, and a grasp of the larger cultural systems with which they and conventional medicine are interconnected. An appendix contains some curriculum materials, guidelines, and exercises applicable to this task.

It is the confluence of vernacular and professional health care activities which comprises the actual range of American health care resources and forms the nexus of health behavior. I submit that both patients and providers will benefit from professional recognition of and response to these facts of American life and health care.

Chapter 1
Defining and Understanding Health Belief Systems

Throughout this century and even before, there has been a general assumption—even a conviction—in the health professions and in academia that folk and popular systems of health beliefs and practices would inevitably decline in modern and industrialized societies, falling away before the forces of modernization and progress to be replaced by modern, Western medicine. Yet this has not been the case. Nonbiomedical healing systems have persisted steadily alongside the burgeoning medical establishment: some waxing and waning in cycles, some holding constant, and some continually gaining in popularity among widening and diversifying circles of proponents. In the past two decades especially, there has been a significant reinvigoration and expansion of nonconventional healing systems of all sorts. As we near the threshold of the twenty-first century, there are an enormous number and variety of health belief systems active in the United States, in addition to conventional biomedicine. Certain of these systems are very closely allied to specific ethnic groups and are largely derived from the group's culture of origin or ancestry. Some systems, whether ethnically identified or not, have a very specific religious or denominational foundation. Others have an appeal that cuts across lines of ethnicity, religion, and social class; and still others are associated almost exclusively with educated, middle-class, "mainstream" groups.

A second prevalent assumption—also misleading—has been the notion that those people who have recourse to nonconventional healing practices are most likely to do so *instead of* resorting to the biomedical system, and this impression has given rise to a good deal of frustration and concern in the health professions. While there are undeniably some belief systems that do discourage use of conventional medical resources, these are relatively few and do not accurately represent the entire range of the pluralistic health care environment of the United

States today. With or without the awareness or acceptance of the health professions, laypeople's health belief systems are integral parts of the psychosocial context of health and illness. They are the sources of an enormous repertoire of substances and actions that are taken for the express purposes of preventive and therapeutic health care, by people of all races, ethnicities, religious persuasions, social classes, and educational exposures. These facts of the current American health care landscape emphasize a need for better understanding of nonconventional health belief systems, whose prevalence and popularity commend them to the attention of social scientists and perforce make them matters of relevance for clinicians. Better understanding requires serious consideration, which in turn calls for a framework within which open-minded studies of nonconventional healing systems can be made. Good studies and enhanced understanding, besides contributing to the advancement of knowledge about the society in which we live, have practical applicability to the establishment of working relationships between conventional medicine and other health belief systems, health professionals' and patients' viewpoints, to the benefit of all involved.

Remapping the Territory

The very first step in this enterprise is to tackle the matter of conceptualizations and definitions, and the values and assumptions they encode. A number of academic disciplines have made studies of, or reference to, healing systems other than modern Western medicine. Too often, these studies have been plagued with prejudgments and value-laden terminology, which have in some cases entirely precluded accurate presentation of information about the systems being studied. Pejorative names such as "superstition" (false belief about causal relations, generally involving supernatural or magical implications), "popular errors" (misconceptions among the laity), "old wives' tales" (silly notions, a term that simultaneously derides the tales and their tellers) and "quackery" (properly defined as medical charlatanism involving deliberate deception) have sometimes been used as polemical devices intentionally to denigrate the beliefs and practices to which they refer. In other cases, they have actually been intended simply to describe, but have carried belittlement into the discussion just as surely. In any genuinely dispassionate inquiry into the nature of nonconventional healing systems, terms must be chosen with precision and care. Conclusions must follow, not precede, collection of data. If the discussion is to be open, descriptive terms whose definitions classify their referents a priori as erroneous, frivolous, or fraudulent must be dismissed as contrary to the purposes of serious investigation.

Other common descriptive terms, such as "primitive," "ethnic," "marginal," "deviant," and "unorthodox" medicine, are factually misleading in many cases, while in others they simply carry an unfortunate connotative load. For example, consensual definitions for "primitive" include archaic, of or resembling a presumed early mental developmental stage, rudimentary, simplistic, and naïve. Use of the term to describe health belief systems outside of the tradition of modern Western medicine implies (1) that such systems are outmoded, simpleminded, or somehow developmentally antecedent to sophisticated thought, and (2) that the people who use them might be expected to show the same traits. This characterization is unsupported by investigation of health belief systems themselves, even when their claims disagree with accepted medical or scientific thought. Such assumptions have contributed to erroneous conceptualizations both of the development of modern thinking and of the meaning, character, and social location of nonconventional health beliefs and practices. Use of the term "ethnic medicine" as a general descriptor for such healing systems gives the twin mistaken impressions that they are mostly found among members of ethnic minority groups, and that "they represent a sort of survival that may be expected eventually to disappear through acculturation" (Hufford 1984:24). "Marginal" means near or beyond the limits of acceptability, and so also implies inadequacy; "deviant" denotes significant departure from an accepted norm but also connotes aberrance; while "unorthodox" carries the ring of oddity, if not of heresy. All three are imbued with suggestions of the devalued and bizarre. Thus each of these terms also puts either an explicit or implicit negative spin on its description, inseparably intertwining evaluative and descriptive functions.

It is difficult to find or forge adequate language in which simply to name and describe, without imposing a connotative judgment. Because the very actions of naming and describing presuppose a particular point of view and often carry moral tone, they frequently go beyond identification to convey a sense of whether the thing named is good or bad.[1] Thus, all general descriptive terms for health belief systems, to be useful as descriptions rather than opinions, must be considered to be *relative* terms whose complete meaning can be derived only from an understanding of their contexts of use and their relationships to one another. In the above-mentioned instances, for example, one would have to ask, "marginal, deviant, or unorthodox compared to what?" The answer implied or stated in much of the academic and scientific literature of the West is "compared to modern, scientific, Western medicine," which in those contexts is commonly taken to be the only correct system of health care and the standard against which other systems may be measured for adequacy.

In much of what has been written on the subject of "other" health belief systems, they have been evaluated on the extent to which they approximate or depart from, or can be recast in terms of, the categories and beliefs of the dominant (Western medical) system. The degree of novelty or incorrectness ascribed to these systems is typically in direct proportion to the extent of their departure from the modern, Western, scientific medical model (Levin and Idler 1981). Such an approach discourages production of the thorough, factual, and unprejudiced descriptions of differing health belief systems needed for practical applications to compare, understand, and facilitate negotiations among various points of view. Further, it fosters a pervasive sense among professional "experts" that nonconventional approaches to health care are probably suspect in one or several respects, and that patients and clinicians alike might be better off if these beliefs and practices were abandoned or stamped out. Such a perspective mitigates against successful intersystem negotiation, and overlooks the salience and significance of nonbiomedical healing systems as resources for coping with illness. To the extent that prior professional and academic inquiry about health belief systems has carried a medicocentric bias, these systems need to be reconceptualized—at least for investigative purposes—and approached as value-neutral. In order to reach reliable conclusions about health belief systems and their contexts of use, we first need adequate and undistorted data. To see all systems clearly—and this caveat holds equally true for the homeopath and the herbalist, the social scientist and the public health researcher, the physician and the nurse-practitioner—it is necessary to avoid looking only through prescriptive spectacles that privilege our own preferences.

Frame of Reference and Definition of Terms

In the United States, as in any complex society, there is an encompassing "official"—that is, authorized and authoritative—culture, which coexists with any number of distinctive cultural subsets.[2] The sanctioned practices, values, and institutions of the official culture are backed by considerable social, economic, and political power. Among these official values is the singular prestige accorded to science and its associated professions, and the sanction of formal education and academically legitimated research procedures (with a strong emphasis on scientific experimentation) as the primary—if not the sole—valid means to knowledge. Among the official institutions is a single authorized and legitimated system of health care.

I use this official system of health beliefs and practices as a point of reference for further definitions and as a counterpoint to the other health belief systems illustrating this study, for the practical reason that the audiences for which this work is intended are most likely linked to it in some way (as its scholars, members, clients, or professional colleagues, and sometimes as its critics), and familiar with its worldview. I do not use the official health care system as a standard against which to measure other systems' adequacy, but simply as a familiar touchstone having the broadest general utility for illustrative comparisons. As culturally elaborated responses to the common human issues of health, illness, and care, both "official" and "unofficial" health belief systems are and should be subject to description and analysis by the same methods and general models. When this kind of "methodological symmetry" (Hufford, personal communication) is observed, inquiry is freest from prejudice, and informational and practical outcomes are most productive.

In general usage, the official health belief system is referred to by a range of terms, of which some very common ones include "biomedicine," "orthodox medicine," and simply "medicine." For my purposes, "medicine" is too broad a term to be restricted to describing a single system, and "orthodox" is too evaluative and doctrinaire, conveying a moral suggestion of especial propriety. "Biomedicine" is a convenient shorthand term, although it is perhaps underinclusive (passing over such fields as behavioral, family, and community medicine which have significant non-biological components—but that is another issue). I have settled on referring to the officially sanctioned medical system of modern Western societies as "conventional" medicine, recognizing that "conventional" is itself a relative and context-dependent term.[3] This designation (though cumbersome at times) has the advantage of moral neutrality, and it accurately describes the position of the official health belief system in the United States and similar societies, with its connotation of that which is widely considered normative, usual, and customary. The conventional medical system enjoys the approval, cooperation, and protection of the country's legal system and other supporting social institutions: government licensing and regulatory bodies, third-party payment systems, preferred access to federal and private research monies, high prestige and social status and their concomitant benefits, including professional associations with substantial lobbying power and professional publications with influential reputations for authority. By contrast, all other health belief systems in the United States are unofficial (Hufford 1988a, 1992a) and can be described collectively as being "nonconventional," especially with reference to individual breadth of membership and to the aforementioned social support structures.

Nonconventional health belief systems are frequently subdivided as "folk" or "popular" in terms of attributes of the system and of its participant groups (Kleinman 1980, 1984; Hufford 1984, 1988a). Generally, systems with constituent groups small enough that they can rely largely on oral tradition and apprenticeship for the teaching of tenets and the training of practitioners, and which are sustained largely in specific speech communities or close associative networks, have been those designated "folk." Examples include the Pennsylvania German powwow tradition, or the *Santería* religious and healing tradition of Afro-Hispanic Caribbean origin. The classification "popular" has been applied to systems relying significantly on print and other media, and frequently having formal institutions and curricula for participant instruction or practitioner training (e.g., naturopathy or chiropractic). These distinctions have utility for some purposes, especially insofar as they can provide a general predictive principle; that is, "popular" systems are more likely to be similar in content from region to region within the country than are "folk" systems, which vary in details of content and meaning according to regional differences in culture as do all folk cultural expressions (Hufford 1984). This predictive principle is useful only as a rule of thumb, for considerable variation also exists among clients and practitioners in "popular" systems; "folk" systems do have stable cores of elements across wide geographic distributions; and the two realms borrow freely from one another (and from conventional medicine).

For general descriptive purposes, all of the nonconventional or unofficial health belief systems and their local, familial, and personal variations can be classed together, in contradistinction to conventional medicine, as constituting a discrete domain in which health care actions occur. I designate them collectively as "vernacular health belief (or healing) systems," taking vernacular to mean native to or firmly held by the people who use the system.[4] This too is a relative, or comparative, term. The analogy is to vernacular language, which, in the sense of "the mode of expression of a group or class," is contrasted with an officially sanctioned, formal, or idealized spoken form: that is, how people *actually* speak, as opposed to how a textbook of grammar dictates that they should properly speak. The perspective is descriptive, rather than prescriptive. By extension, in matters of health and illness, "vernacular" refers not to what people supposedly do or "ought" to do according to an official set of standards, but to what they *actually* do when they are sick, when they wish to prevent sickness, or when they are responsible for others who are ailing. This usage of vernacular (as in the subjects of vernacular architecture or vernacular religion [Primiano 1987, 1990, 1993]), includes values, ideas, beliefs, and the practices associated with them under the rubric of "mode of expression."

Constructing Belief and Knowledge

Central to this study is the concept of the cultural construction of reality (Berger and Luckmann 1967). This is the view, now largely accepted throughout the social sciences, that knowledge and descriptions of reality are culturally shaped; that facts are not "discovered whole" in nature, but are constructed out of selective observations and interpretations, according to shared, often tacit, rules and values.[5] Societies, cultures, and subcultural groups (including academic and professional disciplines) have particular worldviews: intricate, systematic "ways of seeing," of apprehending and defining reality, which are patterned and encoded at all levels of perception and expression (Toelken 1975). Worldviews differ from one group to another to varying degrees—in some circumstances having large areas of congruence, in others diverging radically. Differences in worldview establish fundamentally different conceptions of what constitutes a supportive argument or an adequate explanation, and different conceptions of what appears to require explanation in the first place (Jones 1976). Worldviews determine the character of what is real or true, and how it is reliably to be known.

Recognition of the existence of differences in worldview raises the issue of the distinctions drawn between "belief" and "knowledge," and the means for determining which is which. *Belief* is "a conviction or feeling that something is real or true"; the "intellectual assent to an idea" which is based upon that conviction (Angeles 1981); or the "mental acceptance of a proposition, statement, or fact, as true, on the ground of authority or evidence" (Oxford English Dictionary). *Knowledge* is the "condition of apprehending truth or fact" (Merriam-Webster's Collegiate Dictionary, Tenth Edition), or of "acquaintance with ascertained truths, facts, or principles"; and *fact* is "what has actually happened or is the case; truth attested by direct observation or authentic testimony" (OED). *Knowledge* entails *belief* that particular propositions or assertions are factual or true on the basis of some justification or evidence that sufficiently supports them. The definitions of these terms, far from standing in clear opposition to one another, are juxtaposed and interdependent. Belief and knowledge both involve mental or intellectual acceptance of something as true, actual, or real on the basis of some form of authoritative support for the conclusion. Close inspection reveals them to be more similar than dissimilar to one another in definition and suggests no sure criterion for determining across the board the absolute difference between cases of belief and cases of knowledge.

Belief and knowledge, then, are also relative terms whose meanings

are context-dependent. In practical applications, the difference between them is positional and often political, dependent in part upon
who may exercise the right to say what shall count as information of
one order or another. In common usage, we tend to refer to our own
accepted certainties as "knowledge" and to the claims of others as
"belief" when these are incongruent with or contradictory to our own
categories and claims (see Hufford 1977b). In scholarship, the assumption is that "the cutting edge of the distinction is usually the scholar's
own 'knowledge'" (Hufford 1976a:12): reference to the accepted
canon of an academic discipline or, quintessentially for modern and
complex Western societies, to science. This attitude is inherently ethnocentric, for it takes the accepted beliefs of one's own culture or identity
group to be universally correct or normative, even sufficient in themselves to falsify competing claims without further investigation.

The principle of certainty is usually invoked in an effort to distinguish between belief and knowledge: knowledge is certain and true,
while belief is uncertain and may be mistaken or false. Indeed, many
things are believed that are uncertain and even incorrect. At the same
time, many propositions and theories have been accorded the status of
knowledge for even as long as several generations, and have later been
disproven or discredited and dropped from the canon. Familiar examples include phlogiston theory, phrenology and its use to construct
theories of biological determination of intellect and character, the
theory of miasmas as causes of disease, and the geocentric Ptolemaic
model of the universe. To a certain extent, the validity of defining
knowledge as "certain and true" may be elliptical. That is:

It may be that knowledge is only always certain and true for the same kind of
reason we have for saying that "treason never prospers." We can say it never
prospers, because if it prospers, it is no longer called treason. Similarly, it may
be that we can only say that knowledge is always true because we should decline
[any more] to call it knowledge if it [later] turned out to be false. (Ewing
1951:51–52)

Many modern philosophers (generations of whose predecessors'
efforts have also been devoted to this question) accept a definition of
knowledge as justified and true belief, where "justification" is some
form of logical proof or other evidence offered as sufficient grounds
for substantiating an assertion (Angeles 1981; Clarke 1987). "Our
claims are not so much 'statements that *are* true' as they are 'assertions
that are *believed* to be true based on the evidence.' In a sense, the 'truth'
of our claims is a function of our beliefs, which is [sic] in proportion to
the evidence" (Clarke 1987:29).

For purposes of this study the problem, then, is this: what is accepted
as adequate justification, as proof, as an authoritative source, or as

sufficient grounds for making assertions, are *all* culturally defined and vary considerably from one worldview or belief system to another. For equal applicability of the terms to both "official" and "unofficial" epistemologies, I have operationally defined *knowledge* as any "justified belief" (that is, the grounds for credibility can be logically explicated), and *belief*, within any given system or worldview, as constituting "local knowledge" (that is, accepted as actual or factual by the members of the system). It is in these senses that I will use the terms throughout the book.[6]

A Model for Thinking About Belief Systems

All belief systems produce and support assertions of truth and claims about the nature of reality. In order to describe belief systems sufficiently well to be able to make comparisons among them, I suggest application of a simple structural model, schematized in Figure 1. The model proposes that belief systems (including official systems) have a common basic structure, regardless of the details of their content or the ultimate differences in the specific conclusions they reach and claims they advance. This model is a heuristic device, a tool for thinking, useful with the following caveats: (1) it assumes belief systems that are operating within the bounds of sanity; (2) it is not intended as a literal description of how belief systems are assembled by individuals through particular cognitive, psychological, and other processes; and (3) it certainly does not represent the way that members would experience or describe their own belief systems. It must be emphasized that although the model is depicted graphically in particular spatial relationships and linear sequences, none of the aspects of belief systems identified is necessarily antecedent to any of the others. All the components are related in multiple, complex interconnections. They cross-reference each other and are mutually modifying and mutually reinforcing within the system. The components of belief systems do not typically exist in the awareness of the systems' members as codified "rules" or "parts." Instead, like the tacit rules and structures of a grammar, they simply *function*. It is the scholar of belief systems, like the linguist or grammarian, who observes, elicits, and infers from behavior the components and regulations of a given belief system in order to synthesize a description of its contents, boundaries, rules, and workings.

Givens

Belief systems rest at some points on a body of fundamental definitions and irreducible axiomatic principles, whose truth is accepted a priori: they do not require, and may not be susceptible of, proof. These are

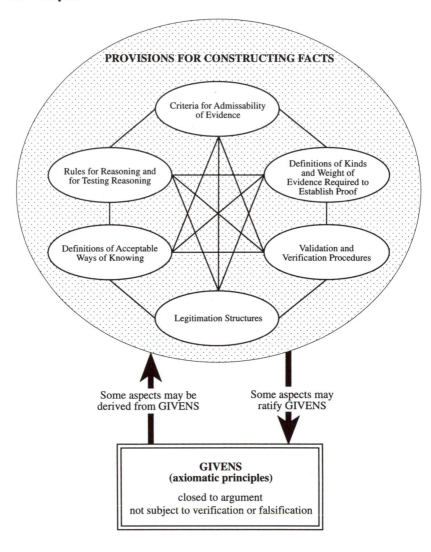

Figure 1: Structural Model for Thinking About Belief Systems.

essentially unassailable or closed propositions within the system, inac-
cessible to argument. Definitions, by their nature, "contain the evidence for their truth in the assertions themselves" (Clarke 1987:30).
Axioms, as "beginning point(s) from which other statements can be
inferred, . . . are not regarded as 'provable' in the same sense as those
statements deduced from them are provable. Their 'proof' is related to

the extent to which they can be used to construct a coherent and inclusive system" (Angeles 1981:22). To avoid confusion with the terminology of formal logic, I refer to these fundamental axiomatic and definitional elements as *givens*.

To illustrate: it is a given in some belief systems both that there is a divine being and that this divinity may influence human events, including the course of an individual's health or illness. For some, it is a given that other supernatural entities or metaphysical forces exist, and also influence health and illness (e.g., spirits of deceased ancestors, for many southeast Asian groups; or the vital force of the body, in homeopathy). Much of a believer's experience and interpretation may continually serve to ratify these axiomatic principles, to confirm by example their veracity and dependability. For instance, within a system in which it is a given that there is a God who is just and merciful, the beauty of a sunset or the spectacle of a birth may be interpreted as a patent demonstration of both the existence and the beneficence of that God. So also may remission of sickness following prayer or the use of sacramental objects confirm divine mercy and reaffirm a conviction of the possibility of healing through divine intervention.

Provisions for Constructing and Legitimating Facts

Belief systems contain provisions for the construction and testing of facts, based on or fortified by epistemological principles that may be implicit or explicit. These principles include definitions and criteria for the admissibility of evidence; definitions of the kind and weight of evidence required to constitute proof; definitions of acceptable ways of knowing; and rules for reasoning that provide both for the proper conduct of reasoning processes and for their evaluation and validation by others. Specific problems of verification are not universal. Since they too are based on culturally substantiated tenets, requirements and means of validation are parts of the belief systems within which they arise.

One of the difficulties that emerges in the meeting of differing belief systems is that criteria for determining the nature and admissibility of evidence, or the proper constitution of proof, may be among the differences between them. Some of these criteria are definitive (given, or axiomatic), and others derived. Some systems may accept as evidence only what they themselves define as sufficient, for example, reproducible experimental results and quantifiable laboratory data. Others may accept in addition, in substitution, and even in preference, personal experiences and convincing accounts of the personal experiences of others—for example, the testimony of the healed. Within

some belief systems, authoritative ways of knowing may include divination or revelation, along with deliberate and structured testing of
disconfirmable hypotheses.

All systems, to a greater or lesser degree, include acceptance of
information on recognized and legitimated authority as a valid means
to knowledge. The nature of legitimated authorities and of authoritative sources, however, can vary among belief systems. These may include, for example, collective sources such as textbooks or scripture or
venerated oral texts, as well as persons recognized as sources of trustworthy and authoritative information: from the parent or grand-
parent, teacher or cleric; to the well-credentialed scientist with a prestigious history of discoveries, publications, and honors; to the shaman
who has become a healer by virtue of recovery from a grave illness or
return from a dangerous spiritual journey during which mystical information and abilities were gained; to the ordinary individual who has
had a clinching or transformative personal experience.

There are innumerable disagreements between systems with respect
to specific content. The differences most likely to prove irreconcilable
are those which proceed from the level of the fundamental assumptions, or givens. Belief systems are impervious to argument at this level
of difference. Denial or disconfirmation of its axiomatic principles
would disrupt the whole system (Angeles 1981). Competing claims at
the axiomatic level call into question the very nature of truth and the
basis of judgment. One system, such as spiritism, may contend that the
dead can and do communicate with the living, both directly and
through the agency of mediums; another, such as Jehovah's Witnesses
or biological science, may assert that the dead are incapable of communication or interaction with the world of the living under any circumstances whatsoever. Other principles derived from fundamental
assumptions, including evidential criteria and categorization of acceptable ways of knowing, may be in conflict as well. What is acceptable as
evidence in one system may be thrown out by another as insufficiently
authoritative, not germane to the argument, or even as not granted
actually to exist.

There is a common assumption among members of the scientific and
related academic traditions that "patterns of thought that reach fundamentally different conclusions from those of modern science must be,
by definition, illogical, irrational, or even nonempirical" (Hufford
1988a:256). This position is frequently advanced in criticism or dismissal of systems making truth claims contradictory to positions supported by scientific thought. But it is a careless critique: the conclusions
reached within a belief system are *logical*, in the ordinary sense of the
term, if they have been derived from the basic principles of the system

together with the evidence that has been adduced, and *rational* if proper methods of reasoning have been followed (Hufford 1984). On the other side of the coin, it is sometimes said in defense of belief systems not congruent with those of Western scholars that they follow "their own logic." This suggestion seems to be offered in defense of the claims of "other" belief systems, an alternative to rejecting them out of hand because of their dissonance with the conventional mode of thought. But this assertion too lacks rigor, for it generally stands unsupported: no models are suggested of alternative processes of reasoning or of different logics and the ways in which they might function. Ironically, the "alternative logic" argument, while intending to be inclusive, buys acceptance at the cost of exoticizing the thought processes involved in reaching conclusions. Both the dismissive and the defensive interpretations of nonconventional belief systems assert or imply that they are somehow categorically different from the officially accepted systems, and that the differences are attributable to the ways in which people think.

Actually, it appears that the tacit rules for reasoning, and for evaluating when it has been properly carried out, are quite congruent among differing belief systems. People of highly diverse persuasions and backgrounds seem to reason to their conclusions in much the same fashion—building stepwise upon their axiomatic foundations and subsequent learning, taking into account their evidence, including observation and personal experience, and testing possibilities and hypotheses: making inferences, and accepting, rejecting, and modifying various propositions as they go.[7] The different conclusions reached within various belief systems do not appear to stem from incapacity to reason, nor from fundamentally different uses of reason. They may simply result from different observations, or differing interpretations of the same observations—exactly as do the respected disagreements within academic disciplines that fuel the engines of endless publication. Or they may stem from quite fundamental, axiomatic differences between belief systems, for "[i]f assumptions, criteria for the admission of evidence and observations differ, then the same kinds of reasoning may lead to very different conclusions" (Hufford 1984:3). My own fieldwork, and the data presented in the discussions that follow, support this contention.

Science as the Paradigm of Knowledge

Although it is now widely accepted as an academic and philosophical principle that knowledge is constructed, and that all systems of knowledge and belief are culturally situated and shaped, it is still the case from within any belief system that its proponents view it simply as a description of the way things *are*, and recognize it as "right." This is true of folk and popular belief systems, as well as of the sciences and medicine, whose constituencies recognize the cultural shaping of knowledge but commonly believe their own enterprises to be largely exempt from these influences. Science is idealized as possessing a clarity of viewpoint and an unimpeachable rigor of method that inherently surmount cultural values and interest-group bias. Scientific knowledge and processes of inquiry are portrayed as genuinely objective and value-free. This claim has of course not gone uncontested, either in scholarship (see, for example, Lock and Gordon 1988; Proctor 1991), or in the public domain (for example, AIDS treatment activists, women protesting underinclusion of female subjects and women's health issues in medical research).

Science and its method are deeply believed by many to have the capacity to provide certifiable knowledge composed only of straightforward distillations of raw and refined facts (Wright and Treacher 1982), and to be the sole means to incontestible and ultimately reliable knowledge. This position has achieved intellectual dominance throughout the official strata of modern Western cultures, and the sciences and their related enterprises have acquired unsurpassed cultural authority. The term "scientific" has taken on an evaluative function, connoting "better" and "more reliable." This evaluative usage has almost wholly supplanted the solely descriptive use of the term, that is, simply "derived or confirmed by scientific methods of inquiry." As a corollary, "nonscientific," meaning simply "derived by means other than those of science," has come to connote inferiority or unreliability, and to function as a critique.

Where scientific claims conflict with claims derived from nonscientific sources—including, for example, experiential knowledge, especially when it is the knowledge of non-"experts"—science (in the official view) has the upper hand. Experimental science is widely regarded as the final arbiter of truth, functioning "as a source of cognitive authority: not only does it provide knowledge and competence, it is required also to evaluate the knowledge-claims and putative competences of those situated beyond its boundaries. Indeed, in modern societies, science is near to being *the* source of cognitive authority: anyone who would be widely believed and trusted as an interpreter of nature needs a license from the scientific community" (Barnes and Edge 1982:2). This viewpoint predominates in spite of recognition that there are many topics to which science does not address itself, and many kinds of problems that are not amenable to investigation by current scientific methods.

Science has enormous rhetorical power in complex modern societies (Zinman 1968), and this continually reaffirms its authoritative status. Because cognitive and cultural authority are densely intertwined with political authority and power (Barnes and Edge 1982), the scientific community and its reputation wield considerable influence well beyond the limits of the direct sphere of inquiry. The extremely high regard in which science as a source and adjudicator of knowledge is held by its members, colleagues, and official social authorities is not necessarily shared, however, in the public domain. While many members of the general populace also esteem and seek scientific information, they do not invariably feel it is the only—or even the best—way to acquire or confirm certain kinds of knowledge. They do not necessarily believe it to be free from bias and corruption, or find its pronouncements trustworthy solely on the basis of their source. Nor do they regard it as the final arbiter of the truth, as much of the remainder of this work will illustrate.

Supernatural and Metaphysical Belief

From the beginning of what we now refer to as the Scientific Revolution of the sixteenth and seventeenth centuries, the new naturalist philosophy was expressly equated with Reason. The replacement of supernatural, and particularly demonic, explanations of illness, suffering, and disaster with natural explanations was even in its early stages represented as the triumph of reason over superstition,[8] a cornerstone of the scientific tradition. In the academic and professional disciplines, and to some extent now in popular usage, "scientific" has come to be equated with "rational," and both to be taken as equal to "true." Conversely, "unscientific" has become loosely synonymous with "irrational," and both of these with "false," or at least "unreliable." Such usages are improper and misleading (Zinman 1968; Hufford 1982b, 1983b, 1985c), but they are quite common and are closely connected with the evaluative functions that have accrued to the terms.

Exclusion of the supernatural from the domain of science[9] imparts to supernatural and other related bodies of belief the evaluative taint of falsity and irrationality, from the point of view of the conventional epistemology. This has significant implications for the interaction of official and vernacular health belief traditions. Most salient are conflicts regarding metaphysical, spiritual, or religious beliefs and their interconnections with explanations and experiences of health and illness. Religious traditions have historically been closely associated with healing practices in societies around the world. Religious and spiritual issues, including questions of morality and of ultimate meaning, are raised by the occasion of serious illness. All religions have something to say about illness, suffering, and death, and some form of healing activity is found in many religious settings in modern Western cultures. In the United States, religious healing has in fact been increasing both in visibility and in range of venues in the last two decades, even extending into or reappearing in denominations in which it had previously been unwelcome (Hufford 1987; McGuire 1982, 1988). Religious, spiritual, and metaphysical health beliefs and practices, since they are excluded from the canon of conventional medicine but are actively maintained by people in their everyday lives and in their self-care, fall by definition into the domain of vernacular health belief systems.

Many vernacular health belief systems have important religious and metaphysical nonmaterial components. These range from a belief in divine or other supernatural means of disease causation and cure; to cosmological influences on the human body and on the growing, harvesting, and preparation of medicinal herbs; to the existence of a font of healing energy (whether divine, cosmic, or marshaled from within) which is tapped by healers. Conventional medicine, on the other hand, does not recognize the operation of supernatural or metaphysical elements in disease etiology or in healing; it does not in fact grant such elements to be real. These differences between conventional and vernacular health belief systems produce disagreement and sometimes conflict between them, on both ontological and epistemological grounds.

Stereotypes Associated with Vernacular Health Beliefs

Nineteenth-century social theories incorporated positivist assumptions of a unidirectional, linear evolutionary process of human thought and human collectivities. These theories portrayed societies as "advancing" through a series of stages characterized by increasing sophistication and accuracy of thought and interpretation. Progress, implicitly defined as "increasing similarity to the culture of the scholar" (Hufford 1983a:307), was considered desirable and, given proper conditions, an inevitable and continuous process. Though this type of evolutionary social model has largely been abandoned in contemporary scholarship, the legacy of the earlier theories is still quite influential. Long-standing acceptance of the concept of inevitable, evolutionary social and intellectual progress has fostered a general expectation that as science and medicine became ever more developed or "advanced" and public education improved and became more universally available, nonmedical and nonscientific health beliefs and practices would die out or be eliminated (and that this would be a good thing). This notion still has considerable currency today, although in actuality its predictions have not been borne out. As a corollary of this point of view, beliefs foreign to or grossly incompatible with modern medical and scientific models are commonly regarded as expressions of isolated surviving popular errors, or as misinformed habits of mind which cultural development and better education will sooner or later eradicate.

This kind of survivalist interpretation implies that differences in worldview or belief system may not be prior conditions but only consequences, that anyone given the "proper" opportunities, education, and information would "think like us." It does not recognize the possibility that nonconventional health care choices might be something other than products of developmental or educational lag, or the results of circumstances of deprivation. It overlooks the point that formal educational systems aren't just teaching knowledge, but also are imparting values. They are designed in part to help create and maintain a common culture (Elesh and Schollaert 1972): they institutionalize specific cultural values and help to induct members into the official worldview. In the United States, this macro-culture and its educational institutions place a high value on scientific knowledge and on conventional medical care (Elesh and Schollaert 1972). As a result, it becomes easy to assume that departure from this model is a consequence of inadequate education or failure of comprehension. This assumption, however, does not stand up to scrutiny a significant percentage of the time.

Evolutionist and survivalist assumptions have given rise to and sustained a series of stereotypes of vernacular health belief systems and their participants as being to some degree socially marginal. The implication has been that they are marginal both to the conventional medical system and to the mainstream of modern society and modern knowledge (Kleinman 1980; Hufford 1984, 1988a). The stereotypes of marginality typically include one or more of the following features: geographic remoteness or isolation (the image of rural Appalachia is frequently invoked); recent immigration or minimal acculturation to core American culture; ethnic minority membership or strong ethnic self-identification or group affiliation; poverty or low socioeconomic status; low formal educational attainment; mental or emotional imbalance; or desperation induced by grave illness or poor outcomes of conventional therapeutic efforts.[10]

These factors are interpreted as producing ignorance of the existence or availability of modern medical strategies and technologies, lack of understanding of disease processes and their relationship to conventional therapeutic responses, lack of physical or financial access to conventional care, or failure or inability to exercise judgment. These conditions in turn are advanced as explanations for the persistence of vernacular health beliefs and practices, and for the failure of individuals or demographically defined groups to make "appropriate" use of conventional medical facilities (with appropriate use being defined from the biomedical point of view). These factors are defined as "barriers" to use of biomedicine, and are perceived to be located in the specific populations they are used to describe—rather than in the *relationship* between differing worldviews (biomedical and nonbiomedical), and differing ways of defining and preferring to address matters of health, illness, and care.

It *is* relatively easy to confirm that vernacular health beliefs and practices are found in association with poverty, strong ethnic or cultural heritage identity, remote rural residence, and so forth. It is not equally easy to confirm, however, that the associations are causal. Historically, research on nonconventional health systems has been carried out among designated "marginal" populations to the exclusion of more "mainstream" groups. The resulting distributional picture is in part an artifact of prior assumptions about *where to look* to find the kinds beliefs and behaviors to which the studies addressed themselves. The enormous extent of recourse to vernacular healing strategies among educated, thoroughly acculturated, "mainstream" groups has only recently begun to be recognized (e.g., Kronenfeld and Wasner 1982; Cassileth et al. 1984; Nations, Camino, and Walker 1985; Lowenberg 1989; Eisenberg et al. 1993). Another long-standing assumption has held that conditions of marginality and the obstacles they actually or ostensibly produce are the principal determinants of nonconventional health behavior. It is demonstrably true that barriers of physical and financial access, for example, do frequently enter into and even govern health care choices for some people. What is not known is the extent to which this occurs, or how these particular factors interact with others in affecting health behavior. There is immense variability of response within groups, and a much more complex set of conditions influences health care choices—even in the presence of obstacles—than has previously been acknowledged in most of the scholarship in this area.

A look at some of the most frequently mentioned specific barriers or obstacles to use of biomedicine raises serious questions about the pervasive assumption that elimination of such obstacles would lead automatically to increased use of conventional medical care. While lack of adequate biomedical facilities in a given location (such as a geographically remote area, or a medically underserved section of a large urban center) may force or encourage use of nonconventional healing resources, the presence of modern facilities does not necessarily reduce the use of these alternative practices. For example, an Iowa study found that use of chiropractors *increased*, rather than decreased, concomitantly with a significant increase in the census of primary care physicians in the county surveyed (Yesalis et al. 1980; Wardwell 1988). A study of self-care in Britain discovered its use to be quite high, even in the presence of the extensive British national health system (Levin and Idler 1981), and another international study of self-care use likewise concluded that levels of self-care are not apparently related to extent and availability of professional care resources (White et al. 1961). Vernacular health care alternatives abound in areas well served by conventional medical care, as a survey of any major metropolitan area in the United States will attest. These resources are used by many people who also respect and use conventional medicine. Indeed, folk or alternative healers may even visit and treat patients while they are hospitalized in large and modern teaching hospitals (Hufford 1988a; Yoruba healer, personal communication).

Finances sometimes dictate avoidance or self-rationing of medical care; familiar examples include a parent's forgoing of care in order to afford treatment for a sick child, or conservative use of physicians' services by elders on fixed incomes. However, it is also common for people—even very poor people—to make great financial sacrifices in order to obtain what they feel is the required care for their conditions. These choices include both conventional and nonconventional resources. For instance, people who are covered for conventional care either by private medical insurance through their places of employment, or by federal assistance programs in the cases of the poor or unemployed, will nevertheless elect for some purposes vernacular therapies for which they must pay out of pocket, and which may even be burdensomely expensive. Medicinal herbs and homeopathic pharmaceuticals are not reimbursable by the prescription plans of third-party payors; the lay midwife who attends a home birth, the shaman whose fees and transportation costs to the home of the patient must be paid, charge their services directly to their patients. To individuals using alternative healing resources in both Britain and the United States, these services usually constitute an additional health care expense (Taylor 1984; Eisenberg et al. 1993). The criterion for choosing among conventional and vernacular healing strategies in innumerable cases is an assessment not of cost, but of benefit: that is, of the perceived appropriateness and efficacy of the therapy or the specialist for the specific health situation.

Without doubt, there are many instances in which people are not aware of specific diagnostic and therapeutic options within conventional medicine, especially when these are very new or heavily reliant on expensive technology which is available only in certain locations (for example, some of the newer imaging techniques such as x-ray computed tomography, or CT scanning, and magnetic resonance imaging, or MRI). Even when well aware, however, people may choose not to use certain modalities out of uneasiness, dislike of the procedures themselves, philosophical concerns over ethical implications of particular technological interventions, preference for the effects of their symptoms over side effects of treatments, and a host of other reasons. This may be the case even when the individuals in question are otherwise thoroughly in agreement with conventional medical thought.

There are innumerable instances in which nonuse of conventional modalities does not result from ignorance (either of available therapies or of conventional explanations of the workings of disease and dysfunction) but represents an actively considered choice. In recent years, we have had the example of states of illness or dysfunction from which many people suffered, but which were not medically recognized as real or treatable diagnostic entities, and are still medically controversial (e.g., premenstrual syndrome, or PMS, and chronic fatigue syndrome, or CFS). Nonbiomedical alternatives were the only recourse for those unwilling to resign themselves to medical disagreement with their experiences. Sometimes different health care choices reflect distaste for conventional care, disagreement with a medical opinion that little or nothing can be done (e.g., in multiple sclerosis, or MS) or a sense that biomedicine is not the best approach for the problem at hand. Yesalis and associates (1980) concluded, for example, that use of chiropractors by people who also used physicians represented a form of self-triage, based on assessment of presenting complaints at any given time. In a study of patterns of use of biomedical resources by urban Gypsies in the United States,

Salloway, impressed by the selectivity and streetwise approach to medical care so visible among the Gypsies, speculated that nonuse of services by disadvantaged groups in effect forms a socially based judgment, rational and purposeful, of the quality of care. The Gypsy network acts to test the efficacy of the care given and offers the individual the support necessary to reject care and go elsewhere. (Levin and Idler 1981:168; see also Salloway 1973)

Explanatory models of illness (Kleinman 1975) that appear from the viewpoint of modern medical science to reflect a misunderstanding of disease processes may instead emerge from wholly different theories of disease etiology and healing (Kleinman, Eisenberg, and Good 1978; Kleinman 1980; Levin and Idler 1981). Examples include homeopathy (see Coulter 1975), traditional Chinese medicine (see Kaptchuk 1983), and the hot/cold theory found in many Latin American cultures (see Harwood 1971, 1981). Where vigorous vernacular healing traditions exist, their use is more often a matter of reasoned choice than of simple ignorance of conventional medical alternatives. Decisions to take one's migraine or chronic back pain to the chiropractor, or a case of soul loss to a folk healer, for instance, are typically based on community and personal experience, and on some acquaintance with what both the vernacular tradition and conventional medicine have to offer to address the particular problem. Their use may as likely reflect disagreement with conventional medicine on specific points (such as whether or not chiropractic is potentially effective for back pain, or soul loss is a possible cause for illness) as misunderstanding of medical explanations and options.

To illustrate: conventional medicine is well known to have limited success in dealing with chronic back pain, and chiropractic is well known to focus its therapeutic attention on the spine. A person could therefore reasonably conclude that chiropractic might be a more successful modality than conventional medicine for treating chronic back pain, irrespective of medical disapproval of chiropractors.[11] Conventional medicine does not recognize soul loss as a cause of illness and so has no appropriate treatments to offer the sufferer of these ills (which are recognized in innumerable cultures around the world, including many well represented in the American population). Medicine's likely response to complaints of soul loss would be a psychiatric interpretation and a recommendation for counseling or drug therapy. Since time is of the essence in treating soul loss before serious sequelae develop, and since psychiatric therapy is not deemed appropriate or efficacious in such cases by those who recognize soul loss, the decision to take the patient to the appropriate vernacular specialist known to be skilled in treating this complaint can be seen as reasonable and expedient.

My fieldwork has repeatedly revealed that vernacular health belief systems have among their central values concerns for appropriate and timely intervention and for seeking the proper specialist. These concerns precisely parallel those found in conventional medicine. In *both* spheres, delays caused by first resort to "wrong" treatments occasion tremendous frustration and concern for the safety of the sick. The physician who worries that use of alternative cancer therapies will produce costly or even fatal delays in a patient's coming to conventional treatment shares a concern with the layperson who worries that psychotherapeutic interventions for soul loss will cause a dangerous or fatal delay in getting a family member to the proper ritual specialist. What differs between these two belief systems is not the depth of their concern for the health of the patient nor their commitment to its prompt amelioration by the best available means, but their conceptions of what treatments are necessary and proper for the presenting conditions and of where the search for relief ought to begin.

Health Belief Systems

There is a persistent tendency to conceptualize vernacular health beliefs and practices as isolated "items," fragmentary or disconnected in
form, and persisting largely through the agency of habit. This is yet
another false impression and impediment to understanding. Closer
inspection reveals vernacular health beliefs more often to be organized
into coherent systems of thought[12] possessing varying degrees of complexity (number of component parts) and integration (numbers and
kinds of interconnections among parts) (Hufford 1983a, 1984, 1988a).
Health belief systems weave together attitudes toward health and illness, and theories of disease etiology and remediation. In addition they
articulate these within a larger cultural framework of other important
beliefs and values—for example, those dealing with religious, moral,
and ethical concerns; with family and community relations and the
requirements of reciprocal responsibility; with the nature of the universe, the world, or Nature, and the rightful place of humanity in
them; with human nature and the capacities and limitations of the
human body, mind, and spirit, and so on (see Kleinman 1973, 1980,
1984; Snow 1974; Egeland 1978; Levin and Idler 1981; Trotter and
Chavira 1981; Hufford 1984, 1988).

Though many of the embedded values and their multiple interconnections remain out of awareness for members of a particular system,
they are in many cases more directly articulated in vernacular health
belief systems than in conventional medicine. In keeping with the
scientific tradition, modern biomedicine has striven to separate itself
from broader cultural concerns and influences (and has considered
itself largely successful in the attempt). It has excluded religious, metaphysical, and philosophical considerations from its explanatory models
of disease and dysfunction and—until relatively recently, when the
rapid proliferation of heroic medical technologies again forced these
issues into salience—also from its treatment decision-making processes. It has claimed for itself a unique value-neutrality and (ironically) valued that neutrality as good. It has taken as simply "the way
things are" its own quite culture-specific value orientation (Kluckhohn
1953), which includes, for example, a strong preference for action, a
belief that humankind can and should dominate nature, a belief in
individual autonomy, a belief that individuals can and should improve
themselves by their own efforts, and a preference for hierarchical
structures of authority (Egeland 1978; Lock and Gordon 1988; Stein
1990a). Its protestations to the contrary notwithstanding, modern biomedicine is, like vernacular health belief systems, profoundly culturally shaped (Payer 1988; Stein 1990a). Unlike vernacular systems,

however, it is greatly divorced from other, quotidian aspects of its surrounding culture.

The systematic and coherent organization of vernacular health beliefs and practices, together with their close interconnections with broader cultural contexts, has helped to account for their persistence and continued vitality. The more complex and the better integrated a system is, the more flexible and stable it is likely to be (Hufford 1983a, 1988a). Likewise, the better integrated a health belief system is within a larger framework of values, the more stable it is likely to be. Tight integration gives a system a functional capacity analogous to that of a generative grammar (Chomsky 1957), enabling participants to incorporate novel input together with familiar material, and to generate responses that remain within the bounds of the system. Observations concerning both successes and failures, together with new information from any number of sources, are readily assimilated to the explanatory models contained in vernacular health belief systems. This process precisely parallels the ease and frequency with which vernacular explanations of both causes and cures are assimilated to medical and psychiatric explanatory models in professional practice and scholarship. The capacity to derive appropriate, system-congruent explanatory responses to novel input on the basis of general organizing principles constitutes a sort of "explanatory competence," analogous to the concept of communicative competence advanced in sociolinguistics (Hymes 1972, 1973). This merely illustrates that coherent belief systems, official and vernacular alike, are self-reinforcing, resilient, and resistant to change by pressure of outside argument when their own internal models will provide acceptable explanations that account for observations and events. These considerations have obvious implications for situations in which differing health belief systems come into contact with each other, especially if there is a need or desire to establish, as it were, diplomatic relations between them.

Vernacular Health Belief Systems and "Mainstream" Populations

Both the stereotypes of marginality and the assumption that modern medical and scientific thought will invariably hold sway with members of the dominant culture have helped to obscure the use of vernacular healing modalities by "mainstream" patient groups. (For purposes of this work, I take "mainstream" to imply—in the case of the United States—English-language fluency, literacy, education through high school or beyond, middle-class socioeconomic standing, and knowledge of and experience with the conventional medical system.) Such uses are extensive, though still relatively little researched. It is largely the college-educated middle class, for example, who are members of the multiplicity of health belief systems that comprise the New Age healing movement (Levin and Coreil 1986). It is this population who fill chartered flights to the Philippines to seek the services of psychic surgeons, and who make up the large majority of the clients of various health and organic foods systems (Hufford 1971a), homeopaths (Taylor 1984; Kaufman 1988),[13] naturopaths, chiropractors (National Center for Health Statistics 1978; Wardwell 1988), and a variety of body-work practitioners and meditative and visualization systems (see Lowenberg 1989; Eisenberg et al. 1993). In the United Kingdom "the upper social classes not only consult the National Health Service more frequently, but are also turning to alternative therapies in significant numbers" (MacCormack 1982:iii; see also Fulder and Munro 1982). Contrary to pervasive assumptions, available data suggest that membership in many religious and spiritual healing groups is also largely middle class and well educated (Levin and Idler 1981; McGuire 1982, 1988; Hufford 1985b). It is also this population who are the heaviest users of over-the-counter medicines for self-care (Knapp and Knapp 1972). Levin and Idler report:

The amount of nonprescription medications may be related to socioeconomic status, the more affluent and better educated purchasing more of them. This appears to run contrary to conventional wisdom that nonprescription self-medication is an attractive option for those who cannot afford, or do not have access to, or do not appreciate the efficacy of, prescribed drugs. It may well be that families of lower socioeconomic status have less access to over-the-counter drugs as well as prescribed drugs; indeed, they have been found to have fewer of both. (Levin and Idler 1981:75. See also Meriläinen, Vaskilampi, and Sinkkonen 1982; Vaskilampi 1982.)

Research efforts focusing on or including mainstream patient groups have been few to date, but among them are a number of studies reporting the presence of nonconventional health beliefs, and use of various vernacular care resources (Saunders and Hewes 1969; Hufford 1971a, 1977a, 1984; Kotarba 1975; Levin, Katz, and Holst 1979; Faw et al. 1977; Snow and Johnson 1977; Helman 1978, Arkko et al. 1980; Blumhagen 1980; Dean 1981; Hautman and Harrison 1982; Kronenfeld and Wasner 1982; Cassileth et al. 1984; Donovan, Blake, and Fleming 1989; Lowenberg 1989; O'Connor 1991, 1993; O'Connor, Lazar, and Anderson 1992; Anderson et al. 1993; Eisenberg et al. 1993). Studies finding widespread mainstream use of nonconventional practitioners or healers probably yield conservative estimates of overall use of nonconventional therapies: a good percentage of vernacular health care does not involve a specialist healer but is handled within the community or the family, as lifestyle choices and actions, or as self-care (Dean 1981; Hufford 1988a, 1988c; cf. Eisenberg et al. 1993). In addition, some studies have failed to consider certain very common vernacular strategies such as the use of prayer or other religious actions taken specifically to promote healing, and so are potentially missing additional significant figures (Hufford 1988a).

A pervasive image in the medical literature is that of fear and desperation as primary motives for the seeking or acceptance of nonconventional therapeutic practices. This stereotype is refuted in a number of the above-mentioned studies. A University of Pennsylvania Cancer Center study of use of "unorthodox" cancer therapies found that a significant number of patients opting for alternative treatment modalities (most in addition to conventional care) began them when they were in early stages of their illness, and many when they were asymptomatic (Cassileth et al. 1984). My field research in the HIV alternative therapies movement has shown a similar pattern (O'Connor 1991; O'Connor, Lazar, and Anderson 1992). Levin and Idler, reviewing studies of religious healing, find that available research shows it to be a misconception that religious healing is sought only as a last resort, in cases of incurable disease, or at disease end-stages (Levin and Idler 1981). They observe in addition that there is no sound basis for concluding that the use of prayers or other sacramental actions for healing purposes is a choice resulting from ignorance, desperation, fear, or exhaustion of other options (Levin and Idler 1981).

Self-Care and Use of Multiple Resources

A number of scholars have reported that the majority of health-related actions in any population are undertaken outside the sphere of the conventional health care system, even by those actively considering themselves to be sick or in compromised health (Elliot-Binns 1973; Levin, Katz, and Holst 1979; Chrisman 1977; Kleinman 1980, 1984; Dean 1981; Levin and Idler 1981). Estimates of health care actions taking place outside the sphere of conventional medicine range from 70 to 90 percent of all care activities (Zola 1972b; Kleinman 1980; see also Hulka, Kupper, and Cassel 1972; Wolinsky 1980). Some stress that laypeople are not merely consumers of health care but are also its primary providers (Levin 1976; Levin and Idler 1981; Wolinsky 1980). In actuality, professionally provided health care is only one of the common resources in "a greater health care system, of which health care professionals are *not* the locus of responsibility for treatment decisions and trajectories" (Kleinman 1984:161). It is in what Kleinman refers to as the "popular sphere" that "help-seeking decisions are made in the lay referral network regarding when to go to a particular practitioner for care, which practitioner to visit, whether to change practitioners or seek therapeutic alternatives, how long to remain in treatment, whether or not to comply with therapeutic recommendations, and how to assess outcome" (Kleinman 1984:142). (See also Chrisman 1977; Chrisman and Kleinman 1983.)

Oral tradition and scientific information learned through the media are parallel sources of knowledge in everyday life (Hostetler 1976). In their decision-making about health care, people draw upon their familiarity with conventional medicine as well as upon popular wisdom, blending the two to forge explanations that inform treatment choices and assist in evaluation of therapeutic outcomes. Far from being inherently contradictory to the pronouncements of science, folk belief and popular wisdom coexist and intermingle with scientific explanations (Levin and Idler 1981), and the two streams of tradition are often complementary in individuals' formulations of interpretations. Indeed, many vernacular health beliefs may be supported and reinforced by contacts with conventional medicine (Helman 1978).

In choosing to use vernacular health care systems, people of every educational and social group make considered decisions in putting together a multifaceted strategy for dealing with health and illness. This strategy commonly involves the serial or simultaneous use of a number of approaches to the health problem, from "common sense" self-care actions such as taking to bed, to therapeutic actions taken at home, to consultation with knowledgeable parties ranging from family or community elders to specialist practitioners. Combined use of conventional medicine and one or more vernacular strategies is extremely common. For example: a person coping with cancer may be following a course of chemotherapy while simultaneously using prayer for healing, together with the application of sacred relics to the afflicted part(s) of the body; following a natural foods diet and taking large doses of vitamins and minerals in an effort to eliminate toxins and bolster the immune system; practicing meditation to reduce stress, and visualization to mobilize the body's healing forces; using botanical or homeopathic medicines to combat the side effects of chemotherapy; and seeing a chiropractor to help restore vitality and proper functioning, or an acupuncturist for pain control or restoration of critical internal balance.[14]

Romanucci-Ross (1969) used the term "hierarchy of resort" to refer to sequential patterns of selection and use of health care resources. The term implies both replacement of prior options by the successive choices and a progression "upward" to increasingly superior options.

While some progressive selections of healing options do entail replacement of prior options, others may be additive. Nor do all such selec-
tions necessarily involve a progression of options from lesser to greater
effectiveness or desirability, in the estimation of those making the
choices. Additive health care selection processes are often a matter
of *combining* selected resources so as to provide an optimal broad-
spectrum response to the health problem. For these reasons, I prefer to
think in terms simply of an "*order* of resort." This usage denotes a
simple chronology in the selection of therapeutic modalities, and re-
moves the implications both of serial replacements and of "upward
mobility" through the therapeutic ranks. The order in which a person
has recourse to various systems of care is changeable, both over time
and in response to the particular condition for which treatment is
being sought; conventional medicine may be introduced at any phase
along the way, neither necessarily as the first resort nor as the final
effort. The ways in which such choices are made and implemented,
and the meaning of the choices in the order of resort, can only be
determined by inquiry on a case-by-case basis.

When used concurrently, the different systems to which an individual has recourse may be selected because each is believed to deal well
with specific features of the health problem. For example, conventional medicine may be used to obtain rapid symptom relief, or for
physical repair or removal of threatening conditions (setting of broken
bones, suturing of lacerations, stabilization following trauma, surgical
removal of tumors, and so on), while a rootworker is used to remove
the hex, a regimen of prayer to expiate the sin, or a change in diet to
correct the imbalance, which is experienced as the underlying cause of
a specific condition. This type of usage reflects a common characteristic
of vernacular health belief systems, many of which view conventional
medicine as addressing only symptoms or treating proximate causes of
sickness, while the vernacular system is equipped to deal with critical
ultimate causes. Some systems, such as homeopathy and naturopathy,
view disease processes themselves as symptoms, expressive of but not
identical with the actual underlying problem.

In the simultaneous use of multiple healing resources, *any* of the
systems in use may be considered by the patient to be his or her
primary therapeutic system, and any other(s) seen as adjuvant therapy.
To illustrate: chemotherapy may be considered primary and chiropractic secondary or supportive in restoring the health and vigor of the
cancer patient, or (as I have often found in fieldwork) a vernacular
system may be experienced as the system actively promoting the healing, with conventional medicine added for diagnostic confirmation or
"mechanical repairs," or used (by virtue of its many quantifiable tests)

as a measuring instrument by which to chart the progress and efficacy of the primary (vernacular) therapeutic modality (O'Connor 1991).

Concerns Addressed by Healing Systems

Vernacular health belief systems tend to address a broader range of concerns than does conventional medicine. This characteristic in many instances facilitates their simultaneous use with conventional care, for the conventional and vernacular systems may be used to deal with different aspects of sickness. Nonconventional systems may place quite different values on particular therapeutic outcomes. For example, vernacular systems frequently undertake to promote "healing," as differentiated from "curing." Just as it is possible to have a disease without a corresponding illness or an illness with no discernible disease (Eisenberg 1977), it is possible to be cured without experiencing healing, or healed without being cured. Curing generally refers to the removal or correction of organic pathology. Healing can encompass such matters as comfort, care, family and community relationships, quality of life, peace of mind, restoration of dignity, acceptance, spiritual growth, and even ultimate salvation. Physical recovery may not be the most important outcome, and healing (at another level) may be felt to have taken place in the absence of physical cure or even of noticeable physical improvement (Hufford 1985d). Vernacular health belief systems frequently include within their purview not just bodily sickness but also mental, emotional, and spiritual afflictions as well as familial, community, and environmental or even cosmological concerns.

Most of these systems recognize medically defined diseases but provide in addition for the treatment of a number of problems not recognized by conventional medicine such as *susto* or soul loss, "nerves," spinal subluxation complexes, imbalances or deficiencies in vital energy, or the effects of witchcraft. Many regard illness as a specific subtype of a more generalized category of misfortune or disharmony which the system may also attempt to redress. Importantly, many vernacular health belief systems address directly the meaning of illness and suffering, offering answers to questions like "why me?" and "why now?" (Hufford 1988a). This is a significant dimension of the experience of illness for which conventional medicine has nothing to offer. Other characteristics common to vernacular health belief systems include a strong empirical, or observational, basis of support for their practices and claims, and a general sense of pragmatism: *that* a therapeutic action works is more important than an explanation of *how* or *why* it works. In systems that include specialist practitioners, these experts may be well versed in the theoretical as well as the practical aspects of the system. Most ordinary members or clients, however, are no more likely to concern themselves with these complexities than are the clients of conventional medicine. Their pragmatism in evaluating therapeutic efficacy is the same in both domains: the beneficial effect of the herb or the acupuncture or the antibiotic is of greater interest and concern than its mechanism of action.

A number of concepts are held in common by a variety of vernacular healing systems as well, although their specific interpretations vary from system to system (Table 1). Among these common concepts are a view of health as entailing harmony or balance (with the corollary that imbalance or disharmony are primary causes of disease), and the importance to health and illness of various kinds of "energy," some of which are transferable. Interpretations of pertinent energies may include a vital force that animates the body and provides the essential condition for health; energies that link individuals to the cosmos or to Nature; energies that flow through channels within the body and whose blockage sets up conditions for disease and dysfunction; negative energies that are sources of disharmony and disease; and healing energies that can be tapped, channelled, or manipulated by healers or by sick individuals themselves. Most of these systems recognize some nonmaterial dimensions of health, illness, and healing, whether supernatural, spiritual, or metaphysical, and hold that restoration of health requires treatment of all dimensions of the illness.

The Health Belief Model

Perhaps the most productive conceptual tool for assessing how and why people make the health care choices they do, and how such choices come to include vernacular healing systems, is the Health Belief Model developed by sociologists of health behavior (see Becker 1974; Janz and Becker 1984). In summary, this model holds that the factors affecting health-related behavior are perceived susceptibility to and seriousness of a given health threat, perceived benefits and barriers to a given course of health-promoting or remedial action, and (internal and external) cues impelling action (Table 2). All of these features are responsive to differences in worldview or belief system, which shape the relevant perceptions and evaluations. Considerations of central importance in one frame of reference may be peripheral or inconsequential in another (Jones 1976). The great analytical and explanatory strengths of the Health Belief Model are (1) that it is applicable to *all* health-related behavior, not only to that involving officially sanctioned system(s) of care (i.e., it is without medicocentric bias); (2) that it assumes the fundamental rationality of health behavior, an assumption for which

TABLE 1. Some Concepts Common to Many Vernacular Health Belief
      Systems.

Distinction drawn between immediate and ultimate causes. Importance of
   addressing ultimate causes in healing actions.

Definition of health in terms of balance or harmony (e.g., innate qualities,
   forces, humors; internal, external, social, spiritual).

Concept of blockage or transference of (some form or definition of) energy in
   illness etiology and in healing.

Disease etiology includes buildup of toxins, impurities, or imbalances (hot/cold,
   yin/yang) in the body.

Vitalism: the body has its own "life force" that promotes health and healing and
   is essential to wellness.

Interpretation of some disruptive states as desirable, for example, rashes as
   indicating impurities or disease "coming out" of the body, or diarrhea as
   indicating purging of impurities or toxins (i.e., some events are not constructed as "symptoms" in the same way as they are by conventional medicine).

Recognition of magical, spiritual, metaphysical, or supernatural causes for or
   aspects of illnesses, with the concomitant requirement for matching aspects
   of healing actions.

Illness as one subtype of a more general category of misfortune; capacity of the
   healing system to address or influence the larger category as well as the
   specific illness.

Contagion or transference in many forms, including magical contagion and
   transference of illness as a "thing," with the implication that the person
   "passing" it no longer has it once the recipient has acquired it.

---

there is considerable empirical support; and (3) that it avoids the
ethnocentric predicament of taking the choice of an unofficial route of
care as being ipso facto an irrational or inappropriate action.

   To begin with, people must perceive themselves to be susceptible to
particular health threats in order to contemplate taking action. For
example, a person who does not believe in the reality of hot/cold or
yin/yang imbalances as sources of sickness will not perceive herself to
be susceptible to these classes of illness; a macrobiotic, by virtue of his
preventive dietary and lifestyle regimen, may not perceive himself to
be susceptible to cancers of the digestive and eliminative organs. A
health threat, once acknowledged to exist, must be perceived as sufficiently serious to warrant active intervention. Asymptomatic hypertension, for example, may by its relative invisibility fail to motivate people
to take prescription medications and follow dietary recommendations.
Gastric symptoms that might in an Anglo American merit only self-
administered over-the-counter antacids or a shift to bland foods for a
day or two might prompt a Mexican American to seek the physician or
curandero. Anglo-European cultural views tend to regard gastric upset
as relatively unimportant; Mexican cultural views by contrast tend to

TABLE 2. Health Belief Model.

Four major variables influencing behavioral responses to health matters*:

1. Perceived susceptibility
2. Perceived seriousness
3. Perceived benefits/barriers regarding any given health action strategy
4. Motivating cues:
    a) Internal (symptoms and other feeling states)
    b) External (cultural and social input)

*This model assumes the fundamental rationality of health behavior.
Adapted from David J. Hufford, "American Healing Systems: An Introduction and Exploration." Hershey, PA: Milton S. Hershey Medical Center, Pennsylvania State University Medical School, 1984. Used by permission.

attach more significance to gastric disturbances, which are perceived to have the potential to develop into more serious conditions if not treated promptly (Schreiber and Homiak 1981).[15]

Perceived benefits and barriers to a given course of preventive or therapeutic action are weighed in the balance. Barriers may include considerations such as inconvenience, fear, pain, expense, embarrassment, risk, or negative side effects. Benefits may encompass such factors as symptom relief, improved life expectancy, noninvasiveness, enhanced wellness or restoration of vital force, spiritual growth or salvation, and consonance with other cherished beliefs and values. Cues to action include internal cues such as experience of symptoms or other feeling states, and external cues such as advice from family and community members, urgings of religious or spiritual counselors, cultural interpretations of the health situation, advertisements of products or services, recommendations expounded in the media, and so on. The Health Belief Model can be applied within any health belief framework, set into any cultural background, to assess how a given individual understands health or illness circumstances and how health behaviors follow from this understanding and from other influences that prompt or inhibit action.

Summary

The long-standing prediction that as science and medicine progressed and education became more generally available, folk and popular beliefs about health, illness, and healing would steadily decline, must now be recognized to be wide of the mark. There is ample evidence, in the United States as elsewhere, that vernacular health belief systems have persisted with undiminished vitality right up to the present day, and that their persistence is not restricted to the ignorant, the desperate, the remote, the deprived, or the unacculturated. They show no signs of dying out, or of being "stamped out." In fact, many vernacular healing systems have experienced an enthusiastic reinvigoration in the past ten to fifteen years, in the United States and in other developed nations (Alver 1982; Hänninen 1982; Hufford 1984, 1988a; Kleinman 1984). In the United States, this resurgence is found at every level of society: ethnic groups have begun to celebrate their cultural heritage and promote a strong ethnic identity and the conservation or reclamation of traditional values and practices (including religious and healing systems); many religious groups have increasingly focused attention on healing; and the middle class generally has fueled a massive self-care and alternative care movement.

It is clear that stereotypes of marginality, ignorance, and desperation are inadequate to an accurate understanding of vernacular health belief systems, and that if used as a finding-aid, they seriously distort the picture both by misrepresenting the systems and their supporters and by overlooking large numbers of users of these pervasive health care resources. It is important now for vernacular health belief systems to be well studied and well understood, since their use has significant implications for conventional clinical care. Such understanding, and the successful therapeutic negotiations to which it can lead, can only be accomplished with the recognition that vernacular health beliefs and practices, like conventional medical care, are systematic bodies of thought which are fundamentally rational, and which are bolstered by lengthy histories of ideas, considerable social support, and reputations for efficacy sustained by experience, observation, and evaluative processes.

Notes

1. An excellent illustration appears in a newspaper account of a Drug Enforcement Agency sting operation, made possible in part by street gang participants: "[The DEA officer] called them 'cooperating witnesses.' They are known on the street as 'snitches'" (Zucchino, *Philadelphia Inquirer* 9 January 1993, p. A8).

2. I am grateful to Dave Hufford for the use of his unpublished 1988 manuscript of stipulative definitions, "A Glossary for Thinking About Belief," which has been helpful to me in formulating several of my own current usages. He observes that "official" is itself a mutable term that can be applied to the "party line" in a number of different settings: e.g., in the case of practitioners of the healing arts, what is accepted and promoted by the American Medical Association, what is accepted and promoted by the International Chiropractic Association, or what is the "official word" of the shaman as to the cause of an illness and the required course of treatment.

3. For example, acupuncture is a conventional therapeutic modality in

China and homeopathy a conventionally accepted system in India and in a number of European countries, but neither is currently considered to be a conventional health care option in the United States generally.

4. Kleinman (1980, 1984) uses the collective term "indigenous healing." I prefer a broader designation, since "indigenous" implies what is native to a group, and many nonconventional health beliefs and practices are acquired through various channels of learning or exposure, including cross-cultural borrowing and adaptation of conventional medical information.

5. This is of course an academic point of view. Proponents of many belief systems outside of the academy might disagree with this contention, since they *do* recognize the existence and authority of knowledge which is discovered whole, and—in some systems—of knowledge which is revealed.

6. Again, these are etic, or outsiders' (academic) definitions. Emic definitions, those from within any given system, would be quite different and would refer back to the principle of certainty. That is, virtually all people will distinguish between things that they say they know (for certain) and things that they say they believe (with conviction, but with less certainty). The mutually referential definitions I propose for the terms belief and knowledge apply in situations of cross-system comparison or description.

7. For a thorough discussion of this issue, see Hufford 1982a, in which he demonstrates hypothesis testing in the reasoning of ordinary people trying to come to an explanation for sleep-paralysis experiences and their attendant features.

8. Early on, it was witchcraft and satanic deceptions that were refuted and rejected as superstitions; "natural" explanations still expressly recognized, and theorists were at pains to reconcile themselves with, a perfect and miracle-working God. Copernicus defended his argument for the heliocentric theory of the universe in part on the grounds that as God was undeniably the perfect architect of nature, it was improbable that He would have created a cosmos as disturbingly inefficient in its workings as the one portrayed by Ptolemaic description (Easlea 1980).

9. See Hufford (1982b, 1985c, 1983b) for discussion of categorical rejection of the supernatural as an academic "tradition of *dis*belief."

10. Desperation is typically invoked by health professionals as a motivator for use of unconventional therapeutic modalities. However, I have heard it from patients as a rationale for entering clinical trials of experimental drugs as well as for other use of conventional pharmaceuticals. One informant with a chronic illness preferred only natural treatments, but in the face of continuing symptoms was contemplating accepting a regimen of prescription drugs which he considered dangerous and toxic. As he explained this temptation, "If you get desperate enough, you'll take anything" (H., personal communication).

11. This association can also be a great frustration to chiropractors, many of whom despair of their public image as "back doctors." Chiropractic aims at preventing disease and ameliorating general health through spinal manipulations intended to restore the proper flow of vital energy throughout the body; it is not self-defined as a system for correcting back problems.

12. It is not the case that all elements of a life or a belief system cohere without dissonance. However, I do think that many elements that appear to be dissonant to an outside observer are not experienced this way emically. When something about a belief system appears to me not to "make sense" or to fit in with the rest of my impression of the system, my first assumption is not that it

actually *is* incoherent, but that I have not yet discovered a higher-order integrating principle used by the person holding the beliefs. This assumption has frequently been borne out in my fieldwork.

13. From the outset, homeopathy enjoyed the support of many prominent people and had its greatest membership in the urban, educated classes. In its current resurgence in the United States, homeopathy's clients are still largely members of well-educated groups (Coulter 1975; Levin and Idler 1981; Starr 1982; Taylor 1984; Kaufman 1988). In the British Isles, Europe, and some parts of Asia, homeopathy was never forced out of favor as it was in the United States, and it remains one of the recognized medical options. In those settings, therefore, it could not properly be classified as a vernacular health belief system but would have to be counted among conventional health care resources.

14. Not all systems are mutually compatible, of course. Homeopathy's theory of pharmaceutical treatment is diametrically opposed to that of conventional medicine, so the committed homeopath would not be likely to use conventional medicine to deal with symptoms. Some forms of religious healing condemn other forms as satanic deceptions, and a few see use of physicians as evidence of lack of faith; the New Age naturopath may regard the root doctor who prescribes plants on the basis of their magical properties as misinformed or actually misleading; the root doctor may feel that the naturopath has access to plants but not to the power required to put them to effective use; and so forth.

15. It is important, in this connection, to reassert the need for caution against assuming homogeneity across belief systems or populations. There is invariably wide intragroup variation in belief and interpretation, and any individual represents an ideally describable belief system only to a certain degree. There is also much intergroup influence, and new information from numerous sources is constantly being incorporated into most systems. Thus one finds powwows who have spirit guides, spiritists who advise meditation and yoga, nurses who practice therapeutic touch and recommend herbal teas and homeopathic remedies, and so on. For these reasons, although knowledge of a cultural tradition tells much about the general cultural repertoire, it cannot be predictive from individual to individual within the cultural group.

Chapter 2
Critical Approaches to Literature and Theories

To arrive at any sort of comprehensive understanding of vernacular health belief systems it is necessary to be able to connect them with a theoretical understanding of belief in general, as well as with an understanding of culture and the cultural frameworks with which all belief systems are interconnected. Belief and behavior are strongly culturally shaped, and definitions of health and illness are cultural products. The most productive approach to vernacular healing systems is necessarily an interdisciplinary effort, for belief and behavior are complex phenomena, and all explanations of complex phenomena are partial accounts. An interdisciplinary or multidisciplinary approach provides multiple reference points and enables differing conceptions to be balanced against and to illuminate each other, providing a more comprehensive view both of the subject and of the various approaches to it.

Several disciplines have either addressed folk and popular health belief systems directly or have engaged in related studies that contribute much to our current capacity to grasp the subject in productive and comprehensive ways. Over time, the regnant social and academic theories and their related concerns and convictions have selectively focused disciplinary attention on particular subjects and objects of interest. These theories and concerns have shaped the scholarship in specific ways. Always at issue, more or less overtly, has been a set of academic beliefs about human nature; about the characteristics of societies or their subgroups; about the nature and production of knowledge and belief; about morals, values, and ethics; and about the relationship of the studier to the studied. In the past twenty years or so this subtext has become a subject of study in itself. This reflexive reorientation has produced a critical inquiry into past approaches, taking into account the cultural shaping of academic and professional knowledge, and articulating the relationships of authority between professional and popular or indigenous ways of knowing.

The Evolutionary Theory of Culture

Late nineteenth- and early twentieth-century investigators of folklore pursued their studies in the well-established atmosphere of antiquarianism, a long-standing intellectual tradition that focused its attentions on all manner of cultural "curiosities," so classified because they were believed to be left over from bygone times. Among these "novel remnants" were included narratives, formulae, manners of dress and performance, and customary practices and observances that were seen as persisting under specific types of circumstances, in spite of a more general social disuse or abandonment. These ostensibly anachronistic cultural outcroppings were typically explained in terms consistent with the social and anthropological theory of cultural evolution. This theory posited the development of peoples and societies by analogy with evolution of plant and animal species, as a linear progression from simpler to more complex, sophisticated, and better-adapted forms over time. It postulated that societies pass through an orderly sequence of developmental phases en route from their most "primitive" to their most "civilized" forms, and equated more civilized forms with the complex and industrialized societies that had produced the scholars and theorizers. These advanced cultures would themselves previously "have gone through the stage of culture now seen in 'primitive' societies. Just as fossils remained in the earth to show earlier life-forms, so cultural fossils might remain hidden in the thought of sophisticated societies, which would show traces of earlier beliefs and customs. The folklore of the people was [considered] just such a survival" (Bennett 1987:3).

A parallel analogy was made to broadly defined developmental stages in individuals, as well. "Primitive" societies were understood to be less socially, educationally, and technically sophisticated than "civilized" societies, and their individual adult members were believed to be—like children—less mentally, emotionally, and cognitively sophisticated than "civilized" or "modern" adults (see, e.g., Black 1883:206). The evolutionary theory of cultures embodied a view of the refinement and perfection of knowledge as both a condition for and a result of social development. In this view, more advanced societies invariably "knew better," both in the sense of having better knowledge and in the sense of having better ways of producing knowledge, than those in earlier stages. Beliefs and practices rejected or left behind by the "official" culture of civilized societies became ipso facto the erroneous products of a less evolved understanding. They were called cultural "survivals." Their study, together with the study of entire cultures still apparently in earlier evolutionary stages (i.e., the primitive[1] cultures of anthropological interest), was embraced by many intellectuals of the period as a valuable archaeology of human knowledge and development, from which significant lessons could be learned for the present (Black 1883:2–4, 214; Wilson 1908).

The circumstances under which vestiges of earlier cultural stages persisted in a generally civilized society were believed to be those which obstructed penetration of the benefits of civilization: isolation, ignorance, poverty, even ethnic difference from the dominant group. A parallel to the evolution of whole societies could thus be found in the social stratification of any given society, with the social elite of the dominant group at the more "civilized" end of the continuum, and the poor and peasant classes at its more "primitive" end. Social class stratification could readily be interpreted as a natural taxonomy of types which resulted from the sorting of people by inherent cultural developmental qualities. Since the leading edge of cultural development was located in the upper social strata, it followed that knowledge and progress must originate there as well. The hypothesis of *gesunkenes Kulturgut*, or "sunken cultural materials" (see Yoder 1972) depicted a society in which new ideas and knowledge poured forth like a spring among the upper classes, with the runoff eventually making its way down the social hill. Nicknamed the "trickle-down" theory, this hypothesis posits the cast-off beliefs of the social and intellectual elite as the source of much folk belief ("we" are sophisticated and now know better; "they" are simple and naïve, and cannot discriminate as well as we between correct and incorrect ideas). Information gradually filters down to the masses, but since this process takes time, the knowledge is outmoded by the time it arrives. The corollary assumption is that the masses lack the capacity to assess these tardy arrivals, and simply accept their content wholesale. The lower classes thus inevitably lag behind the elite in the validity and currency of their knowledge.

Cultural evolutionism as a theory of culture is now generally academically discredited on grounds of gross oversimplification and, worse, of parentalism and ethnocentric bias. Nevertheless, this intellectual history has left a pervasive and often damaging legacy. "Folk belief" has continued to be implicitly or explicitly defined as that body of belief and knowledge which is contradicted or superseded by modern or scientific knowledge. This presumption in turn has conditioned approaches taken to the subject, as would be expected of any subject defined at the outset by its investigators as "incorrect." Evolutionist and survivalist assumptions about culture, cultural processes, and belief and knowledge have until very recently focused the attention of scholars of folk belief almost exclusively on nondominant groups, defined by virtue of their social position and difference from the dominant culture as "the folk." These definitions do much more to invoke the authority of the scholars who generated and continue to sustain them than they do to accurately or usefully represent unofficial belief or its social distribution.

Guided by these views, investigation of folk belief and of the specific subset identified as folk medicine has been carried out, until recently, only in those groups of people recognizably different in some way from the identity groups of the scholars. (Note that this is also the direction currently being taken by most investigations of "culture" and health beliefs and practices. The cultural shaping of the health professions, or of the health beliefs and practices of the investigators, though addressed by some disciplines, is still largely left out of the account.) Because researchers have found in these groups what they were looking for—namely, "old-fashioned" propositions they did not themselves believe and practices in which they did not themselves engage—the skewed definitions have been reified, stereotypes solidified, and investigative attention locked onto only a segment of the researchable field. Whole populations as well as their individual members have been described, by virtue of their difference from the investigators, as "picturesque" (Noall 1959); "eccentric" and "very odd characters" with "peculiar ways" (Rosenberger 1958); "childish . . . crones" and others with "untutored mind[s]" (Hand 1961); "curious" (Davis 1969); and "irrational" (Hand 1961; Tillhagen 1976 [quoted in translation by Holbek 1977]). This has been as true of scholars who did not mean to cast aspersions on their informants as it has been of those who fully intended to disparage anyone who claimed as current, true, and functional those things which "progress" and "modern knowledge" dismissed as outmoded, trivial, or false. Such intentional and unintentional pejorative interpretations persist up to the present and continue to distort the picture of the nature, distribution, and significance of much unofficial belief and knowledge.

Evolutionist assumptions, together with kindred positivist impulses, have obscured recognition of the varying means of production of valid knowledge in all social groups, again reinforcing stereotypes. Knowledge produced through institutionally trained cognitive and technical ability, and application of increasingly sophisticated technologies not accessible to the general public, has the highest status in modern Western societies. The facts of access (to schooling, to credentialing processes, to research funding, etc.) do indeed concentrate these kinds of technical effort in the upper social classes. This situation appears to ratify the trickle-down theory, when it is actually an artifact of the social structure itself. Knowledge is indeed produced "at the top," but largely because only some kinds of knowledge are highly valued and no one else is permitted the same kinds of access to their modes of production. Knowledge produced through lived experience and through ordinary observation of and response to the surrounding environment—the common currency of most people's lives, and the basis of much folk belief and knowledge—has lower status. When it competes or conflicts with officially sanctioned knowledge (and knowers), it is readily dismissed. None of this is to suggest that there is no mistaken information classified as knowledge or that there or no false beliefs. It is rather to say (1) that these, together with accurate information and correct beliefs, exist in both the folk cultural and the official canons; and (2) that whole systems of thought by which millions of people productively guide their lives should not be dismissed out of hand, either because they are not produced or held by the "right" people, or because they actually or apparently contradict official and professional belief and knowledge (see Hufford 1982b, 1983b, 1985c).

Relating to the "Other"

Until quite recently, cultural investigation has typically focused on the "other" (often on the *extremely different* other).[2] This focus derives in part from the same impulse that underlay cultural evolutionism, namely, an ethnocentric bias that one's own ways are normative and speak for themselves, whereas those of "others," insofar as they differ from one's own, are strange and invite explanation. Explanations have then typically been rendered in terms of the nature and causes of otherness. This position easily camouflages "normalcy" and "strangeness" as inherent qualities of thoughts and actions, rather than highlighting them as measures of the familiarity and propriety of thoughts and actions *to specific persons, or set in specific contexts, established by specific cultural custom*. The search for explanations of otherness proceeds from a perceived separation between the researcher (me) and the research subjects (not-me), but also reifies that separation. It focuses attention on difference to the near exclusion of interest in (or notice of) commonality. This orientation has shaped the directions and therefore the findings of research in folk belief and folk healing, by selectively directing scrutiny first to "different" populations, and second, to only those parts of their cultural repertoires which are "different." It has helped to entrench a sense of separation between expert[3] and layperson (or in health care, provider and patient), and has produced a predetermined portrait of the social location of "belief" (layperson: not-me) as opposed to "knowledge" (expert: me). It has obscured the large areas of congruence that exist between folk belief and official belief, for example, such convictions as "that corn is good to eat, that quinine relieves malaria symptoms, or that camels are useful as desert transport" (Hufford 1988d:4), which are found in both repertoires and may be arrived at either experientially or by formal instruction or experimentation. Too frequently it has produced analyses that are beset with overt or implicit invidious comparisons of the culture, beliefs, and intellectual attainments of the study population to the culture, beliefs, and intellectual attainments of the investigator.

It has long been a rule of research that investigators should maintain distance from their subjects (especially their human subjects) in order to promote objectivity in observation. When quantitative methods are used, the methods themselves are generally accepted to promote objectivity, or the "ability to make an evaluation of a situation without being affected by feelings, emotions, and preconceived notions" (Angeles 1981:193), partly by helping to maintain, through their technically specialized character, the distinction of and distance between expert and layperson, me and not-me. (We must leave aside as too knotty for consideration here the proposition that any research method can be free of preconceived notions.) When the methods are qualitative, pressure is increased to maintain distance, not to compromise "objectivity" by identifying too closely with the researched: proper subjects have traditionally been in the not-me category. Violations may result in forfeiture of credibility, especially in controversial topic areas such as folk belief or vernacular health beliefs and practices.[4] Examples include the investigator's "going native" while in the field (i.e., becoming a member of or convert to the culture or belief system being studied); or being a member of the subject group to begin with. Questions of credibility arise especially if the studied group does not have significant cultural authority, or if it espouses views not accepted in the official canon or challenges official authority in some way. For example, it is much more likely that the analytical objectivity of a member of a religious group studying that group's beliefs and practices will be challenged by outsiders than will, say, that of a neurosurgeon studying the beliefs and practices of his or her profession.

In the past ten to fifteen years, as reflexivity has entered many disciplines and as other cultural forces have called into question the utility of certain kinds of "objective" measures, qualitative research methods such as ethnographic studies and focus groups have gained increasing respect and wider application. Quantitative and qualitative studies are beginning to be used to illuminate each other. Recognition is steadily growing of the important contribution of "insider" interpretation of data, especially in matters of values, belief, and behavior which are so readily subject to analytical distortion by the biases of the analyst. Researchers studying not-me groups more frequently include members of the group in the study design and the research team. Researchers who are members of the groups being studied now have in some ways an interpretive edge: their viewpoint is seen to be culturally authentic and accurate, because they have knowledge that can only be gained by experience. (There is of course a danger of oversimplification and stereotyping in this assumption: *all* cultures are diverse, and a cultural insider *may* be just as unfamiliar with important aspects of the worldview as an outsider may be.) Even in quantitative studies, members of the study population in some cases have gained new roles in determining the appropriateness of the definition of the research problem, and of the study design to the population. (The highest-visibility example is the inclusion in the past five years or so of HIV-positive persons on HIV treatment research advisory and review boards.) This narrowing of the gap between me and not-me is now well accepted in qualitative research, which in this era derives its explanatory power from accurate descriptive representation of the insider's point of view.[5] It is still quite controversial in quantitative research, however, and it does call into question the distribution of recognized "competence to make judgments about the nature of reality," that is, of cultural authority (Hufford 1988c:5).

Translating the "Other"

Some efforts to explain the "other" do so by imposing constructs which have the effect of translating insider (emic) claims and explanations into more professionally familiar and acceptable (etic) terms. The implicit or explicit suggestion is that the trained outside observer (me) is better equipped than the cultural insider (not-me) to decipher what is "really" going on. Functionalist and psychoanalytical interpretations offer two examples. Functionalist theories explain the existence or persistence of cultural traits such as folk belief and practice either *as a function* of a given set of social circumstances or constraints, or in terms *of the social functions* of the belief traditions themselves , or both. Functional analyses have produced many important insights and have led to the formulation of innumerable productive research questions. The approach has two inherent dangers, however: (1) it is very often selectively applied (on the basis of the not-me principle), and (2) it frequently advances a descriptive *interpretation* as if it were a sufficient *explanation*. The two are interconnected, and if not guarded against, they skew the resulting image.

For example, the presence of witchcraft beliefs and practices in a given cultural group is often "explained" by the observation that the witchcraft complex (interrelated beliefs, prohibitions, behaviors, sanctions) serves the social functions of allocating responsibility and blame for certain kinds of misfortune and of linking punishment with specific orders of social transgressions. This must account for its presence (implication: otherwise, why would people believe these things that modern knowledge has rejected?). Indeed, it does do these things. Official systems of jurisprudence and legal codes established by written charter and sustained by social and cultural authority also serve these social functions. Yet no scholar would seriously suggest that these functional outcomes solely or sufficiently explain the existence and structure of a legal system or of the judiciary branch of a government. The inadequacy of such an "explanation" is apparent. By extension, neither can social functions properly be said wholly to explain the existence of witchcraft traditions—especially as they are commonly found in societies that *also* have legal and judiciary systems.

With regard to nonconventional health behavior, explanations of people's recourse to vernacular healing traditions (and especially to heavily magical or religious traditions) have commonly been offered in terms of these systems' socially integrative function in bringing family members together in support of a sick person, and their psychological function in reducing anxiety in the face of illness. The taking of antibiotics by persons convinced of their efficacy in fighting infections also serves an anxiety-reducing function (Hufford 1988a). Hospitalizations can serve a socially integrative function in rallying family and community members to the aid of a patient. Neither of these indisputable functions, however, can adequately explain the use either of antibiotics or of hospitalizations in responding to episodes of sickness and in seeking to restore health. Neither can strictly functional expositions adequately explain recourse to vernacular healing systems.

Psychological and psychoanalytical theories of culture and behavior share characteristics with functionalism. Each focuses varying degrees of its explanatory attention on latent functions. But while functionalism locates the functions of folk belief and attendant behaviors within the social system, the psychological and psychoanalytical approaches locate them within the needs and drives of individuals. This often has the unpleasant effect of portraying the individuals (or whole populations) being observed as in some way emotionally, cognitively, or psychologically impaired: driven by excessive anxiety for which they have no other coping mechanisms (Mullen 1969); unable to distinguish actual from illusory events (Honko 1964; Ward 1977; de Vries 1982); frankly neurotic (Charles 1953); or even, in some cases, schizophrenic (Stevens 1982). This type of interpretation has been liberally applied to folk belief, to nonbiomedical healers, and to members of vernacular healing systems. I do not mean to suggest that such interpretations are never appropriate. Rather, I want to observe that they have been grossly overapplied, sometimes producing significant and damaging distortions as when applied, for example, to healing traditions or to religious experience (for the latter, see Cartwright 1982:65; Havens 1960:82–83).

Explanations in terms of latent social or psychological functions tend to be offered for the existence of only certain classes of the total range of beliefs and behaviors described for a study population. This selective application generally involves beliefs and behaviors not in the scholars' own cultural repertoires of positively valued options (which may be the very reason they have attracted attention in the first instance, and have been classified as standing in need of explanation). For example, Mullen (1969), in a study of the lives of commercial fishermen, notes that beliefs and behavior patterns have both instrumental (overt) and psychological (covert) functions: "instrumental functions are designed to handle problems not subject entirely to empirical control," while psychological functions provide relief from anxiety and stress related to the built-in risks and uncertainties of people's lives (p. 216). To illustrate, he cites certain magical beliefs and practices of fishermen, noting that they are part of a "complex system of devices that function as instrumental aids to the fishermen," a system that also includes "products of modern technology" such as electronic communications and navigational devices, the latest fishing and boating equipment, and up-to-the-moment professional meteorological forecasts. Both magical and technological beliefs and behaviors are identified as having instrumental intent. However, only the magical beliefs and behaviors are "explained," and the explanation is rendered in terms of their covert or psychological functions (derived from psychological theories).

In support of his analysis of functional reasons why magical beliefs and practices form a part of the work lives of the fishermen, Mullen quotes Malinowski: "Wherever there is danger, uncertainty, great incidence of chance and anxiety, even in entirely modern forms of enterprise, magic crops up" (Malinowski, 1931; reprinted in Lessa and Vogt, 1965). No doubt this observation is correct. However, it is equally correct to observe that wherever there is danger, uncertainty, great incidence of chance and anxiety (even in *non*modern forms of enterprise), a proliferation of logistical and technological responses crops up. Surely the uses of modern technology, no less than the uses of weather charms and good-luck practices, necessarily function among fishermen to relieve the anxiety of a risk-laden work life and are wishfully employed to promote success in their business ventures. Nevertheless, one would hardly would posit that *this* range of responses arises out of "acute psychological need" (Mullen 1969:224) or that the individuals who "have the greatest need will internalize [their acceptance of them] to the greatest extent" (p. 219). Neither with respect to folk belief and practice any more than with respect to scientific and technological belief and practice can interpretation in terms of latent functions (social or personal) constitute a full and adequate *explanation* of the existence of the beliefs and behaviors in question.

Functionalist and psychological theories lean toward constructing otherness as the product of the stresses of special social circumstances (e.g., limited resources, acculturation processes), of combined social and personal stresses (e.g., occupational anxieties, role adaptation), or of personal attributes (e.g., ignorance, reduced coping ability, wish-fulfillment or projective ideation, perceptual or interpretive deficits). Such influences upon human behavior are not trivial, but their explanatory value is limited to the situations in which they can actually be determined (not assumed) to apply, and overextension of their application is misleading. When selectively applied to beliefs and actions in which the scholar does not participate (and especially to those which the scholar explicitly rejects), such theoretical orientations imply that the beliefs to whose analysis they are applied are false, and the actions those beliefs inform "really" accomplish something other than what the actor intends and believes them to do.

This stance assumes "*a priori* that [the investigator's] view fits more correctly with the objective reality of the situation" (Scott 1993:17) than that of the investigatee. Without substantiation of this assumption, however, such analyses remain essentially theoretical. They are acts of translation into terms congruent with academic belief (and with academic "traditions of disbelief"; see Hufford 1982b, 1983b). As with all translations, their final accuracy of reflection of the original material depends upon some capacity to "check back" against the original, and to assure that nothing critical has been lost in the translation process. It is essential to evenhanded study of belief traditions to recognize that such translations constitute "shift[s] in perspective" but cannot be taken at face value as "correction of [a subject's] errors" (Cartwright 1982:65). It is not necessary to agree or to exoticize in order to describe and comprehend belief traditions. It *is* necessary, however, to avoid oversimplification or premature judgment.

Effects of the "Lens" upon the View

It is evident that particular theoretical orientations, particular sets of assumptions, condition the ways in which a subject is approached. It is increasingly well recognized too that assumptions, theories, and methods influence what is and is not observed or taken into account about the subject, and may even dramatically shape what are taken to be the actual contours of the subject itself. That is to say, what is seen and how it is seen may be (to varying degrees) artifacts of the lens used to do the seeing in the first place. (This caveat is expressed more pungently in the modern proverb, "When all you have is a hammer, the world looks a lot like a nail.") This is an important notion to bear in mind when exploring the literature, especially in dealing with complex or controversial topics such as unofficial belief and vernacular healing practices.

The extent of theoretical influence is well illustrated by an example from two approaches in folklore scholarship to a body of oral narratives that recount the protagonist's being physically oppressed by some unseen force (Hufford 1982a). Central features of these narratives are typically that the victim is resting or sleeping when the attack begins, that s/he feels pressure on the chest and perhaps has difficulty breathing, and that s/he is unable to move or to cry out while this usually very frightening event is going on. Such features figure prominently in all of the narratives and help to define them as a class. Additional features of the narratives may include variable details about the critical event itself, interpretations of the event, details about the protagonist or the setting or the actions and outcomes, appeals to various sources of verification or legitimation of claims, and morals to the story. The attacks are frequently interpreted in these narratives as some form of supernatural assault.

One approach that folklore scholars have taken to this body of narratives is that of genre analysis, a well-established academic tradition for classifying and explicating the enormous variety and quantity of material in oral traditions. This approach treats oral traditions as significant forms of artistic expression. The genre orientation has worked together with certain definitions of folk belief to classify narratives of supernatural experiences together in a single broad category, with topical subdivisions such as ghost stories, witch riding, and so forth. Categorical subdivisions were based on other traits: those told in the first person, for example, and therefore alleged to be firsthand accounts, received the classification "memorate" (von Sydow 1948;[6] Honko 1964). The particular narratives to which our example refers, owing to variations in the narrative voice, settings, and interpretations they reflected, were parceled out among the subsets of supernatural stories. The recognizable themes and descriptive elements that linked the stories together (the particular event as subject, features such as oppression, inability to move, etc.) were readily cross-checked with important reference works of folktale themes and motifs (Thompson 1955). Their repeated appearance in certain clusters helped to classify the tales as types of supernatural tales, while widely variable elements were lumped together as ancillary but unnecessary details, idiosyncratically supplied by storytellers as must have seemed to suit the occasion of the telling. Other contents, such as preventive or remedial actions mentioned in the narratives, would be parceled out into separate categories of "folk belief" and "folk remedies," assumed to be naïve, false, or fictive. First-person accounts could be accepted as the believed reports of persons who had had experiences conditioned or even produced by their cultural knowledge of the traditions (Honko 1964; Ward 1977).

In sharp contrast is the experience-centered or phenomenological[7] approach to supernatural narrative and belief, originated by David Hufford in his studies of the "Old Hag" tradition of Newfoundland and its cross-cultural counterparts (Hufford 1974a, 1976a, 1976b, 1982a). This approach is founded on the considerations that experiences commonly give rise to narratives, and that narratives that contain supernatural elements or interpretations are not ipso facto confabulations that emerge from artistic, fictive oral traditions. Pursuit of the possibility that the reported paralysis experiences might be actual—that is, not products of imagination, perceptual errors, or cultural modeling—led to Hufford's discovery that behind these particular memorates indeed lay an identifiable experience of transitory recumbent paralysis common to roughly one-quarter of the members of any randomly selected population (Hufford 1982a, 1988b). This experience is usually (but not always) identified in the medical literature as a form of sleep paralysis. In folk traditions, it is identified in variable ways, including (but not restricted to) supernatural assault of the victim (for a full treatment of the phenomenon and its varieties of official and folk interpretations, see Hufford 1982a). A phenomenological approach recognizes that experiences affect and even produce belief, and demonstrates that the connections between experience, belief, narrative, and practice are complex and multidimensional.

The central recurrent features of these narratives are those of the experience itself. Since these have been widely observed among people who have had the experience, they also figure prominently in its description and can be intersubjectively validated by others who have had the experience. Put simply, they appear so frequently in the narratives not because that is the way stories are told in this culture or that, but because that is what *happens* to the people who have the paralysis experience. They are also oral traditional motifs. This *does* mean that they are motifs that have been widely recognized in and collected from oral tradition (in many types of narrative frameworks), but it *does not* therefore mean that they are by definition fictional elements. Variable features and individualistic details, which genre analysts have classed as "unnecessary" details in memorates, turn out in this case to be details of personal observation that vary according to individual circumstances at the time of the paralysis attacks. These details are furnished and even stressed in the narratives because narrators use them to emphasize the accuracy of their observations, and to diminish any impression that they may have been mistaken or confused in their perceptions at the time of the experience (Hufford 1976b, 1982a). They are not dramatic devices, but evidential submissions (see Cartwright 1982). Far from being somehow "dispensible" (Honko 1964), the personally variable details are as central to the accounts as the traditional motifs, both of which link them reliably to actual experiences. Preventive and curative measures reported in the narratives are not interjections of some other genre of lore, but reports of efforts made and found effective, central elements of the whole accounts.

The phenomenological approach to belief does not reject out of hand the possibility that narratives of believed events may be reports rather than fictions, *even if* their subjects or their interpretive frameworks are contrary to the accepted ontological categories of academic, professional, or scientific belief. It is possible and productive to assume this investigative stance regardless of the investigator's degree of acceptance or skepticism of the material itself. It is an approach that can be applied as productively to accounts of nonbiomedical healing as to the narratives cited in this case example. An experience-centered approach calls for suspension of disbelief or judgment until all of the data are in, and it opens the investigation to orders of data that narrative or genre analysis excludes (data, in this case, that have also been excluded by many social or psychological functional theories; see Hufford 1982a). It takes fully into account the narrator's claims or point of view. By separating the informants' *interpretations* (e.g., supernatural assault) from their *observations* (e.g., paralysis, feeling of pressure on the chest, inability to vocalize, fear), this approach pursues the reported experience and its sources with as much interest as the interpretations and their sources. It takes account of all of the data (as opposed to rejecting some a priori and discounting other parts as superfluous), and derives theoretical analysis *from* the data, as opposed to applying it *to* the data. The analogy to health care settings, and to full and careful consideration or patients' beliefs and points of view, should be apparent.

Overview and Summary of Literature

A number of disciplines have dealt with vernacular health belief systems, and an interdisciplinary search is essential to finding the full range of available material. A great store of information, together with a variety of theoretical and methodological orientations, is found in the combined literatures of folklore, anthropology and its subset, medical anthropology, sociology, nursing, public health, and biomedicine. Also relevant to aspects of this complex phenomenon and its interconnections with other parts of human experience and culture are the literatures of religious studies, philosophy, history of medicine and public health, international public health, ethnobotany, pharmacognosy, communications, counseling, international business (intercultural communications and negotiations), and conflict resolution, among others.

Because the material has been differently classified and interpreted across disciplines and through time, there is an abundant variety of index terms that lead to the topic. Study of the terms and their changes and distributions by discipline and decade of scholarship is fascinating in its own right and shows that the index, far from being the neutral finding-aid that we generally assume it to be, is itself a revealing rhetorical device. Indexes to literature and databases list material on non-biomedical healing under such diverse keywords and search terms as "folk medicine," "ethnomedicine," "traditional medicine" (which in other contexts refers to modern scientific medicine), "primitive medicine," "unorthodox medicine," "herbal medicine," "botanical medicine," "marginal medicine," "healing," "alternative medicine," "cults," "medical anthropology," "occult medicine," "lay health care," "self-care," "unproven remedies," "health belief," "health behavior," "quacks and quackery," "health education," and "popular errors and misconceptions," among many others.[8] Searches should also include terms specific to particular systems (e.g., moxibustion), to particular diseases or syndromes, and to specific populations. The latter will turn up references to many populations but cannot be used to find distribution of alternative healing modalities in populations of no specific identity-group affinity, because they are not a "listed group." Variation of search term combinations will produce different yields, even when terms appear synonymous.

Across the literature, evaluations and descriptions have encompassed—with varying degrees of precision and adequacy—questions of efficacy, theories of health and illness, modes of achieving therapeutic results, reasons why systems are believed and used, motivations and personality types of healers and clients, longevity and popularity in communities of believers and patrons. Approaches taken in one time period or in one discipline should be compared with those of other time periods and disciplines, and all should be read thoughtfully and analytically for their particular assumptions and biases. Literature-based research should not be confined to academic sources, for this subject has also received extensive coverage in the popular media, including critiques, explanations, popular reference works, self-help guides, how-to publications, and advocacy literature of many types. Some of these sources give the most thorough and detailed explications of the theoretical bases and practical contents of nonbiomedical health belief systems. They are excellent resources for understanding how clients may see the systems, for they are typically the identical sources which clients use for information and reference. As with the academic literature, this literature should be read analytically, with an eye to bias and underlying assumptions, so that the fullest understanding of the approach to the subject can be gained.

Owing to the enormity and complexity of these bodies of pertinent literature, only selected disciplines will be reviewed here. The reviews are necessarily simplified, general, and cursory, highlighting only a small selection of the relevant points and significant publications. Generalizations refer to well-represented trends within the scholarship as a whole or within referenced subsets; there are of course exceptions to all of them. Every discipline has its general orientation, its biases, and its collection of viewpoints. I have tried to identify some of these, sometimes as critiques but always as information pertinent to understanding an additional and very important dimension of their findings. Members of various professional disciplines frequently publish in the journals of other disciplines, and authors seek the outlet that will put their material before the eyes of the audiences to whom they find it most pertinent or useful. Many journals are interdisciplinary in nature and are organized around specific problems or issues, rather than disciplinary background, orientation, or membership. The disciplinary divisions I have used are conventions reflected in the literature but do not necessarily reveal the specific training of individual contributing authors.

Folklore

Folk Belief

The antiquirian impulse and the perspective of survivalism led for many decades to avid collecting of "surviving items" of folk belief. These were generally defined as being cultural "remnants," ideas and modes of thought that no longer had currency in academic and professional or "educated" portions of society (Noall 1959; Hand 1961, 1964; Barrick 1964; Byington 1964a; Kirtley 1964; Hatch 1969; de Vries 1982). The survival of these modes of thought was thought to be accounted for by such factors as geographical isolation or a general backwardness and credulity in the people who maintained them as traditions. This position assumed, among other things, an equation between education and schooling, and often an equation between schooling and intelligence (biases still alive and well today).

The "item" orientation developed from assumptions that the various propositions discovered were isolates, "nuggets" in an otherwise quite differently constituted cultural matrix. This view pitched folk belief naturally into genre studies, where it was classed as a "minor" oral genre (i.e., short utterances or statements, vs. complex narrative forms), along with jokes, riddles, proverbs, and other traditional locutions, all dealt with according to literary and linguistic or philological theories. Comparative studies have produced extensive collecting over both historical and geographical ranges and have resulted in the publication of numerous regional and ethnic collections (e.g., Puckett 1926; Brendle and Unger 1935; Randolph 1947; Browne 1958; Dundes 1961; Hand 1961, 1964; Byington 1964; Hyatt 1970). Though these are largely listings, with little or no contextual information, they are valuable comparative finding-aids and reference works, especially where annotated.

For most of the history of its study, folk belief has been reduced to "superstition," and to categories of supernatural or magical belief (Hand 1961; Honko 1964; Blehr 1967; Mullen 1969), with the remainder of popular wisdom unstudied in any comparable depth. Incorporated into this definition is the presumption of falsity (inherent in the term "superstition") which is the legacy of cultural evolutionism and positivism. Others have added as definitive criteria that folk belief "must have a function different from [its] avowed instrumental intention" (Mullen 1969:216), or that it is "always illogical" (Tillhagen 1976, quoted in translation by Holbek 1977:143). Problems of classifying "popular beliefs and superstitions" turned on definitional debates, and most of the definitions dealt not with qualities of "the material itself but rather with *opinions* about the material" (Dundes 1961:26, emphasis added). As a result, much of the explicative literature (in folklore and in other disciplines) has centered either on falsification of believers' claims or, later, on their explanation in terms quite different from those used by the believers themselves but purporting to be what they were "really" about (the majority being psychoanalytical or functional analyses). These tendencies were perhaps exacerbated by the concentration of collecting effort and analytical interest on the two broad subcategories of folk religion and folk medicine, departments of belief in which feelings run high and official authority has long been firmly established.

The genre approach for decades diverted academic attention away from folk belief as active, systematic, dynamic, and interrelated with numerous facets of people's lives and of their surrounding cultures. Only since the 1960s has this veil been lifted, and description expanded to include complex traditions and systems of belief, rather than "beliefs," as items. The example was set in the sixties for description and analysis of folk belief *as it actually exists* on the cultural landscape: thoroughly enmeshed in entire ways of life, in complex worldviews, and in systems of thought and values touching upon all aspects of life (Yoder 1965, 1972, 1974; Hufford passim). Compartmentalization was recognized as a creation of the academy, and its contribution to misrepresentation of the subject began to become clearer. Increasingly, scholarship has called for social and cultural contextual information (Goldstein 1964; Pentikäinen 1965; Yoder 1972, 1974; Hufford 1974, 1976a, and passim), as well as for precision in recording and reporting informants' exact words along with their explanations (Goldstein 1964; Hufford 1974, 1976a), in order to assure that academic interpretation not precede full collection of the data (Hufford 1976a). These requirements are central to an ethnographic approach to the study of belief.

Belief began to be recognized as dynamic, variable by circumstance and through time for a single individual, as well as variable across populations of believers (Goldstein 1964; Yoder passim; Hufford passim). By the 1970s scholars began to define belief not as a "thing," but as an attribute or quality that cuts across genres and activities—quilting and farming and pottery-making no less than telling legends and tales or reciting proverbs to invoke a moral in a specific situation (Dundes 1971; Yoder 1972; Hufford 1974; 1976a). Folk belief began to be defined not in terms of incongruence with academic belief or of social location (i.e., in specific populations, "the folk") but in terms of kinds of processes contributing to its formulation and support—observation, experience, and informal modes of teaching and learning (Yoder passim; Hufford passim). As such, folk belief coexists with official belief in the worldviews of all kinds of people, from all kinds of cultural backgrounds, and of all degrees of formal educational exposure. These recognitions guide much of the current work on folk belief.

Most influential in shaping current belief scholarship have been the theoretical and methodological contributions of David Hufford. In the 1970s he began to challenge existing notions of folk groups and folk belief (1971, 1976a), and to insist that the study of belief be pursued with the same accuracy, thoroughness, and rigor of description as the study of any other aspects of culture (narrative, technology, architecture, foodways, etc.). The subject, in other words, is a serious subject, which must be taken seriously and treated seriously. In this pursuit, as in any other act of scholarly investigation, thorough description must *precede* judgment and form the basis for analysis (1976a). Questions of truth or falsity cannot be antecedent to the study of belief. Often truth or falsity are moot, or cannot be demonstrated with certainty either way using academic theoretical tools (e.g., much supernatural belief). It is not necessary to agree with the belief system in order to obtain a detailed description, and description in emic terms does not imply endorsement (1976a, 1982a).

Hufford explicitly challenges assumptions that have informed the bulk of prior study of folk belief. He identifies academic and scientific belief, as well as their "traditions of disbelief" (1982b), as inviting investigation and explication equally with traditions of folk and popular belief. Academic and folk belief are open and amenable to the same modes of inquiry (1983b). Any belief system can productively be studied in terms of its contents and worldview, its cultural shaping, and its complex interconnections with all aspects of the lives of its members. All can be investigated in terms of their reasons for credibility, answers to the question "why is thus-and-so believed to be true (or false)?" Factors such as observation and the accumulation of empirically based supporting evidence; acceptance of tenets on the basis of recognized authoritative status of their source; use of inductive and deductive reasoning; and grounding in personal experience are processes that official and unofficial belief systems have in common.

Using ethnographic methods and a phenomenological framework, Hufford focuses on the connections between belief and experience (both personal and collective). This approach by no means excludes recognition of cultural, social, and psychological influences on the development and reinforcement of belief, nor does it fail to recognize that belief traditions serve significant social and personal functions and that analysis of these functions is illuminating and important. But it does reject such analyses as sole and sufficient explanations (Hufford 1976b, 1982a, 1985c). Hufford establishes three methodological minimum conditions, radical in relation to prior research in this area: (1) that the perspective of the believer be weighed equally in the balance with the perspective of the scholar, and that each be identified *as* a perspective; (2) that the belief systems of scholars be answerable to the same questions as those applied to the belief systems they study; and (3) that the community of scholars not subject the belief systems it studies to types of interpretation (or other considerations) from which it holds itself to be exempt. This approach is readily transferable to all interactions between health professionals and their patients (e.g., for each of the three points above, substitute "provider" for "scholar") in which it is important properly to understand and consider the patient's (layperson's) point of view.

Folk Medicine

Folk medicine has been dealt with, until very recently, primarily as a subset of folk belief (and its attendant practices). This is at least in part appropriate, given that a full understanding of vernacular healing traditions cannot be achieved without accompanying knowledge of the ways in which all manner of beliefs about health, illness, and healing are integrated into broader cultural frameworks and larger systems of belief and values. It has been damaging, however, in that the "bad" reputation of folk belief in general—assigned to it by its scholars—has been contagious, and study of folk medicine has suffered accordingly. The same presumption of randomness and silliness has been applied to folk healing traditions, with the same detrimental effects. There is a pervasive impression among writers on folk healing (and this holds in all disciplines) that when these systems achieve their intended thera-peutic ends, they do so only serendipitously—having apparently been based on no application of prior knowledge, pragmatic principles, or gathering of data through observation—and that it is only by fortune that they do not cause widespread harm.

"The history of the study of folk medicine has followed the same general pattern as other aspects of folk culture, first the literary or philological approach, followed by the sociological or functional ap-proach" (Yoder 1972:194). That is to say, the focus of attention has ranged from genres and collectanea (or "items") with emphasis on their historical and geographical derivations and distribution, to analy-sis of causes or contributing factors of patterns of occurrence and distribution. The latter interest has been propelled largely by the un-derlying assumption that any former practical utility these cultural elements may have had must have been superseded by modern tech-nological and scientific developments. It is related as well to the long-prevailing sentiment that folk belief is by definition outmoded or in-correct. In the United States, folk medical "items" have consistently appeared in the general collectanea of "popular beliefs and supersti-tions" as well as in small collections of exclusively folk medical focus. Such collections are, like folk belief collections in general, largely ag-gregations of snippets and statements (e.g., "to cure x, do thus-and-so") lacking accompanying contextual information—including verification of whether the items collected were actually believed and used, or simply familiar (perhaps only as remembered phrases) to those from whom they were collected. This "collections" approach both proceeded from and reinforced, by its presentation, the survivalist position, which conditioned a view of folk medicine as consisting largely of random, isolated, or at best loosely aggregated ideas and practices.

Articles and notes in the folklore literature have until quite recently centered primarily on enumerations: "remedies" or "cures," statements about how people come to have healing knowledge and abilities, brief observations on the healing properties of particular plants and other substances, and recipes for home remedies specific to certain conditions or ailments. Varying combinations of these topical foci frequently appear together, but seldom with any explication of the ways in which they are interconnected in tradition. Collections tend to be regional or ethnic in focus (e.g., Hansen 1959; Hand 1961; Lathrop 1961; Barrick 1964; Byington 1964b; Anderson 1968; McIntosh 1978). The folklore journals of the southern states in particular publish a great number of pieces dealing with their own regions' traditions, especially as they are found in rural areas. This pattern may reflect not only the regional interest and regional pride characteristic of the South but also the "rural assumption" that has long been a part of the stereotype of users of nonconventional medicine in all parts of the country.

The Centennial Index of the *Journal of American Folklore* lists "medicine" as a subhead of "belief systems" and contains seventy-two entries for this single journal in the one hundred years it covers (1888–1988). Of these, a mere thirteen articles provide any significant amount of contextual information or describe a folk medical *system* used by a person or group. The item/genre approach is still very much in evidence in folk medical articles of recent vintage (Hand 1985; Ashley 1986; Muzzy 1986). In spite of their informational shortcomings, collectanea are not to be entirely disparaged. They do collectively form a compendious account of the range, prevalence, and distribution of folk medical *propositions*. They make good comparative references, and they do give some idea of the historical depth of the presence of such propositions both regionally and nationally (e.g., when a particular remedy or proposition is reported in a turn-of-the-century collection and is still reported in a very recent one).

Prior to the 1960s there are relatively few descriptions in the folklore literature of healing traditions in context, or of healing traditions as they are actually put into practice. Notable early exceptions are the studies of Brendle and Unger (1935) and Simmons (1955). These studies are also exceptional in placing their primary emphasis on the nonmagical components of the systems they describe. In addition, Simmons's article is an early example of "applied" interest, as he considers the implications of the local folk medical system for responses of Peruvian and Chilean indigenous peoples to proposed widespread introduction of conventional medical clinics in their homelands. Since the 1960s, published descriptions of healing practices or of health belief systems have increasingly included contextual information (e.g., Firestone 1962; Gunda 1962; Barrett and Vogt 1969; Stekert 1970;

Hufford 1971a, 1974a, 1976b, 1977a, 1982a, 1984, 1985d, 1987, 1988a; Brown 1973; Reimensnyder 1982; Graham 1985). Barrett and Vogt (1969) and Hufford (1971) give descriptions of the belief systems of primarily educated, middle-class groups, and Reimensnyder (1982) of a tradition (Pennsylvania German powwowing) that cuts across educational and social class lines within a particular cultural heritage group. Stekert (1970) demonstrates with clarity and detail how domestic public health measures can fail as a consequence of incompatibility with the beliefs, values, and needs of a specific population of intended beneficiaries. Hufford (passim) and Graham (1985) stress the intragroup diversity in personal acceptance of specific health belief systems, and Hufford (passim) also addresses belief traditions which cross ethnic, cultural, and socioeconomic boundaries.

Special issues of *Keystone Folklore* (Vol. 9[3], 1964) and *Western Folklore* (Vol. 44[3], 1985) have been devoted to folk medicine in recent decades. Of closely related interest and relevance are also special journal issues on folk religion (*Western Folklore* 33[1], 1974) and on the study of belief (*New York Folklore* 8[3/4], 1982). The Anglo-American folklore literature contains as yet very few studies of individual folk healers, which would be most useful additions. This gap in the scholarship no doubt proceeds from the long-standing orientation to folk medicine as a genre, rather than as an active and integral aspect of folklife and folk cultural studies. Perhaps it does at any rate appropriately reflect the considerable percentage of folk healing that does not involve specialists or practitioners but is carried out as self-care, or within a nonspecialized family or community setting.

Academic classification of vernacular healing systems or their specific practices has commonly divided them into two subcategories, one containing material and one nonmaterial elements. Practices based on physical interventions and on botanical and other substances are sorted into the material category, also called "natural" or "rational." Those involving the influence of planetary or cosmic forces, or uses of magical actions, sacramental objects, "charms, holy words, and holy actions" (Yoder 1972:192) are classed as nonmaterial, also called "magical," "magico-religious," "irrational," and occasionally "occult" (e.g., Bø 1963; Hand 1976, 1980, 1985; Alver 1982; see also Yoder 1972). Folklorists have tended to overconcentrate their attention on the "magical" category, its apparently inherent greater interest deriving from the long-standing equation of folk medicine and folk belief with "superstition" and from the association of superstition, magic, and other "survivals" with specific populations or "folk groups."[9]

The binary classification model is not indigenous to the vernacular systems themselves.[10] They are "outsider" (or etic) classifications that reflect traditional academic categories and derive from application of the standards and criteria of conventional medicine to the evaluation of other healing traditions. Principles congruent with those of scientific knowledge—such as the belief that plants and other substances may be used to relieve symptoms and promote healing—are classed as "rational." The underlying assumption is that these applications "might actually work," and therefore constitute rational responses to sickness. Principles which conventional medicine and science have rejected— the spiritual, cosmological, metaphysical, and supernatural elements—are labeled "irrational."

The binary model misrepresents the systems it is used to study, and frequently creates descriptions of healing systems that are actually descriptions of the model's way of seeing. On examination of health belief systems as wholes, the model breaks down rather quickly (see Hufford 1983b, 1984, 1988a; Alver and Selberg 1987b). The majority of vernacular healing systems integrate material and nonmaterial elements in a unified healing practice and philosophy: for example, combining herbal medicaments with charms to insure their efficacy and prayers for swift relief; harvesting and preparing medicinal herbs according to astrological signs or principles of sympathy; recognizing both naturally and supernaturally or spiritually caused classes or aspects of sickness, each with its distinct requirements for healing. Medicaments may or may not be used pharmacologically: they may be taken for other kinds of healing properties. Physical interventions may or may not not be used for physical remediation: they may be intended to promote redistribution of energies or to stimulate the body's vital force. Classification of the elements of vernacular healing systems in terms of etic categories and theories thus obscures the complexity and integrative connections of the whole system and overrides or even omits the system's own explanatory theories.

Successes of vernacular healing systems are academically evaluated in light of their plausibility within a scientific framework. (This approach is common to all disciplines that have addressed the subject of folk medicine.) Botanical remedies are considered to be actual or potential "objectively effective medicines" (Honko 1963:291) whose efficacy, if any, is pharmacological.[11] Some medicinals are asserted to achieve their effects through placebo responses. Successes of nonmaterial interventions are attributed either to placebo response or to some mechanism analogous to psychotherapeutic processes, since they are presumed to have no objectively real basis (Hufford 1983b; see e.g., Lathrop 1961; Dillner 1963; Honko 1963; Meñez 1978; Forssén 1982; Vuori 1982). Folk illness categories are assimilated to psychological states or psychiatric diagnostic categories (Hufford 1988a), with which they are not identical or isomorphic. Some of these interpretations, in some instances, may prove well supported if adequately tested. The problem is, at present, they are seldom the results of testing but rather the assertions of a predetermined position. They contain much strong feeling, but little actual information. They are good research *questions*, posing as answers.

The study of folk medicine in folklore, as in other disciplines, has long been dominated by evolutionism and survivalism. These influences have helped to perpetuate several inaccuracies. Prominent among these are (1) a view of unofficial forms of healing as illuminating "earlier and more primitive stages of man's development," or indeed of surviving from such stages (Hand 1983:252); and (2) the notion that these traditions consist largely of leftovers from earlier periods in the history of conventional medicine (e.g., Honko 1982). These interrelated assumptions have contributed profoundly to the stereotyping of folk medicine or nonconventional healing as residing only in the "marginal" subcultures of any society. The stereotype in turn, with its implications of ruralism, poverty, and lack of education and understanding, is easily reinterpreted as causal in the persistence of folk medical traditions. The image is clear in statements such as these: "Folk medicine thrives in rural areas where doctors are nonexistent or, if they do exist, are too expensive for the low-income family to call except in dire emergency" (Barrick 1964:100). The statement may be fairly accurate as to the vigor of folk medicine in rural areas, but it is shaped by (and contributes to the perpetuation of) the marginality assumption, several of whose images it invokes in a single sentence: ruralism, poverty, and lack of conventional medical resources. As we now know with certainty, folk medicine (by which we mean broadly all "unofficial" forms of health care) also thrives in both rural and urban areas where doctors are plentiful; where income levels and insurances (even for the poor, e.g., medical assistance programs) may not prevent access to conventional medicine; and where other considerations besides determination of emergency enter into decisions to seek help from a doctor, or to use any of a wide array of other health care means.

Folk medicine often gives the appearance of supporting survivalism, as well as the trickle-down theory of knowledge. Vernacular health belief and practice do in fact actively retain a number of elements that were once current in official medical thought but have subsequently been discarded in that domain.[12] Examples include the principle of vitalism, humoral models of health and illness, the doctrine of signatures in herbalism, and such healing practices as cupping and bloodletting, purging with cathartics or emetics, application of blisters and plasters, and pursuit of healing actions or substances according to astrological principles. These elements, however, are not survivals in the sense implied in evolutionary cultural theory. That is, they are not "primitive" elements, shown through cultural progress to be worthless, yet somehow still present in some social strata as intriguing cultural fossils. Rather, they are active elements of vigorous and adaptive systems that continually incorporate new knowledge and undergo dynamic change, and are held and used by intelligent and reasonable people in all social strata. They survive from an earlier *historical period*— as does a large portion of the content of any culture—but not from an antecedent *developmental stage*. Healing traditions, like narrative traditions or material cultural traditions, continually undergo processes of dynamic evaluation and selection, and elements that have no further utility, or that no longer appear effective, drop out of the mix. That causal relations are differently attributed by conventional medical explanation and folk medical explanation does not alter the fact that observation has supported a sense of both the efficacy of particular therapeutic measures and the predictive and explanatory utility of theories of illness and healing within folk medical tradition.

The relationship between folk and official health belief is a great deal more complex and interactive than trickle-down notions suggest, and the flow of information does not always move in one direction. Conventional medicine has learned and can still learn much from folk tradition, as a number of standard drugs demonstrate, and as the current (and well-funded) interest of pharmaceutical firms in folk healing traditions as potential sources of new drugs attests. Many similar or identical techniques have been separately developed in different healing traditions. Early historical sources note, for example, that Aztec healers practiced bloodletting and sweating, administered herbal purgatives and cathartics, sutured, and set broken bones (Murdock 1980). These techniques were virtually identical with the healing practices of the European physicians of the day but were well established on this continent before European contact. Historically a good number of explanatory models of illness and healing have also been common to both professional and popular belief, just as germ theory is current in both domains at present. Very wide divergence between conceptions in the professional and popular spheres is a recent phenomenon (Rosenberg 1979). Even with the current divergence spurred by increasing technical specialization of knowledge, medical ideas and terminology become rapidly available to the public through various media and are selectively incorporated into unofficial traditions. Further, ideas and practices from the popular sphere gain attention, spark experimentation, and give rise to treatment programs in conventional settings (examples include acupuncture, meditation and visualization, and relaxation therapies).

In the early 1970s it began to be observed that official and unofficial medical traditions share the ground (i.e., their use is not mutually exclusive) and that the clientele of nonbiomedical healing systems encompasses a wide variety of groups and individuals (Yoder 1972). It can no longer be presumptively identified with peasant cultures and uneducated segments of society. Following the lead of European folklorists and the folklife approach, Yoder notes that "folk" is best defined "not in terms of class or cultural level in society but as a way of thinking within the individual, always combined today with other levels and types of thinking" (p. 193). Folk medicine is best conceived as the "viewpoints about sickness and health [that] people possess on the ground of their own thinking" (Erich and Beitel, quoted in translation in Yoder 1972:193–194).

Yoder's definition marks the beginning of an important shift in American folk medical scholarship in the early 1970s. A quantum leap was made by Hufford's development of the "health belief systems" approach, which places folk medical traditions in their full, working, cultural and personal contexts (Hufford 1983a, 1988a). The systems approach includes healers, patients, theories of disease causation and cure, *materia medica*, and therapeutic techniques within its purview. It takes into account cultural influences, personal interpretation, intra-group variation in belief and practice, and the dynamic aspect of belief (its variability through time, across changing circumstances, and from person to person). Health systems are assessed in terms of their degrees of complexity (number of parts) and integration (number and kinds of interconnections among parts) (Hufford 1983b); their sources and media of transmission of ideas; their relationships with other healing traditions, including conventional medicine; and their connection to other aspects of cultural life, such as religion, narrative traditions, and so forth. It is an approach consistent with the more encompassing *folklife* branch of the discipline (Hufford 1992b; Scott 1993), with its attention to the intricate connections of people to their creations (knowledge and belief, aesthetics, material culture) and to each other (values, identity, community).

Medical Anthropology

Anthropologists and folklorists have long studied folk medical belief and practice. While folklorists have tended to work within their home cultures and countries, it has been a hallmark of anthropology until quite recently to work in countries and cultures distant from the scholar's own. Thorough description of host cultures has long been the aim of years spent "in the field," and health beliefs and practices have always received attention in those descriptions. The current subfield of medical anthropology began to take shape in the early 1950s (Caudill 1953) and gathered momentum throughout the 1960s and 1970s to become a well-grounded professional specialty. Like its parent discipline, medical anthropology has historically focused its attention on tribal societies and on the cultures of non-Western countries and developing nations. Particular interest has centered on the intersection of physical, environmental, and cultural factors in health and illness (Scott 1993), and on what happens to health and health behavior (along with other facets of culture) under conditions of acculturation and far-reaching change (Chambers 1985). As anthropologists have extended their researches into complex societies in recent years, their emphasis has largely remained on indigenous or precolonial peoples and on relatively unassimilated or minority, ethnic, and immigrant groups (Romanucci-Ross et al. 1983; Chambers 1985). The literature of medical anthropology is replete with ethnographic studies and cross-cultural comparative analyses of indigenous medical systems, referred to as "ethnomedicine." Topical foci include illness and disease etiologies of various cultures, studies of indigenous practitioners and their roles, descriptions of specific healing systems or complexes of healing practices and of local *materia medica*, "social construction and cultural interpretation of health and illness" (Bletzer 1980:1), management of health and illness within different cultures, and the relationship of processes of cultural change to changing health status and practices of affected groups (Bletzer 1980). Special issues of the anthropological section of the journal *Social Science and Medicine* have included "The Comparative Study of Medical Systems" (Vol. 12B[2], 1978), "The Transcultural Perspective in Health and Illness" (Vol. 13B[2], 1979), and "Parallel Medical Systems" (Vol. 13B[3], 1979).

Anthropology has a long history of interest in the nature of the relationship between culture and individual psychology in shaping behavior and worldview. The "culture and personality" approaches that arose early in this century questioned whether inherent biological or psychical forces in particular peoples might be determinative of cultural pattern, and whether or how cultural patterns might be determinative of individual personalities and their expressions in society. On a related tack were the psychological and psychoanalytical approaches to cultural interpretation that gathered momentum between the 1930s and 1950s. The latter posited human psychological universals, based largely on a Freudian model, and interpreted individual and cultural behavioral patterns accordingly. In contrast, the culture and personality school had a greater interest in seeking culturally determined variability in the configuration of personality (Stein 1990b). Prior to

1950, much of the health-related interest of anthropologists had to do with these sorts of questions, and many publications appear in psychiatric journals (Foster and Anderson 1978). There is a sizeable body of literature focused on these themes, but the analysis is in large measure theoretical in nature (Foster and Anderson 1978). Its analytical views are often views less of the subject than of the theory itself. In the end, the culture and personality trend collapsed because scholars were unable to encompass the actualities and variations in both individual and group behavior in any single coherent theory (Foster and Anderson 1978; Scott 1993). Psychological and psychoanalytical approaches persist, and they have both ardent supporters and energetic detractors in the ranks.[13]

Application of the psychiatric model to the study of indigenous healing systems has been very influential and has shaped the scholarship in several ways. Healing systems are frequently interpreted as "ethnopsychiatry" or folk psychiatry (e.g., Kiev 1964, 1968; Frank 1974; Koss 1975; Harwood 1977a, 1977b; Lemoine 1986). This is especially common when the systems involve extensive use of verbal measures such as prayers, incantations, and charms, but is not restricted to such situations. Healers are defined and evaluated as psychologically deviant or abnormal personalities who have found adaptive ways to reintegrate themselves into society (e.g., Devereux 1961; Fabrega and Silver 1970; Foster and Anderson 1978). Local illness categories or illness etiologies are reinterpreted in psychiatric, psychological, or emotional terms (Cannon 1942; Gillin 1948; Rubel 1964; Harwood 1977a, 1977b). All of these moves rest on the assumption (or conviction) that indigenous views that differ from Western academic views are incorrect, and that the scholar is in a good position to determine, with the "objectivity" provided by training and distance, what is "really" going on. Recent challenges to this position come from experience-centered approaches (e.g., Turner 1992), which tackle the cultural construction of academic theories and acknowledge the validity of indigenous ways of thinking and knowing (Wagner 1983; Stoller 1984; Turner 1992; see also Scott 1993). Academic and indigenous thought are subject to the same evaluative processes, and it does not go without saying which may be "right" about a given phenomenon.

Anthropology has a long-standing interest in the relationships between culture and the incidence and manifestations of mental and emotional disturbances (Hasan 1986), and in the cross-cultural study of behavioral disorders. Many aspects of folk healing systems have been assimilated to this interest through interpretation in psychological terms. As in folklore scholarship, healers and healing systems have commonly been classified according to a material/magical heuristic division. Those classed as "magical" are those most often assimilated to the Western psychiatric model, since this model offers explanations which are culturally acceptable in Western medical terms for classes of events (spiritual, metaphysical, or supernatural aspects of health, illness, and healing) not recognized in the Western nosology. Extensive studies have been made in many cultural settings of shamanism, witchcraft and sorcery traditions, healing cults, spirit possession, and spirit mediumship. While descriptively rich in many cases, these studies have until quite recently been almost exclusively psychological or psychoanalytical and functionalist in interpretation. Assessments of healers or their clients in terms of psychiatric instability or motivation by neurosis or anxiety, and interpretations of indigenous categories of illnesses as being "really" psychogenic in origin, are *not* value-neutral. They are stigmatized in many cultures, including those of most of the scholars, and their application additionally implies epistemological inferiority of the culture of the "studied" to the culture of the scholar. Where the subject peoples become aware of them (as has happened with some Native American and Alaska Native groups, among others), these theories have understandably engendered resentment and distrust.

Folk illnesses or the so-called culture-bound syndromes (e.g., Yap 1969) have been a major interest in anthropology. These are kinds of sicknesses that particular cultures recognize and treat, but which are not recognized as disease categories by conventional Western medicine. These illnesses have conventionally been interpreted (etically) as behavioral or psychiatric disorders, or as culturally specific behavioral manifestations of varying kinds of distress. Accumulating evidence of the occurrence of several of these syndromes outside the cultural groups with whom the illnesses were first associated[14] has recently initiated a re-evaluation of the propriety and accuracy of their classification, and therefore of their evaluations as well. New questions have been raised concerning the kinds and extent of causal factors that may be involved in addition to cultural shaping and psychological input, such as neurophysiological and other biological factors, and environmental influences (Simons 1980; Hufford 1982a, 1988c). The definition has been broadened to include a range of illnesses varying "from syndromes not thought to exist at all outside a certain cultural group to cases in which cultural shaping is seen as bringing about a distinctive manifestation of symptoms of a recognized [medical] diagnostic entity" (Hufford 1988a:251). Current debate questions the very utility of the category of culture-bound syndromes itself (Simons and Hughes 1985; Hufford 1988b). In addition, there is a growing recognition that in some cases the vernacular belief traditions surrounding these illnesses "contain substantial information about these states that is not a part of

medical knowledge" (Hufford 1988a:251) and much of which is clinically relevant (see, e.g., Simons 1980, 1983a, 1983b; Hufford 1982a,
1988b; Simons and Hughes 1985). This realization serves as a correc-
tive to overapplication of behavioral-medical or psychological explanations and to the "explaining away" of indigenous knowledge.

In recent decades in medical anthropology (and in all of the social
sciences), increasing emphasis has been placed on the critical importance of the "insider's" point of view to an adequate understanding of
health belief systems (Murphy 1976; Kleinman 1975, 1980; Trotter and
Chavira 1981; Rubel, O'Nell, and Collado-Ardón 1984). Awareness has
increased of the value of vernacular healing systems as genuine health
resources for those using them. Psychiatric and social-functional interpretations still prevail with respect to systems having significant magical
or spiritual elements (e.g., Harwood 1977a, 1977b).[15] Nevertheless, as
scholars have become less theory-bound and ethnocentric in their
assessments of vernacular healing systems, the image of the indigenous
healer has been "rehabilitated" (see, e.g., Jilek 1971). Some mental
health services in areas heavily populated with a specific cultural heritage group have initiated cooperative programs between conventional
mental health services and folk healers (Kreisman 1975; Ruiz and
Langrod 1976a, 1976b; Garrison 1982), who may even be recognized by
staff as "paraprofessionals" in the field.[16]

Several recent publications address vernacular health belief systems
in the United States. Collections of ethnographic descriptions of current American systems of health beliefs and practices include those by
Spicer (1977), with a southwestern regional focus (subdivided by ethnicity, and including one essay on Anglos), and Harwood (1981), a
hefty collection of essays each treating a particular ethnic group in the
United States and integrating ethnographic and epidemiological information. Two thorough studies of a specific health belief system are
Harwood's (1977b) study of the Puerto Rican spiritist religion and
Trotter and Chavira's (1981) superb treatment of Mexican-American
curanderismo. (A comparison of Trotter and Chavira's descriptive study
with an ethnopsychiatric interpretation of the same system [Kiev 1968]
gives a very useful sense of the ways in which approaches to the subject
determine the type of portrait that emerges.) Klein (1976) studied the
use of both professional and popular health care resources in a rural
American community, which he made a point of selecting because its
"mainstream" population differentiated it from the ethnic groups typically studied by anthropologists. Helman (1978, 1982), a physician-
anthropologist, discusses vernacular models of health and illness commonly found among middle-class, non-ethnically identified patients in
the British National Health Service, and demonstrates ways in which

their contacts with physicians may in actuality help to reinforce those models.

Much of recent medical anthropology stresses clinical applications and relevance, and includes the multiculturalism of complex societies in its purview. Kleinman (1975) introduced the concept of the explanatory model of disease. Demonstrating how explanatory models can differ between patients and health professionals, and what the consequences of those differences, if unexplored, can be for communication, diagnosis, treatment, and outcomes (Kleinman 1975, 1980; Kleinman, Eisenberg, and Good 1978; see also Good 1977; Good and Good 1982), anthropologists have helped to focus professional attention on the significance of the patient's point of view. In 1985 the journal *Medical Anthropology* published a special issue, "The Client's Perspective in Primary Health Care" (Vol. 9[1], 1985). Current scholarship stresses the cultural construction of health and illness in both official and unofficial belief, or what Kleinman (1977b) calls the "cultural construction of clinical reality" (see also Kleinman, Eisenberg, and Good 1978). Increasing attention is focused on actual patterns of use of health care resources in the United States and other complex, industrialized societies, patterns that encompass many resources outside of the professional health care system. Kleinman (1984) suggests defining the entire spectrum of health care resources as a single complex system, encompassing folk, popular, and professional "sectors." Each of these sectors has its own referral network and accepted therapies, and copes with particular types of illness or aspects of the lived experience of ill health and its consequences (Chrisman and Kleinman 1983; Kleinman 1984). The utility of this practical knowledge of the "lay of the land" in patients' health care practices should go without saying. Helman (1984) has also summarized approaches and research in medical anthropology, with an emphasis on their "practical relevance to both medical care and preventive medicine" (Helman 1984:vii).

Of potential value to improved understanding, to productive reshaping of provider-patient relations, and to public health and preventive medicine, is the enormous corpus of anthropological work on planning and implementation of professional (Western) health care services in developing nations and non-Western settings. These efforts and their supporting research began to gather steam after the Second World War (Foster and Anderson 1978). Through time, international public health efforts (especially under the aegis of the World Health Organization) have become less intent on promoting wholesale substitution of professional Western values for values and practices indigenous to the host cultures, and more focused on implementing health services in ways that are consonant with local cultural mores and established health beliefs and behavior. WHO now favors incorporation of indigenous healers into the staged introduction of conventional Western medicine in developing countries, and promotes scientific evaluation of traditional medical practices, rather than rejecting them out of hand (Vuori 1982). Many of the lessons of the international public health effort are generalizable to the domestic public health arena—which no less frequently involves great differences in values and worldview between planners/providers and intended beneficiaries, and which still tends strongly to impose outsiders' definitions of both health problems and solutions upon prospective patient populations (see Saunders 1954). Accounts of both the successes and the failures of international health efforts are generalizable to client-sensitive and client-responsive health care planning in any setting.

As anthropologists' reflexivity has expanded, their sense of affiliation with health professionals and the medical agenda has altered. Cross-cultural studies of healing systems and of the relationships between nonbiomedical systems and conventional Western medicine have shifted in perspective. "When anthropologists operated from within the framework of biomedicine, relationships between western medicine and nonmedical systems were seen to involve issues of development and education. When both biomedical and nonmedical systems came to be seen as cultural systems, those relationships were reframed as involving issues of cultural authority, the social construction of reality, and political and economic dominance" (Scott 1993:14). Recent anthropological interest has turned to models for restructuring the conventional Western health care system (Bletzer 1980), and to studying that system both as a cultural artifact subject to the same types of analysis historically reserved for "other" healing systems (Hahn and Gaines 1985; Baer 1987; DiGiacomo 1987; Lock 1987; Lock and Gordon 1988; Rhodes 1990) and as itself a complex culture (Stein 1990a).

Medical Sociology

Medical sociology addresses itself to a range of interests in the complex web of the healing professions, their patient populations, and patterns of interaction within and between these spheres.[17] One branch of medical sociology (referred to as sociology *of* medicine) devotes its efforts to the study of medicine itself. Topics include the social organization of provider education and service provision, socialization to professional roles, professional interaction patterns, and related concerns. Another branch (referred to as sociology *in* medicine) looks primarily at the patient populations and their relationships with health and illness and with the health care system. Topics include health and illness behavior; patient-provider relationships; the effects of illness on social systems such as marriages, families, and communities; conditions associated with relative health and illness in specific population cohorts; and so forth. The focal range of many sociological studies is of whole populations or groups, frequently delimited by social roles or social class (see Levin and Idler 1981). Study of illness from within this frame of reference is typically at the level of social patterns: sociopolitical conditions such as poverty, racism, or community crisis which broadly affect selected populations; lifestyle factors or stressful life events seen in terms of their statistical tendencies to promote or contribute to morbidity and mortality; adaptive group responses to the stresses of members' illness; or patterns of illness behavior. Interpretation in these studies is typically in terms of social functions of institutions, roles, behavior patterns, and the like. As in other disciplines, functionalist approaches come under criticism for their conservatism and for the unexamined assumptions they embody. Criticism from within sociology derives from several sources, notably the social constructionist tradition (Berger and Luckmann 1967), critical theorists, and the symbolic interactionist and sociology of everyday life perspectives (Lowenberg, personal communication; and see Lowenberg 1993).

Medical sociology has made several influential conceptual contributions both to the study of health care as a social system and to the worldview of the official health care system itself. These have included the interconnected concepts of sickness as a form of social deviance (i.e., deviance from the norm, which is defined as health and productivity); of the "sick role" (Parsons 1951, 1975); of the social mechanisms of entrance into this role and subsequent reintegration into normative social roles; and of the social functions of support systems, healers, and healing institutions. Most influential of these is the concept of the sick role. This is defined as a set of expectations socially provided for people who are sick, which both legitimates their exemption from certain aspects of their ordinary obligations and social expectations and prescribes appropriate attitudes and behaviors for the sick to promote their return to ordinary life conditions and role fulfillment. In summary the sick role theory proposes that society does not hold individuals responsible for sickness and suspends their responsibility for their usual obligations during sickness, at the same time that it expects sick persons to find their condition undesirable and to engage competent help in getting better. A corollary is that there is a certain benefit, called "secondary gain," that accrues from the exemption given to sick persons. The role requirements of desiring to get well and seeking competent help in doing so keep the secondary gain from governing the sick person's behavior.

The sick role constructs have become increasingly controversial since their formulation and, although very widely accepted, have been criticized on several grounds from both inside and outside their parent discipline (for reviews see, e.g., Foster and Anderson 1978; Wolinsky 1980). It has been noted repeatedly that the construct applies more usefully to acute illness than to chronic illness, to physical illness than to mental illness. It fails to take account of the significant extent to which Americans do in fact hold one another accountable for their states of health—from assigning blame on the basis of behavior (smoking, going out in the cold without a wrap, engaging in dangerous activities or disapproved sexual behavior) to stigmatizing illnesses and those who suffer them (e.g., tuberculosis, epilepsy, cancer, chronic fatigue, AIDS). It reflects the middle-class values of the dominant culture, including (1) the assumption that one is *able* to be exempted from everyday obligation (not likely, for example, for the primary responsible parent [usually mothers], or for those who work on a wage rather than a salary basis, or who have no sick-time arrangements with their employers); and (2) that one should strive diligently to overcome obstacles, including the obstacle of ill health. It takes no account of cultural differences in defining health and illness or appropriate behavior with respect to either. It omits consideration of the significant portion of illness behavior that is governed by the physical facts of the illness itself. It assumes secondary gain universally, though many illnesses and their consequences are sufficiently dreadful that it is difficult to make the case for secondary gain; and many individuals' socialization is such that they do not *experience* secondary gain (even if it ostensibly comes with the territory). It omits the point of view of the patient and reflects a professionalist bias in the assumption that seeking "competent help" means seeking a physician. Use of alternative practitioners, self-care, or the caring services of family or community members—all very common in actuality—are not accounted for in the model. In short, the sick role model contains many weaknesses that seriously limit its utility for adequately describing or explaining many aspects of actual and common social and individual responses to illness.

The role theory aspect of sociology deals with roles (as sets of obligations and expectations), not with persons, and concentrates its study on relationships between social roles and their functions. Nevertheless, the sick role and sickness-as-deviance constructs have lent themselves quite easily to reinterpretation as qualities of *persons* who occupy the roles, rather than as features of roles and role theory per se. The theory is about social provisions for managing sickness, which is potentially disruptive to society. It is ostensibly *descriptive*; that is, it posits that certain things *do* happen when sickness befalls. In everyday application, however, it often becomes *prescriptive*, amounting to a catalogue of what *should* happen. At the same time, it departs from roles and attaches to sick persons. It then shapes evaluative judgments of sick individuals and imparts to such judgments quite a strong moral tone. This sort of reinterpretive shift is common, though often unintentional, in everyday practice in the professional health care system, and in studies of patient behavior. The theoretical norm reflects the professional point of view, not necessarily the patient's. Individual patients' incongruence with this norm (seen as "departure" from the norm, not as a lack of fit between the theoretical norm and those it purports to describe) becomes the basis of judgments about the propriety of the patient's behavior and motives (e.g., the "good patient," cheerful and active, "compliant," eager to get back to work, versus the "malingerer," worried about "trivial" things, reluctant or fearful to resume activities, variable in follow-through with medical advice). Such prescriptive shifts fail to take account of the fact that social roles, including the sick role, are academic constructs which, like all heuristic devices, are limited to a certain range of utility only: in this case to modeling behavior at the *societal*, not the *individual*, level of complexity. It obscures the fact that a *role* is not a *person*. This usage confuses the map with the territory, the model with actuality. And when the two do not match up, it is often the actuality or the territory, not the model or the map, that is thought to be amiss! More seriously consequential than the reification of the constructs, however, is the ease with which this misapplication leads to approval or disapproval of individuals (e.g., particular patients) on the basis of their degree of conformity to roles we (academics and health professionals) have constructed, and to which we ourselves have assigned them. That degree of approval in turn affects professional attitudes, provider-patient relationships, the patients' experience of care, and the quality of care itself.

More recent developments have given rise to what may more properly be called the sociology of health (Wolinsky 1980) or the sociology of health and illness (Conrad and Kern 1986, 1990), as opposed to classical "medical" sociology. This more inclusive framework still attends to the relationships between illness and care structures and broader social factors (such as economic and political forces, distribution of and access to resources, and power relations within society and between patients and care providers) which are the hallmarks of sociology. It incorporates as well a greater attention to the relationships between health and illness and various forms of social interaction: the experience of illness, the "positive health effects of social support and social integration" (Levin and Idler 1981:20), forms of patient decision making that affect health behavior, recognition of cultural influences and cultural difference, analysis of familial and patient-provider face-to-face interaction, and the social and cutural construction of the realities of health, illness, and care patterns (Conrad and Kern 1986, 1990). This intellectual climate has nurtured the formulation and refinement of the Health Belief Model (Kasl and Cobb 1966; see also Becker 1974; Janz and Becker 1984) for the interpretation of health-related behavior. This model, unlike sick role theory, does accommodate cultural influences and differences in worldview. It applies to the behavior of individuals and seeks to discover and understand the point of view and rationales of the sick person in his or her own terms.

Sociologists have recognized that self-care and nonconventional modalities constitute the bulk of health care interventions (Zola 1972b; Wolinsky 1980; Dean 1981, 1989c). A recent topical focus on self-care represents an important addition to efforts to describe and understand health behavior, and increases attention to the roles of culture and belief in health care and health behavior. The journal *Social Science and Medicine* has devoted a special issue to this topic (Vol. 29[2], 1989). Sociological studies of the experience of illness, and of the meaning of health, illness, and care in the lives of specific persons affected have addressed issues such as definition (or redefinition) of self (Davis 1958; Schneider and Conrad 1983; Charmaz 1991), self-management of illness states and effects (Schneider and Conrad 1983; Charmaz 1991), and patient management of medical recommendations (Conrad 1985; Trostle, Hauser, and Susser 1983; Trostle 1988) to make treatment regimens more congruent with individuals' values, self-definitions, and the requirements and paces of their lives. The self-care and experience of illness studies incorporate the patient's point of view in defining health and illness and in shaping treatment actions and decisions. Another branch of sociological studies of the patient's point of view deals with interactions between patients and physicians in conventional health care settings, illustrating the substantial differences between professional and patient conceptions of the nature of the medical problem, the goals for the clinical interaction and for treatment, and the actual topics of concern (Fisher 1986; Todd 1989; Anspach 1990; Mishler 1990). Todd (1989) demonstrates how this conceptual mismatch, together with ineffective communication, can compromise the quality and appropriateness of medical care. Some of these studies suggest that the missed communications, lack of shared meanings, and resulting conviction on the part of patients that adequate care has not been delivered may prompt people to seek alternative practioners (Lowenberg 1989), just as failure to achieve desired therapeutic outcomes from conventional physicians may (Kotarba 1975).

Academic awareness over the past two decades of an international growth of popular interest in "alternative" health care is likewise reflected in sociology and is stimulating research to "help to explain why people in relatively affluent industrial countries seek therapies other than those provided by the medical profession" (MacCormack 1982: iii). Sociologists have undertaken studies of nonconventional healing systems and their participants (e.g., Kronenfeld and Wasner 1982; McGuire 1988; Lowenberg 1989), as well as addressing the relationships of nonbiomedical healing systems to biomedicine and the medical models of illness and of care giving (Kotarba 1975; Lowenberg 1989). A special issue of *Social Science and Medicine* on "Traditional and Modern Medical Systems" (Vol. 15A[2], 1981)[18] deals with interactions between conventional biomedicine and other systems of healing in a different perspective, concentrating attention on developing nations, on unacculturated groups within complex societies, and on complex societies (e.g., China, India) that have made government-level efforts to integrate "traditional" and "modern" medicine in their total health care systems.

Medicine

Coverage in the medical literature of vernacular health belief and of cultural issues in health care is relatively sparse and focuses on their manifestations in clinical settings and their implications for both clinicians and patients. Editorials tend either to lament or to marvel at the tenacity of vernacular health beliefs and practices, often continuing to characterize them as vestiges of the past that will (and should) eventually give way before advancements in medical science and public education. Substantive descriptions of health belief systems and their underlying theories are rare in the medical literature, although several good examples may be found (e.g., Harwood 1971; Snow 1974; Trotter 1985). Two special issues of the *Western Journal of Medicine* deal with a broad range of considerations in cross-cultural provision of medical care (Clark 1983; Barker 1992), and a recent special issue of the *Journal of Medicine and Philosophy* deals in some breadth and depth with the epistemologies of a variety of nonorthodox medical systems (Clouser and Hufford 1993).

The significant percentage of medical articles dealing with cultural issues and nonbiomedical health beliefs highlight racial and ethnic minority groups, particularly those who are recent immigrants or in lower income brackets (e.g., Kimball 1970; Harwood 1971; Snow 1974; Chesney et al. 1980; Yeatman and Dang 1980; Hoang and Erickson 1982; Glassbrenner 1985). These populations have high visibility in clinical settings, as the medical profession identifies them as "different," and they may present challenges to the system and its dominant-culture values. (Other populations just as likely to have very different views and health practices tend to be overlooked because of prevailing stereotypes about what "difference" consists of and where it is located.) They have sometimes been identified as "difficult patients."[19] The implication of the label is generally that the "difficulty" resides in the patient, rather than in the coming together of divergent sets of views and expectations in situations in which professional authority and control are the norm.

The medical literature reflects a steadily growing awareness of diversity of health beliefs and practices in the American population, and of their significance for clinicians (e.g., Harwood 1971; Yeatman and Dang 1980; Trotter 1985; Buchwald, Panwala, and Hooton 1992; Eisenberg et al. 1993). Vernacular healing practices are still overassociated with ethnicity, cultural heritage, and socioeconomic "marginality" in the medical literature. There are notable recent exceptions to this stereotypical view, however (e.g., Cassileth et al. 1984; Curt, Katterhagen, and Mahaney1986; Greenblatt et al. 1991; Anderson et al. 1993; Eisenberg et al. 1993; O'Connor 1993), and these have contributed a more accurate picture of the prevalence and distribution of nonbiomedical health care modalities. Folk and popular, or alternative, healing practices are typically presented in a context of physician concern for their potential as sources of problems for patients' health (e.g., Hatch 1969), or for the success of the conventional therapeutic regimen. On the basis of these rationales, strong opposition is often expressed to patients' use of vernacular healing practices, even when supporting evidence for the authors' claims is not offered. As much of this literature is based on uncontrolled observation by clinicians (Hufford 1988c), this type of categorical objection is made on essentially theoretical grounds. It expresses a combined concern with medical unknowns and with challenges to medical authority, and often has a strong emotional and moral tone.

Individual case studies and aggregations of cases do report documented harmful effects of particular substances or practices (e.g., D'Arcy 1991; Smitherman and Harber 1991; de Groot and Weyland 1992; Dunbabin et al. 1992; Nightingale 1993) and issue important general alerts based upon these documented instances. These reports call attention to the possibility of adverse reactions and toxic effects, but they do not provide any means of actually assessing risk, since the total number of exposures across the population is not known. The adverse reactions and failures may come to medical attention (though it is also not known what proportion of these do so), while successful or uneventful use remains clinically invisible. What is missing from the research, and thus from the literature, are well-designed and well-executed studies of prevalence and distribution of a range of vernacular healing practices against which to balance known adverse reactions in order to adequately calculate risk. Studies of efficacy of vernacular healing practices are also few, though the National Institutes of Health Office of Alternative Medicine is currently funding a small number of pilot efficacy studies (National Institutes of Health 1993). These subjects have not heretofore been a significant part of the research agenda of medicine, science, or industry, and they will be as costly and time-consuming to investigate with appropriate rigor as is any other research subject.[20]

Articles addressing the importance of physician-patient communication increasingly articulate the need to be aware of cultural and ethnic diversity in health beliefs in order to enhance communication, though "cultural factors" are almost invariably assigned only to the patient's side of the equation. Increasingly they emphasize intracultural as well as intercultural diversity, cautioning against the assumption that all members of a cultural group subscribe to the same beliefs and values. A few suggest that providers be willing and able to "modify treatment regimens to accommodate the patient's unique perspectives" (Johnson, Fenton, and Stein 1986; see also, e.g., Harwood 1971; Glassbrenner 1985). These attitudes are gaining proponents in medicine but also still meet with formidable resistance. They are especially likely to have support in medical specialties that place more emphasis on the importance of psychosocial aspects of health and illness, and which are more receptive to modifications of provider-patient relations that entail reduction or alteration of physician authority. Considerations of cultural and individual values, of nonbiomedical healing practices, and of modification of professional health care routines also appear as central elements in the developing literature on patient-centered care, which encompasses all aspects and branches of medicine and reintroduces the patient's perspective as an authoritative voice (Boumbulian et al. 1991; Delbanco 1992; Reiser 1992, 1993; Gerteis et al. 1993; Hufford 1993a).

Recently the medical profession has begun to recognize the diversity of health beliefs and practices among members of dominant cultural groups or "mainstream" patient populations. Much of this awareness came about through studies of cancer patients, among whom there is very widespread use of nonbiomedical therapies (Cassileth et al. 1984; Herbert 1986; Brigden 1987; Danielson, Stewart, and Lippert 1988; McGinnis 1991). These are generally referred to in the medical literature as "unorthodox," "unproven," or "questionable" therapies, and occasionally as "alternative" therapies. Cassileth and associates (1984), in a survey of patients' uses of nonconventional cancer therapies, were among the first medical authors to challenge the prevailing stereotypes of users of alternative cancer tharepies. Patterns of use of nonconventional therapies in their study population inverted this stereotype, proving greatest among patients who were white, well educated, and in middle income brackets. This observation has since received considerable support in other sources (Curt, Ketterhagen, and Mahaney 1986; Levin and Coreil 1986; Kaufman 1988; McGuire 1988; Wardwell 1988; McGinnis 1991; Eisenberg et al. 1993).

The medical literature expresses a number of primary concerns about alternative therapies: that they are incorrect and unfounded; that they will cause direct harm; that they will delay or replace use of conventional medicine, thus causing indirect harm; and that they are perpetrated by quacks and frauds motivated by profiteering impulses (e.g., Cobb 1954; Brody 1980; Glymour and Stalker 1983). The standard medical article on the subject of "unproven" therapies has until quite recently been almost formulaic: it briefly describes the therapies in question, then concludes with suggestions for dissuading patients from their use and admonitions as to their perils. However, relatively few of the practices have been subjected to rigorous investigation to determine if these conclusions are warranted on the basis of medicine's own methodological principles. This has only recently been identified as a shortcoming by medical writers. In an unusual statement, Curt and colleagues note:

There is a need to establish procedures by which unproved and unorthodox treatments are formally evaluated for safety and efficacy so that current and reliable information can be obtained by both physicians and patients. [. . . Physicians now use] the lack of peer-reviewed publications supporting the treatment or the lack of scientific credentials among those offering the treatment . . . to discredit the therapy. This passive approach is unlikely to convince those patients who seek out alternative therapies, since they are generally intelligent and inquisitive. (Curt et al. 1986:507)

Interestingly, the indignant tone and the stringent concern and urgency to dissuade patients from alternative therapies that pervades much of the literature on cancer alternative therapies are absent from most of what has been written about uses of alternative therapies for HIV disease. Indeed, a number of the latter take quite a matter-of-fact position with respect to HIV alternative therapies and urge physicians and other care-givers to be aware of them and to maintain attitudes that will above all else keep open the lines of communication with patients (Abrams 1990; Glazier and Glazier 1990; Greenblatt et al. 1991; Kassler, Blanc, and Greenblatt 1991; Rowlands and Powderly 1991; Anderson et al. 1993).

Medical writers pay particular attention to alternative therapeutic practices provided by specialist practitioners, that is, those which replicate the clinician-patient model. This emphasis overlooks the fact that a significant percentage of folk and popular medicine consists of self-care practices, or the ministrations of family and community members (Hufford 1988a). This selective notice, shaped by a medical practice model of health care, contributes to underestimation of the actual rates of use of vernacular healing modalities. It is also a factor in overestimation of the prevalence and threat of "quacks" or fraudulent practitioners (see Hufford 1988c). In both cases, the misrepresentations make it more difficult to accurately assess actual rates and distribution of usage of nonconventional health care practices and to understand both "their clinical importance and . . . the patient behavior involved" (Hufford 1988c:102).

Nursing

The nursing literature has in common with medicine a focus on clinical manifestations and implications of diversity in health belief and practice, especially as these are represented in specific ethnic and cultural heritage groups (e.g., Kay 1973; Rocereto 1973; Anderson and Tighe 1976; Branch and Paxton 1976; National League of Nursing 1976; Tripp-Reimer and Friedl 1977; Powers 1982; Flaskerud and Rush 1989; Rempusheski 1989; Flaskerud and Calvillo 1991; Galanti 1991; Spector 1991). By virtue of its professional orientation of engagement with patients, nursing shows a much greater interest than medicine in increasing both awareness of and responsiveness to patients' needs and preferences. The professional mission of nursing is the provision of *care*, which by definition encompasses attentiveness to individual needs, as defined by those who experience them. By virtue of their respective roles, nurses much more often than physicians experience extended contact with patients and their families, and this exposure has long since heightened nurses' awareness of the significance of cultural issues and health beliefs to the provision of nursing care (MacGregor 1967; Taylor 1973; Tripp-Reimer, Brink, and Saunders 1984).

Since the early 1970s there has been an active subspecialty of "transcultural nursing," which integrates anthropological and nursing concepts to stress provision of culturally responsive and culturally appropriate care (Leininger 1970, 1977, 1978; Branch and Paxton 1976; Brink 1976; Orque, Branch, and Monrroy 1983; Tripp-Reimer, Brink, and Saunders 1984; Tripp-Reimer and Afifi 1989). In formulating its models for care delivery, transcultural nursing theory emphasizes differences in worldview and the cultural construction of clinical reality in both folk and scientific explanatory systems (Tripp-Reimer 1984). A special issue of the *Journal of Nursing Education* in the mid-1970s was devoted to the topic of "Cultural Diversity in Nursing" (Vol. 15[2], 1976). Since that time there has been an enormous proliferation of nursing literature on this topic, including theoretical works, assessment and skills training techniques, and descriptive articles focused on specific health belief systems, specific populations, and the management of specific health problems and life stages in differing cultural frameworks. Many nursing curricula now include transcultural (or, in other terms, cross-cultural) content as a part of the core curriculum, and most offer elective material in this area. A specialty professional journal, the *Journal of Transcultural Nursing*, began publication in 1989.

In the past decade there has been an increasing emphasis on a holistic approach in nursing. The journal formerly entitled *Topics in Clinical Nursing* was renamed *Holistic Nursing Practice* in 1987, reflecting this emerging concern. The professionalization movement of the past three decades in nursing has contributed to the development of a body of theoretical literature and of qualitative research in nursing that stresses a holistic perspective, individuation of care, and cultural or worldview awareness as distinctive features of the professional orientation of nurses. In this philosophical and intellectual climate there have emerged several descriptive studies of health belief systems, which have included use of nonconventional therapies in "mainstream" populations (e.g., Hautman and Harrison 1982; Strawn 1989; Sanders 1989) as well as of health belief systems associated with specific ethnic and cultural heritage groups (Powers 1982; Flaskerud and Rush 1989; Flaskerud and Calvillo 1991; Flaskerud and Thompson 1991).

Awareness of the existence and importance of varied cultural worldviews and systems of health belief and practice has long been a common theme in the nursing literature. In medicine the dominant approach to such awareness has been to lament these phenomena and work to change the patient. In contrast, the response of nursing for the past thirty years has increasingly been to accept the phenomena, even to find them interesting and challenging, and to work to change the attitudes and routines of the providers, along with working for selective change in belief and behavior of patients (to the extent these are considered potentially harmful). Nursing is inclined to explain the "culturally different" so-called "difficult" patient in terms of differences in belief and expectation that involve *both* provider and patient: difficulty arises in the interaction, and sometimes in providers' misunderstandings (e.g., Powers 1982). This view differs significantly from the common medical response in which cultural difference is presumed to be a characteristic of the patient, and is offered as an explanation of what makes such a person "difficult." An excellent example is offered by Powers's (1982) description of the health belief system of an African-American patient who is simultaneously using conventional medicine and seeing a root doctor. This study stresses the need for nurses to be aware of the possibility of simultaneous use of differing health care resources and to grasp the rational nature of the integration of these two systems on the basis of fundamental principles that may differ markedly from the basic assumptions of many health professionals. Powers additionally points out the great range of intracultural variation in belief and stresses the flexibility and adaptability of folk health belief systems.

Summary

Folk medicine and belief and health-related behavior have been objects of fascination to health professionals and academics for generations. Since the 1960s the study of health beliefs and practices, and their complex connections to larger social and cultural frameworks, has been a growing interest in a number of disciplines with varying theoretical foundations and concentrations of interest on selected facets of the phenomena or applications of the knowledge. Interdisciplinary efforts have proliferated, as the productivity of combining perspectives and specialized expertise has become more and more apparent. An example is the exceptional two-volume work by Crellin and Philpott (1990), which contains both an ethnographic and biographical study of herbalist Tommie Bass (Volume 1) and a compendious treatment of each of the items in his *materia medica* (Volume 2). This remarkable piece of scholarship, jointly authored by an M.D./medical historian and a botanist, is one of the most thorough studies of a living folk healing tradition available. Other recent interdisciplinary efforts include edited collections of articles on "unorthodox medicine" (Gevitz 1988) and current "traditional healing" (Kirkland et al. 1992) by authors from a range of academic and professional backgrounds, including folklorists, anthropologists, physicians, historians, behavioral scientists, sociologists, and ethnobotanists. The literatures of public health, behavioral medicine, and the behavioral sciences, by their very constitution interdisciplinary fields, have frequently addressed aspects of these complex phenomena.

The most comprehensive understanding of health beliefs and practices, and of their sociocultural contexts, can only come with cross-disciplinary reading, with interdisciplinary efforts. Each discipline has a particular theoretical lens (or set of lenses) to turn on the subject, and each has a different focal range. The holographic image, with the greatest dimensional completeness and clarity, can only be assembled by incorporating a variety of views, *and* by taking into account the orientations that produced them. Recent approaches in terms of systems of belief and knowledge—taking laypersons as rational people making choices for ordinary and comprehensible reasons, and giving weight to the insider's description and explanation along with the researcher's perspective—have been very productive of informative detailed descriptions, as well as of theories which stand up well to empirical testing.

Across the literatures, certain cautions pertain. Assumptions about the causes and the social locations of nonconventional health beliefs and practices have led to misrepresentations of the prevalence and distribution of the phenomena, as well as of the intelligence, character, and motivations of participants. A persistent tendency to concentrate research on lower socioeconomic groups, on specific ethnic and cultural heritage groups, or on the intersection of the two, has skewed findings and reinforced the prior assumptions that defined the boundaries of the inquiry. Scholars in all disciplines have "found unconventional health beliefs and practices only where they looked for them, and then interpreted the distribution of their own efforts as the distribution of the beliefs and practices themselves" (Hufford 1988c:24). Now that researchers are casting a wider net, several facts have come clear: that folk and popular health care systems remain quite vigorous today in most complex societies; that they have adherents at all levels of educational and economic attainment and in all races and ethnicities; that people have recourse to them for a wide variety of reasons; that they are quite frequently used alongside conventional medicine; that they are flexible systems which readily accommodate new input; and that new variants are continually developing.

It is now apparent that these systems serve as valuable resources to patients, and that conventional biomedicine does not and cannot provide many things that people need to cope with illness or to maintain their own sense of optimal health (Hufford 1988a). It is becoming clear that patients often assess their own situations and make important decisions about their care on the basis of their own priorities and beliefs, and on the authority of their own experience. These realizations suggest that conventional health professionals would do well to be aware of parallel healing traditions and to develop ways to interact with them in providing patient care. The health systems model provides a framework for understanding (and further exploring) vernacular health beliefs and practices and the conditions that have helped to assure their continuation with undiminished vigor up to the present day.

Notes

1. The very definition of "primitive"—"little evolved" and "characteristic of an early stage of development" (Merriam-Webster's Collegiate Dictionary, Tenth Edition)—derives from the evolutionary view.

2. There are, of course, exceptions to this general rule. Sociologists have frequently studied members of their own cultures and social classes, especially in the sociology of medicine. Notable anthropological examples include Lloyd Warner's studies in Newburyport and Kansas City; studies of American culture by Margaret Mead and Clyde Kluckhohn; and Ray L. Birdwhistell's study of a Kentucky county.

3. Where expertise is defined as the product of formal technical training.

4. Honko, for example (1964, 1965), asserted plainly that the investigator of (supernatural) folk belief *is not able* him-/herself to "see spirits."

5. Interested readers are referred to the extensive literature, spanning several decades, debating the proper stance of ethnographers to their informants or field consultants, and chronicling the changes in that stance and their rationales and justifications.

6. Von Sydow's original 1934 article was written in German; it first appeared in English in 1948.

7. Phenomenology, in this sense, means simply that "reports of subjects of their conscious experiences are taken as [primary] data" (Havens 1960:80).

8. My basic search list consists of fifty-two terms, *exclusive* of the names of specific systems, actions, health conditions, or populations. Different combinations of terms, even when close in meaning, yield different citations, even from the same database. For example, I have found one set of references using the combined set "HIV and alternative therapies," but turned up additional ones on each move substituting "AIDS" for "HIV" and "unproven" and "complementary" for "alternative."

9. Ethnobotanists, on the other hand, have concentrated their efforts on analysis of pharmacologically active ingredients in *materia medica*, dismissing other explanatory and contextual elements as "cultural baggage" (Hufford 1984).

10. Some may recognize a difference in indications, technique, and outcomes for healing on a "material level" as opposed to on a "spiritual level" (e.g. Trotter and Chavira 1981), but they typically stress the importance of working with both, and view the aspects as mutually supportive and interinfluential.

11. But note that an entire *materia medica* is also frequently disparaged on theoretical grounds (i.e., without testing or evidence) as being "at least harmless" (Lathrop 1961:22; Hatch 1969:163) or as having "no effect whatever" (Honko 1968:293). Remarkably, Honko's statement appears in an article whose opening declaration is, "The therapeutic effectivity of popular or 'primitive' medicine cannot be judged solely from the point of view of modern medicine" (Honko 1963:190).

12. Although it is important to note in this connection that the elements "derived" from any period in conventional medical history account for only a small portion of folk medical tradition.

13. The journal *Culture, Medicine and Psychiatry* deals with all manner of health belief systems (including biomedicine) from many cultures. While its contents represent a wide variety of interpretive approaches, its title reflects its origins in this branch of anthropology.

14. They were first associated with particular cultures by anthropologists. Their apparent distribution or restriction to these cultures was a reflection of the extent of anthropology's cross-cultural knowledge at a particular time, not necessarily of the actual distribution of particular syndromes.

15. Although these healing systems treat physical illnesses as well as psychical and spiritual ones, the conventional health care system's theoretical and experimental acceptance of their utility does not yet extend recognition beyond the sphere of mental health.

16. There have of course always been some anthropologists who regarded indigenous healers as the analogues of Western health professionals and did not diminish their stature with psychiatric labels. As early as 1947 Warner, Kluckhohn, and Birdwhistell were among those who urged the physicians attached to the United States Bureau of Indian Affairs to develop collegial relations with Navajo and Sioux healers, and to bear in mind that these healers were prestigious notables in their own societies who should be approached as peers (Ray L. Birdwhistell, personal communication). This is a significant step farther than granting "paraprofessional" status, and one that has yet to be made, even in most cross-cultural cooperative settings. Such accommodation will come with difficulty to the tightly hierarchical world of the health professions.

17. Also germane to inquiry into health belief systems, and to the interaction between official and unofficial knowledge, are works in the sociology of science and the sociology of knowledge.

18. The journal is no longer divided into its former disciplinary subsections (Medical Anthropology, Medical Geography, Medical Economics, Medical Psychology, and Medical Sociology), but intermingles these approaches and interests in each issue. This shift reflects the significant overlap in interest among the disciplines and recognizes both their utility to one another and the impossibility of maintaining strict subject divisions when topics, methods, and theories overlap.

19. When scheduling a recent presentation to a department of an urban northeastern hospital, I had given my presentation title as "Cultural Issues in Health Care." When I arrived on the day of the event, I found the title listed on flyers and schedule boards as "Managing Difficult Patients: Cultural Issues in Health Care." This revealing, and entirely unwitting, shift naturally made an excellent starting point for the discussion!

20. It is important to recall, in this context, that definitions of benefit of given health practices from the point of view of patient populations differ considerably from medical or scientific definitions of benefit, which typically hinge on efficacy, or the capacity to produce a narrowly defined effect. This means that scientific research that does not demonstrate specific efficacies is not necessarily pertinent to patients' concerns and does not necessarily falsify their perceptions of benefit.

Chapter 3
Hmong Cultural Values, Biomedicine, and Chronic Liver Disease

In the past decade, scholars of many disciplines concerned with health care in complex societies have paid increasing attention to the importance of matters of culture and worldview in health care delivery. The education and training of health professionals in the United States, however, does not yet incorporate much of this information or routinely teach the skills for evaluating and responding to significant differences in worldview between patients and providers. As a result, many providers remain unaware of the extent to which such differences can affect clinical interaction and outcomes, and are badly hampered in cross-cultural encounters. The case history recounted in this chapter illustrates the possible extent of the complexities of this meeting of very different views of health and illness. It highlights the great variety of values, beliefs, and cultural considerations—not merely those directly related to health and illness—which may have bearing on both patients' and providers' responses to illness and to care. Mr. L., the patient in the case, is a young Hmong refugee who was resettled in Philadelphia in 1979.

Historical Background

The Hmong are an ethnically distinct southeast Asian group whose origins are generally traced to central China, during the second millennium, B.C. (Chindarsi 1976; Geddes 1976).[1] In the middle of the eighteenth century large numbers of Hmong were forced out of China and began a decades-long peregrination that resettled the majority in Laos and Vietnam by the early to mid-nineteenth century, with smaller numbers migrating into northern Thailand. In these adoptive homelands the Hmong were mountain dwellers, as they had been for centuries in China, inhabiting the forested ridges at altitudes several thousand feet above sea level. The Hmong have traditionally been an agrarian people. In promising mountain sites, they established settlements, typically of some thirty to forty households, and practiced swidden agriculture. Villages generally remained stable for the duration of land fertility. When land became unproductive, or if infectious sickness or other misfortune overcame a village, the houses would be abandoned and the village moved to a fresh site.

Throughout their history of continual resettlement the Hmong have remained culturally separate and ethnically distinct from other southeast Asian peoples. A powerful sense of cultural identity has led throughout their history to a quite deliberate maintenance of ethnic unity within Hmong society, and of separateness from surrounding peoples. Although engaging in trade and other economic relations with them, Hmong seldom socialize significantly with other groups in their countries of residence, and very rarely marry non-Hmong (Chindarsi 1976; Geddes 1976; Lemoine 1986). The strength of the Hmong sense of ethnic identity and solidarity has been undiluted by hundreds of years of migration and a wide diaspora.

Those Hmong who resided in Laos in the mid-twentieth century became entangled, by virtue of their location, in the political machinations of the Indochinese wars that began in about 1945, with resistance to French domination in Indochina led first by the Japanese and later by the Viet Minh and Pathet Lao (Dao 1982). Laotian Hmong villages tended to be located in places well suited, and thus susceptible, to guerrilla warfare. The Hmong began to be displaced, often with violence, by local opposition forces. In consequence they allied themselves for protection with the French and the Royal Government of Laos. This alliance in turn made them targets of Viet Minh and Pathet Lao eradication efforts. Following the withdrawal of the French from Indochina in the mid-1950s, many Hmong continued to fight in the ongoing Laotian battle against North Vietnamese occupation forces in the northeastern parts of the country.

The United States government began in the early 1960s to support the Royal Laotian government and its allies (which included the Hmong) in the fight against North Vietnamese forces in Laos during the American military engagement in Vietnam. This alliance helped to set the stage for the later exodus and relocation of the Hmong as the Western effort in Vietnam began to collapse. A mass exodus of Hmong from Laos to Thailand began in 1975. Enormous refugee camps were established in Thailand to receive the influx, and resettlement efforts were handled out of these camps. Countries of relocation included the United States, France, Australia, Canada, Argentina, and China (Dao 1982).

The first Hmong refugees began arriving in the United States in the spring of 1976 (Dunnigan 1986). Some 100,000 Hmong had been re-located abroad by 1982 (Dao 1982), including roughly 50,000 in the United States. U.S. census figures for 1990 list a Hmong population of 84,823 in the United States. The Hmong community in Philadelphia numbered approximately 3,000 at its peak of population in 1982–1983. Further migration within the United States has reduced its current number to some 500 people (local figures supplied by the Southeast Asian Mutual Assistance Association Coalition and the Hmong Association of Philadelphia).

Biographical Sketch

Mr. L. was born in Laos, in Xieng Khouang province. He grew up principally in the large and stable town of Muong Chiang, where he participated in farming activities at the outskirts of town and attended school until he reached the age of sixteen, in 1975. Mr. L. estimates that close to a thousand families lived in Muong Chiang, giving it a population of approximately ten thousand. (A similar estimate was provided by Bruce Thowpaou Bliatout, personal communication.) The typical Hmong mountain village, by contrast, might have thirty to forty families, or some three hundred to four hundred inhabitants. By 1975, Laos was well penetrated by North Vietnamese troops. Muong Chiang was largely abandoned by its citizens as North Vietnamese moved into the territory and the town, and Mr. L.'s family lived "in the jungle" for some three months. During that time his parents and one of his three brothers were killed. The occupation forces' policy obliged all captured Hmong to serve either as soldiers in the North Vietnamese army or as forced laborers in their camps and supporting enterprises. Having lost many family members, and wishing to avoid conscription and servitude, Mr. L. and several friends in similar circumstances decided to leave Laos.

A large-scale exodus of several thousand Hmong from Laos to Thailand had taken place two months previously, and Mr. L. and his companions determined to follow the route this group had taken to northern Thailand. They estimated that this trip would take them about two weeks on foot. Fifteen people made up his escape party, and they managed, in spite of extreme hardships along the way, to escape undetected to Thailand. There, Mr. L. met relatives in the Nong Khai refugee camp, where he stayed for a year. At that time, most Hmong refugees were transferred to Ban Vinai camp, where Mr. L. and his relatives remained for another four or five months before he and one "brother"[2] and sister-in-law came to Philadelphia, where they joined other clan relatives.

First Emergency, Hospital A

In October 1987, Mr. L. became ill suddenly and began to vomit blood. Family members took him to the emergency room of a large local teaching hospital. He was shortly diagnosed as being in incipient liver failure as a result of liver tissue damage caused by chronic hepatitis B. He was admitted to the hospital on an emergency basis. His bleeding (hematemesis) was the result of distended and thinned veins in the esophagus (esophageal varices). These in turn were the consequence of localized blood-pressure increases owing to liver tissue damage, which decreased the capacity of blood circulation through the organ. He showed considerable fluid buildup (ascites) in the abdomen and extremities. Mr. L. was recommended for evaluation for liver transplant. Arrangements were made for air-ambulance transport to Pittsburgh, the nearest center with a well-established liver transplantation program, for evaluation within six or seven days.

The presence of the esophageal varices called for two immediate medical responses: (1) restriction of intake by mouth to clear liquids only, to prevent irritation of the varices by swallowing of food, and (2) direct treatment of the bleeding varices by injections of hardening solutions, done through an endoscope (sclerotherapy). Mr. L.'s treatment team consisted of a senior gastroenterologist, two much younger residents, and a number of nurses from the service. There was a considerable sense of urgency on the floor about the gravity of his condition, the importance of controlling his episodes of esophageal bleeding, and the need to secure his consent for the air-ambulance transport to Pittsburgh. At the time of this emergency admission, Mr. L.'s physicians estimated that without transplant, his chances of survival did not far exceed three or four months.[3]

Under any circumstances catastrophic illness, hospitalization, and invasive treatment procedures in an atmosphere of urgency make difficult ground for physician-patient interactions. In Mr. L.'s case, all of the interactions were greatly complicated by cultural differences between conventional medical and Hmong views: of the nature of sickness and of emergency; of the locus and time requirements of decision making; of the means of selecting appropriate times for action; of the requirements of nourishment; of the definitions of proper treatment and of risk; and of the nature of acceptable handling of the body. The nature and extent of these complications understandably were largely opaque to the medical and nursing staff, who were unacquainted with Hmong culture. At the same time, Mr. L. had never before been in a hospital. He and his family were entirely unfamiliar with biomedical culture: the protocols, procedures, and expectations of the medical model of disease and treatment, and the stratification, scheduling, and workings of a hospital.

While Mr. L. and his family were very alarmed at his bleeding episode, they tended to interpret it as an isolated serious incident of unknown cause. They knew it needed to be stopped quickly, before harm occurred; and they acknowledged this goal to be beyond the scope of Hmong medicine, which has no immediate curative strategies for bleeding freely inside the body (F. L., personal communication).[4] They were unconvinced by the American physicians' diagnosis that the bleeding was symptomatic of a serious underlying disease of long duration, which had finally done enough damage to cause this outward manifestation. For the Hmong, as for people of many cultural backgrounds, the development and presence of disease are indicated by the presence of symptoms or other physical signs. Symptoms short of intense pain or incapacity tend to be borne stoically or perceived as minor ailments:

The Hmong consider illness a condition that renders an individual incapable of eating, drinking, or getting out of bed. An individual who can still force himself or herself out of bed is hardly considered ill. Thus a person is sick only when he or she cannot perform or fulfill his or her social tasks and responsibilities. (Thao 1986:367)[5]

Mr. L. had no prior knowledge of having had any liver disease or dysfunction and had no reason to suspect its presence. His only complaint at the time of his crisis, other than the hematemesis, was fatigue. He had no pains, did not feel ill, did not look especially bad. He did have substantial fluid retention (ascites) as a result of his liver dysfunction, and this distended his abdomen and caused some swelling of his extremities. Such signs are subject to a variety of interpretations within the Hmong cultural framework (Xoua Thao, M.D., personal communication). In Mr. L.'s case, members of his immediate community had tended to interpret these visible effects as "fat." These manifestations had not occasioned alarm, although they had been visible for some days, as fat is regarded as one of two essential elements (together with blood) that provide vitality to the body. Mr. L. was not at all incapacitated until the vomiting began. Even afterward, he maintained his appetite and was distressed that he was denied food. The previous day he had been competing in the community soccer games, and he was successfully pursuing a demanding schedule of schooling and a job. On the whole, he was leading a life indicative of considerable vigor.

Within the Hmong outlook, the emergency consisted only in Mr. L.'s uncontrolled bleeding. Family members agreed with the physicians that the presenting problem was life-threatening. However, since they did not at the time concur with the notion of a long-standing and invisible underlying condition, they were unable to come to terms with the physicians' insistence that this underlying condition itself was life-threatening. The need to take drastic measures other than those involved in controlling the bleeding was neither self-evident nor especially convincing for Mr. L.'s family. As a consequence, they could not accept the urgency of decision and action to which the physicians were so committed.

The Role of Family and Community

For the Hmong, as for most southeast Asian peoples, it is not the individual but the *family* that is the locus of identity, action, care, and decision making (Tung n.d.). The self is collectively developed and conceived, within the structure and mutual obligations of multigenerational family relations and clan affiliation. In traditional Hmong terms, there is no equivalent to the willful, self-interested, and individuated self that is so deeply ingrained and idealized in contemporary American culture. The consent form that Mr. L. would have to sign for transport and evaluation for liver transplant could indeed be signed by him. But the act of consent that could occasion this signature had, in fact, little to do with him personally. Within his cultural framework, momentous decisions can only be made collectively, by a meeting of all relevant family members. Each family member has the right and duty to express his or her thoughts on the matter, and the opinions and concerns of all then form the basis of a general discussion.

The decision-making process includes consideration of effects of actions upon individual members and upon the entire family network. When critical health problems are involved, the meanings of individual physical life and a wider concept of the *social* life in which individuals are inextricably embedded inform this discussion, as does the Hmong conception of the life-cycle with its sense of delicate balance between the states of life and death (Xoua Thao, personal communication). In the end it is the male family elder (or elders) who brings together all of the sentiments expressed and comes to a decision by which everyone will abide. The person whom the decision will most directly affect (as seen from the individualist American perspective, or as encoded in the bioethical principle of patient autonomy) does not have private rights in such matters that can override an elder's decision.[6]

The Hmong trace family and lineage membership patrilineally. Fathers pass on to their sons important familial and ceremonial connections and their attendant rights to authoritative speech and action. A special closeness is inherent between (sibling) brothers:[7]

The principle on which the lineage is formed is that of the family extended through its male members. Of particular importance are the bonds between father and children and between brothers. So long as either of these bonds persists, all descendents of the male line of the persons so linked will consider themselves to belong together in a group with special obligations to one another. (Geddes 1976:53–54)

In Mr. L.'s case this equation was complicated by the additional factor that he was orphaned in the war in Laos. Here in the United States he has family ties only at the level of clan membership. Since Hmong identity and obligations derive entirely from family and clan affiliation, Mr. L. was understood to be in the care of his clanal family, to whom he owed an asymmetrically greater obligation of respect, deference, and obedience.

Mr. L.'s family in Philadelphia consists of members of his patrilineal clan, who have the same surname. Over the course of the first four or five days of his hospitalization, this group of some seventeen people met several times to debate the complexities of the problem and to propose possible solutions. Two brothers in Ohio and a sister in Wisconsin offered their thoughts and opinions by telephone. In addition, the president of the Philadelphia Hmong community was present at some of the family meetings. This important leader is not a member of Mr. L.'s family or clan but represents a higher authority within the community as a whole. Following the traditional Hmong pattern of arbitration, when elders at the family and clan levels are not able to satisfactorily settle a question, or when the consequences of the matter at hand are too great for lesser authorities to be comfortable in adjudicating it alone, the matter is referred to the community leader.[8] He is expected to bring together all considerations of the case, acting to promote consensus and function as its authoritative voice, though by virtue of his position he also has final power of decision should consensus not be achieved (Geddes 1976). The president's presence in the family meetings about Mr. L. signaled the gravity of the situation and the significance of Mr. L.'s illness as not merely a personal, family, or clan incident, but a matter of community-wide concern: "An individual's *disease* is a community *illness*. If death should occur, the whole community would be prepared to grieve" (Xoua Thao, personal communication; emphasis in original).

These clan and community members constituted the decision-making body. Mr. L. alone did not have a voice in the initial decision-making process. Though his own opinions, impressions, and preferences were solicited in the discussions, Mr. L. was very cautious about his responses. He felt that it would not have been proper for him to express a strong preference at the height of the crisis. His family members were all very distressed for his sake, and he worried that they might be swayed by emotion if he made an appeal one way or the other in this difficult process (B. L., interview, November 1989). In addition, he felt that since the problem centered upon himself, he could not trust the clarity of his ideas about it in the way that he could if he were helping to solve a problem of another person; he was confused by its proximity and immediacy (B. L., interview, November 1989). Deference to family and community decisional authority also has the social function of helping to assure that individuals will not be isolated during or after the crisis (Xoua Thao, personal communication). Individual Hmong are socialized not to attempt to resolve grave problems for themselves but rather to turn to the collective judgment of their extended families; consultation is the norm in all situations of any consequence and is virtually synonymous with decision making. Individuals are not held personally responsible for decisions in critical situations, nor are they socialized to consider individual decision making desirable (or even possible) in such circumstances, unless one is utterly alone and hence without consultative resources. In illness, it is traditionally Hmong *families* who "seek cures for sick family members, rather than the sick person seeking a cure for himself or herself" (Bliatout 1986:361).

The oldest male member of Mr. L.'s family, himself a leader of considerable stature in the Philadelphia Hmong community, had the right and responsibility to interpret all opinions and render a decision—a process that requires considerable time and care of deliberation in matters of such gravity. In this instance, he was charged with making interpretations between radically conflicting views and explanations of how ill Mr. L. truly might be and why, in order to arrive at a proper decision. The information supplied by his own cultural background provided no final explanation and suggested no known treatment for the obviously serious problem of vomiting blood. The information supplied by the American physicians seemed dubious for many reasons—yet it merited profound consideration for its portrayal of the illness, as well as the very passage of time in coming to decisions about it, as matters of life and death.

Mr. L.'s family members consulted and discussed among themselves over the course of days, often meeting in his presence in Mr. L.'s hospital room. A diviner consulted by the family soon after Mr. L.'s admission to the hospital had determined that the auspices of the day on which his crisis occurred did not foretell insurmountable danger (B. L., interview, November 1989). This pronouncement helped to quell somewhat the sense of urgency and impending doom that the medical opinions tended to promote. During these family deliberations, the physician team, in earnest commitment to their own beliefs, exerted considerable pressure both for a timely decision and for a decision in favor of the medical recommendations. Unable to recognize that what they were asking was literally not possible for him to provide, they continued to press Mr. L. for his personal opinions and individual consent.

Proper Treatment of the Body

Mr. L.'s inpatient therapy continued, with solid food restrictions and endoscopic treatments to control the bleeding varices. Both of these practices caused additional alarm to Mr. L. and his family. For the Hmong, rice is the primary nutrient and the centerpiece of the entire diet. It carries enormous symbolic and ritual significance in addition to its nutritive value; it is their "staff of life." It is considered essential to have rice at every meal, and "even [if] you have nothing else, if you have rice, you have a meal" (B. L.). It is always bad not to have rice. It is worse not to have it when one is ill and in especial need of nourishment to restore health and vigor, and to fuel and foster the life within the human body. While the Hmong do recognize conditions of illness in which food intake must be restricted, in such cases the *primary* nutritive and medicinal food is rice. In these circumstances, rice is boiled in extra water until it is reduced to a thin gruel that may also be pureed to remove any particles, so it can easily be drunk by the sick person. So centrally important is the regular consumption of rice that in the midst of the frightening and unfamiliar events of Mr. L.'s emergency hospitalization, when he was asked if there was anything he needed that American friends in particular could help him with, his first (and very distressed) response was, "I want to eat rice." (In retrospective conversations, Mr. L. has continued to emphasize the critical importance of his having been denied rice in the hospital—a practice he and other Hmong find baffling, insulting, and dangerously foolish.)

Within Hmong culture family are always present in the diagnosis and treatment of the sick, and family aid is profoundly relied upon in times of crisis. Mr. L. had been terrified when he was taken alone to his first endoscopy. At his request, one of his brothers was permitted to accompany him for the second and subsequent treatments. This accommodation occasioned both family gratitude and additional shock, as there was insufficient explanation from the medical staff to help Mr. L.'s brother either to anticipate what he *would* see, or to interpret what he *had* seen as anything other than a hideous ordeal. The procedure entails the introduction of a long tube into the mouth and down the throat and the esophagus. This allows direct visualization of the varices and permits them to be individually injected with the sclerosing substance, so that they harden and are not as likely to bleed again. For such procedures, the patient is sedated and a tubular, hard rubber bite-block is inserted between the teeth, to permit introduction of the endoscopic tube while preventing the teeth from clamping shut. Though the patient is essentially unconscious during the procedure, the gag reflex is still active, and sounds of gagging and choking, together with reflexive reaching with the hands to stop the tube, typically accompany the introduction of the tube into the throat.

Stories circulate in Hmong communities, both in the United States and in the resettlement camps in Thailand, telling of barbaric practices in which American medical doctors engage—practices such as the cutting up of dead bodies; the removal of organs and other body parts from both living and dead bodies; and the excessive withdrawal of blood, a critical vital element of the body's health and well-being (Hurlich, Holtan and Munger 1986). Such narratives are based on observation and experience of common medical procedures such as surgery, autopsy, and blood sampling (which is sometimes repeated at short intervals or entails the withdrawal of multiple tubes of blood). Interpreted in Hmong cultural and religious terms, these phenomena can pose spiritual dangers[9] and quite reasonably give rise to other fears. For example, a Hmong American woman who visited Ban Vinai refugee camp in the early 1980s as part of a U.S.-based medical research team was asked:

"When Hmong people die in the United States, is it true that they are cut into pieces and put in tin cans and sold as food?"
"After you die, why do American doctors try to open up your head and take out your brains?"
"Do American doctors eat the liver, kidney, and brain of patients?"
"Why do American doctors draw so much blood from patients?" (Hurlich, Holtan, and Munger 1986:433)

Misunderstood or unfamiliar invasive procedures are readily assimilated to this existing body of narratives and occasion a great deal of outrage, anguish, and dread.[10] In addition, there is a shared suspicion and fear among many Hmong that Western physicians will use Hmong patients for purposes of experimentation, or for practicing techniques actually uncalled for in their particular medical circumstances (B. L., Pang Xiong Sirirathasuk, Xoua Thao, personal communications). In this initial hospitalization, members of Mr. L.'s extended family were disturbed by a "very big suspect that some of the doctor[s] might try to do something to my people" (B. L., interview, November 1989).[11]

The Hmong have an active tradition of magically invasive procedures, manifested in the intrusion by sorcery of disease-causing agents such as tiny stones (about the size and shape of a grain of rice), bones, nails, or small bits of cloth or red thread,[12] and likewise their removal (by a specialist) by magical means. Apart from the probing of wounds to remove embedded foreign objects (a practice that gained considerable currency during the Indochinese wars when bullet and shrapnel wounds became commonplaces), there is no concept of physically invasive procedures, equivalent to those of biomedicine, as a part of diagnosis or healing. The core concepts of healing, for many southeast Asian groups, are concerned mainly with invisible fluids and energies, and with immaterial elements that need to be helped to reach proper balance (Tung n.d.; Thao 1986). This is never accomplished by physically invasive means. For the Hmong, in addition, disease etiology is essentially spiritual or supernatural (Chindarsi 1976; Bliatout 1982a; Mottin 1984). There are recognized categories of natural causes, such as illnesses associated with climate or seasonal change. Organic causes, such as general weakness occasioned by a person's "lack[ing] something in the body" (Thao 1986:371), are also recognized, but these causal events do not necessarily rule out spiritual or supernatural factors: "Sickness . . . may be recognized to have a natural cause, especially in the case of accidents, and can be treated on this basis by medicines and the removal of the immediate cause. But even in such 'natural' cases there remains the question, 'Why did it happen?' or 'Why did it happen to this person rather than another?' Supernatural selection of the victim is implied" (Geddes 1976:97).

There is also no Hmong indigenous practice of surgery or any equivalent. In addition the Hmong share with many southeast Asian peoples a general horror of bodily mutilation, linked in part to a belief that mutilation prevents the departure of the spirit to join its ancestors prior to rebirth (Sherman 1988). If these considerations make endoscopy shocking, they render transplant surgery virtually incomprehensible, as it entails not only the cutting open of a living body but also the complete removal of critical parts. What is more, a spirit deprived of release from earthly confines owing to bodily mutilation (as would be the case, for instance, if a person died during surgery) becomes an imminent source of danger to others (Chindarsi 1976; Bliatout 1982a). Earthbound spirits may afflict family members with illness and other sorts of misfortune. These intranquil spirits require costly ceremonies and sacrifices to secure their propitiation or to bring about their hoped-for release from earthly confines. In addition, if body parts have been lost in life, a person's ghost may return after death to the place(s) in which bodily losses were incurred and to the people involved. It will be seeking to collect all of the body's original parts, so that it may go whole to its destiny and thus avoid being reincarnated with serious physical defects (Pang Xiong Sirirathasuk, personal communication). These ghosts are a source of fear and danger to the living.

The religion native to Hmong culture has a lengthy tradition, but it has no formal orthodoxy or doctrine. It is not standardized, nor is it separable as a social institution from other features of everyday life or from the general worldview; it is as intrinsic to ordinary actions as to special devotional or propitiatory actions.[13] Hmong religious tradition is what scholars of religion call animistic, recognizing many types of spirits in Nature and in buildings and dwellings. It includes the worship and propitiation of ancestors. Its broadest, most general form is roughly the same across the culture. However, specific variations in practice, belief, and cosmology follow family and clan lines, since it is the male head of household who is responsible for the carrying out of religious observances and who teaches them to his sons (Chindarsi 1976; Bliatout 1986).[14] Indeed the lineage group, in addition to being an affinal and consanguineal community, "is a spiritual community united by the fact that all its members worship the same set of ancestors" (Geddes 1976:52) and observe the same set of ceremonial occasions and practices. Extended families sharing clan membership share religious bonds as well, which are interdependent and of equal importance with other bonds of kinship:

> The interests which the clans serve are security and prosperity in the wide world of natural and supernatural forces. They do so by providing combinations of persons united in spiritual strength and cooperating in mutual help. . . . As their religious aspect is fundamental to their conception, we may define the clans and their sub-divisions as essentially religious associations conferring rights of community upon their members through the spiritual bonds between them. (Geddes 1976:57)

In the Hmong cosmology, spirits in Nature may cause sickness in response to having been either purposefully or inadvertently angered or mistreated. Since these spirits are numerous and invisible, occasions for provoking them abound: they may accidentally be stepped on, hit by hunting implements en route to their intended quarry, struck by rocks thrown into the river in play, spattered with offal being tossed out, and so on (Chindarsi 1976). Ancestors may also cause illness and other misfortune if their worship is neglected or improperly carried out, or if they are simply in need in the afterworld. (Chindarsi 1976; Geddes 1976; Bliatout 1982a; Lemoine 1986). Life and death are complementary in the Hmong worldview. The needs and demands of the afterlife precisely parallel those of earthly life: food, clothing, shelter, money, work implements, seed for planting, and the like. Ancestors lacking in food or money, for instance, may cause sickness or misfortune to living family members as a signal (for they have no voices) to call attention to their need for an offering of those goods. The recently deceased are more likely to trouble their survivors in this way than are those who have long ago passed on (Chindarsi 1976; Geddes 1976).

Special Considerations Associated with the Liver

In addition to the general cultural dissonance between Hmong and conventional Western medical interpretations of health and illness and their attendant behaviors, there are very significant cross-cultural complications in the specific instance of liver disease. For the Hmong (as for some other southeast Asian cultural groups), the liver is invested with the special symbolic and functional significance with which we in the United States invest the heart (Bliatout 1982b, 1986). It is the locus of feeling and personality, of one's very character and motivations. Anglo-European cultures describe persons as being hard- or softhearted for cruelty or kindness, bighearted for generosity, flint-hearted (or having a heart of stone) for meanness and stinginess, stouthearted or faint-hearted for showing courage or trepidation, pure-hearted for unimpeachability of motive, warm- or coldhearted for warmth or coldness of character. Moods may be heavyhearted or brokenhearted for deep sorrow, lighthearted for gaity or frivolity. The heart may be "lost" in love, ache in grief, and "go out" to others when empathizing with their hardships. In contrast, it is the liver that determines a person's motivations, moods, and character (in Mr. L.'s words, his "kindness") in Hmong culture. The very admirable Hmong person, showing exceptional purity of motive, "is considered to have a 'white liver'" (Bliatout 1986:350).

The Hmong recognize categories of mental and emotional illness and distress, in addition to physical illness. In Hmong culture, such problems are linked to the liver. Some specific categories of these types of illnesses have the translated names of "ugly liver," "difficult liver," "short liver," "murmuring liver," "rotten liver," and "broken liver" (Bliatout 1982b, 1986).[15] Bliatout asserts that the "'liver terms' [used to refer to mental and emotional health problems] do not in any way imply a physiological problem with the liver, but are purely idiomatic" (Bliatout 1986:350). Physicians' attempts to explain to members of Mr. L.'s family the concept of chronic, largely asymptomatic, liver disease appeared at the outset to have been interpreted as references to some sort of ultimately nonphysical problem relating to the liver. (This is not surprising, given that the Hmong concept of physical disease requires the presence of active, physical symptoms.) But Hmong knowledge of the categories of liver-associated mental or emotional illnesses and their specific symptomatologies would then disconfirm conventional medicine's assertion that an ongoing, but not physically manifest, liver disease could be present: Mr. L. had none of the behavioral symptoms associated with any of the well-known "liver" categories. The very description of his problem defied cross-cultural consensus.

Among the most serious of the Hmong cultural influences upon this case were the religious and spiritual considerations. Prominent among these is a belief, held to varying degrees by members of the Hmong community, that the liver is a possible anatomical location of one of a person's major souls. According to Bliatout, "[t]he Hmong believe that each person has three major souls.[16] One soul lives in the head area, one in the torso area, and one in the legs area. It is believed that upon death, one comes back to live with the descendants, one remains at the grave site, and one goes back to heaven and may eventually be reborn" (Bliatout 1986:351).

Even in the absence of these religious beliefs, liver transplant is an ominous prospect: one's personality and motivations might be removed and replaced with others unknown. What sort of person might such a procedure create? Who would one be? When the religious considerations are added to these concerns, the metaphysical perils of liver transplant become even more critical than the already considerable physical risks of organ transplantation. The risk of death on the operating table is significant and may occur after the removal of the liver, leaving a mutilated and soulless body and placing surviving family members in jeopardy from an earthbound spirit. Even granting physical survival, it is horrifying (if not impossible) within a system recognizing reincarnation to contemplate the potential surgical removal of a major soul to an unknown and disconnected domain. Far from being ameliorated, this horror is compounded by the thought that such an excision will be followed by implantation of some anonymous soul whose "karmic debt" and other attributes one presumably then inherits.[17]

Soul Loss and Its Consequences

Loss or removal of body parts and the souls that animate them greatly complicates the passage of a deceased person's spirit to the afterworld. Unusual, untimely, or violent death likewise generates serious obstacles to a smooth transition between this world and the next (B. L., interview, November 1989). Any of these circumstances may create dangerous spiritual sources of sickness and affliction for others. In addition, loss of a soul or souls is a significant cause of illness for the person losing them (Chindarsi 1976; Geddes 1976; Bliatout 1982a, 1986; Lemoine 1986; Thao 1986). Souls are conceived of as being fairly loosely attached to the bodies they animate and protect. Of special significance is the fact that they are susceptible of separation during life, as well as at death. Geddes (1976:98) observes that "[i]n the majority of cases of sickness, soul separation is believed to be a factor"; and Thao (1986) reports that while the Hmong recognize many causes of illness, soul loss is the primary cause. Souls wander forth from the body during sleep, producing dreams (Chindarsi 1976). They may fail to return or may become lost or transmuted (Thao 1986) on their way home. Separation may be the result of a curse (Bliatout 1982a, 1986); of "crossing a snare for souls" set up by malicious spirits in the environment (Geddes 1976); of a wandering soul's having entered another form of life, such as an animal (Thao 1986) or a human or animal embryo at the instant of conception (Chindarsi 1976); of a sudden fright (Chindarsi 1976; Bliatout 1982a) or other strong emotion (Thao 1986); or simply because of a soul's lingering in pleasure at a lovely place while its owner continues on (Bliatout 1982a). So likely is it that souls will become separated from bodies that

wherever they go [the Hmong] usually utter words to say that it is time to go home, and the soul, wherever it is at that moment, must return too. When the Hmong are at an unfamiliar place, or even when they are on a picnic, they rarely return quietly. Parents would call loudly to their children's souls. Individuals can also call their own souls. If the parents fail to summon the souls back, their imprudence dooms their children to eventual sickness. (Thao 1986:368)

"[T]he longer one has been separated from one's soul or souls, the more severe the symptoms of illness become" (Bliatout 1986). Failure to reunite the body with the missing soul or souls can result in death (Thao 1986). Clearly, within this framework, a proposal to slice open a living body and remove one of the very dwelling places of a major soul can hardly be embraced as a course of action likely to result in anything resembling a cure for the patient.

Predestination and Life-Sustaining Measures

Notwithstanding the major conceptual differences between the Hmong and the biomedical systems' views of the nature and extent of the problem, and of the acceptability of the proposed solutions, Mr. L. and his family did agree with the medical team that what was happening to him was very serious, and that it was (at least in certain of its aspects) life-threatening. They did not agree, however, that any and all conceivable efforts should be made to save or sustain his life. Nor did they hold

equivalent views of the risk/benefit ratios of the interventions suggested. Certainly some of the medical proposals were rejected because
of the spiritual peril they implied, and others because they made no
cognitive sense across the cultural gap. For example, the community
president expressed a withering doubt that a dead thing removed from
a dead person and sewed into a living one could itself be made to live
again. Mr. L. summarized this view: "just try to stick together only dead
part[s], it won't work." Many members of his family were convinced that
if he should have the transplant he would be bound to die *sooner*, since
his living, if damaged, liver would be replaced by a dead one (B.L.,
interview, November 1989). In their view, such an exchange clearly
involved "trading down."

The Hmong view of the predestination of human lifespans constituted another telling factor in the decision process. Hmong religious
beliefs about reincarnation include the belief that the length of each
soul's lifetime in a given incarnation is predetermined by a limited
license or spiritual charter for that life. Bliatout (1982a:18) refers to
this spiritual charter as a "'visa' to enter earth," Chindarsi (1976) as a
"license," and Thao (1986) as a "mandate." Mr. L. refers to it as a "pass"
(B.L., interview, November 1989). Just before reincarnation, each soul
is allowed

to take, without looking at it, one license from a supply of licenses which have
different expiry dates. The length of time on the license determines how long
the soul can live in the world of men.

   When his license expires a Hmong dies. . . . (Chindarsi 1976:30)

Some episodes of illness are part of the soul's charter, and these may
include fatal sickness if and when "death is due" (Thao 1986:370). A
Hmong shaman may, in a diagnostic and healing ceremony, seek to
bargain with the spiritual powers for an extension of a patient's expira-
tion date, when the time for death is determined to have arrived.
However if the extension is denied, nothing further can be done on the
patient's behalf. This view of the ultimate governance of the arrival of
natural death[18] has a definite influence upon the lengths to which
Hmong might go to try to extend a life, as well as upon the sense of
which sorts of interventions might actually be likely to accomplish such
an extension. For example, interventions regarded as having potential
for success in extending the charter of life would *not* include those
(such as transplant surgery) which themselves carry a significant risk of
causing death. Though not without anguish at the prospect, Mr. L. and
his family showed an understanding resignation in the face of the
possibility that Mr. L.'s time, in spite of his youth, might have come.

Leaving the Hospital

Mr. L.'s initial critical episode and hospitalization ended with the family's decisions to reject the option of liver transplant, and to refuse transport to Pittsburgh for further evaluation. Though some of the younger men in the family felt that the evaluation itself could do no harm, the older men (and in general the majority of the decision-making body) felt that pursuit of the evaluation would involve a significant risk of being coerced into the transplant itself: "since . . . they are the doctor[s], right?; so they say things; scare us, right?; . . . to make [us] decide to say yes" (B.L., interview, November 1989). Family members decided instead to remove him from the hospital against medical advice, and to take him home for family-based care. All of the factors discussed heretofore figured into these conclusions. Also contributing were two additional concerns: a strong dislike of the intense pressure for rapid and compliant decisions the family felt from the medical staff of the hospital (experienced as coercive, and therefore intensifying feelings of distrust); and uneasiness about the youth and relative inexperience of the resident who had primarily handled hospital interactions with Mr. L. and his family. Because the Hmong strongly associate wisdom with age and experience, and respect for age is emphasized throughout the culture (Geddes 1976), it was difficult for Mr. L. and his family to feel comfortable acting on a young person's opinions in matters of such gravity and consequence. There were persistent worries that the resident might be "too young to know" (B. L., interview, November 1989). The relative unavailability (and thus, apparent lack of involvement) of a senior physician also provoked concern that Mr. L. and his problems were not being taken sufficiently seriously, which implied additional risk. The medical response, on the whole, was regarded as inadequate, mystifying, and potentially dangerous.

Hmong Healing Strategies

Once home, Mr. L.'s regimen of care included medicinal, physical, spiritual, and dietary therapeutic measures. He was treated by family members and especially knowledgeable women in the community with traditional herbal medicines and health-promoting foods, and subjected to specific dietary combinations and restrictions as well. Some of his herbal medications were ingested, some used topically, and others used to make healing infusions in which he bathed himself. As soon as Mr. L. was home from the hospital, a shaman was called in to determine the cause of his illness. She divined, as contributing factors, that his parents were in need of food and shelter in the spirit world; and that his grandmother was restless and unhappy because another grave had been placed directly above her own and as a consequence of this crowding she wanted her body to be moved. Part of this information corroborated a communicative dream Mr. L. had had two days before his bleeding episode, in which he had seen his parents living a "cold life" (B. L., interview, November 1989).[19] They had been asking him for help because they had begun their farming far too late in the season to have a successful outcome.

The Philadelphia shaman interceded on Mr. L.'s behalf with the spirits of his parents, explaining that he was young and alone in a strange country, and was therefore without the means both to earn his own living and to provide fully for them. She urged them to be understanding of his plight and to lessen their demands to conform more closely with his means. Mr. L. conducted a propitiatory ceremony for his ancestors, with special attention to his parents, inviting them to eat with him. Later, with the aid of a sister-in-law in Wisconsin who is a shaman, he burned spirit-money, fashioned into the form of a house, for his parents. The burning of spirit-money is a sacramental act, connecting the natural and supernatural realms; the smoke carries the money or other goods represented from this world to the spirit world, where it can be used by those to whom it is sent to better their conditions.

Shamanism, found in numerous cultures around the world, includes religious or spiritual healing arts in which specialist practitioners deal directly with various forms of culturally defined supernatural entities in their healing activities.[20] The Hmong shaman, or *txiv neeb*, translated roughly as "father (or master) of [helping] spirit" (Lemoine 1986),[21] is a male or female healer whose expertise lies in entering and communicating with the world of souls and spirits to discover the sources of health problems and the requirements for their amelioration. Causes of illness that the shaman may discover include spirits of ancestors who are angered at having had their ceremonies neglected or improperly carried out or who are in need of something in the spirit world that their living relations can provide for them;[22] or soul(s) of the sick which have escaped or been frightened away, become lost or transmuted, attempted to return to the sky, or been trapped by offended nature spirits or wantonly malicious entities.[23]

The shaman is brought to the home of a sick person, where s/he conducts the diagnostic and healing ceremonies. The shaman's work is done in a state of trance, during which s/he is assisted by a personal helping spirit to enter the spirit realm. There s/he can consult with ancestral spirits who may have been offended to determine what they need from their living family members, bargain and struggle with wild spirits who may have captured a sick person's soul, or locate lost souls and either entice them back or forcibly return them to their owners in the material world. The shaman has two essential obligations to a patient: "restoring the self" by bringing back lost or captive souls; and literally taking over the patient's struggle for life (Lemoine 1986), for often the healing effort requires a pitched battle in the spirit world, from which the shaman may return "dripping with sweat" (Mottin 1984). The helping spirits of shamans are of differing powers and abilities. If one shaman proves unable to help, a family will typically consult another whose resources are more powerful. The shaman's ceremonies are quite expensive and may consume a significant portion of a family's resources, especially if second or third opinions are sought.

In many resettlement countries, there are fewer shamans per group of Hmong than was typical in Laos, because shamans frequently "were excluded from the resettlement list[s] as useless religious practitioners," (Lemoine 1986:346)[24] or were regarded by some Christian missionary resettlement groups as undesirables. As a result of the relative scarcity of shamans in the United States, the expense of the shaman's services is often greater here than it was in Laos—for it now frequently entails the additional cost of paying airfare to transport a shaman to a community that does not have its own. It is worth noting here that when the services of a shaman are indicated, the family will pay whatever is within their collective means to obtain them, even if it is a hardship to do so. This fact argues against the erroneous stereotype of vernacular healing systems as fall-back strategies used by people who cannot afford conventional medical care. In Mr. L.'s case, his educational program provided him with excellent health insurance coverage for conventional medical treatment, but the shaman's not inconsiderable expenses had to be paid out of pocket. Far from being a compromise option adopted out of economic necessity, the shamans engaged were the practitioners of choice (i.e., the proper specialists) for treating certain critical aspects of Mr. L.'s illness.

The Second Medical Opinion

In addition to actively pursuing numerous culturally familiar healing strategies, Mr. L. and his family strongly desired a second medical opinion. Their example underscores the fact that much of the use of vernacular healing systems *accompanies*, rather than replaces, the use of conventional, Western medicine. This is frequently the case even in ethnic cultures that are largely self-contained, and dramatically different from the culture of conventional medicine. As a coincidental mutual acquaintance of both patient and doctor, I was able to introduce Mr. L. to Dr. O., a hepatologist at Hospital B, a second major teaching hospital in the city. Dr. O. was willing to accommodate many of the salient cultural aspects of Mr. L.'s case, in the knowledge that his care would require some adjustments of medical expectations and occasionally of established procedures. Dr. O. approached Mr. L. conservatively, using extensive laboratory work to establish baseline data and to confirm and monitor initial impressions. He outlined a much longer time frame for decision making than the rush toward transplant Mr. L. had experienced in Hospital A. Mr. L. and his family felt substantial trust in Dr. O.'s judgment, at least in part because of his apparent lack of haste. In addition he had made clear his intention to give due consideration to *all* important aspects of the illness, to the best of his ability. Recognition of his efforts to be accommodating to their own concerns made Mr. L. and his family more willing to regard Dr. O. as an authority to be respected, for relationships of authority in Hmong culture entail precise expectations and demonstrations of reciprocal responsibility. Dr. O. showed respect for the Hmong worldview and in return the family gave careful consideration to his suggestions, even when these were confusing or distasteful within the Hmong conceptual framework.

Following Mr. L.'s initial evaluation in his outpatient therapy, the hepatologist recommended a continuing program of sclerotherapy on a periodic basis (initially, every two to three weeks), to monitor the esophageal varices and to treat them directly. In addition, Mr. L. was to take prescription medications to maintain lowered blood pressure, and to control the formation of ascites. All of these recommendations were aimed at preventing a recurrence of bleeding from the varices. This regimen, though straightforward from a conventional medical perspective, was difficult for Mr. L. to follow. He had a deep dread of the unpleasant and invasive endoscopic procedures. At that stage of his illness, each sclerotherapy treatment itself provoked some amount of bleeding and required medical monitoring during a distressing and uncomfortable recovery period of several hours. Mr. L. felt that the procedures seemed to cause difficulties rather than prevent them. The procedures were made more dreadful by the fact that initially Mr. L. was admitted to the hospital for a day and an overnight stay each time he received a treatment. In part this strategy assured the medical team that Mr. L. would be available far enough in advance of the endoscopy for medically required preprocedure laboratory testing to be done. From the Hmong point of view, the linear-time, American sense of strict punctuality with which patients are expected to meet hospital appointments is a notion without currency. The Hmong concept of time is extremely flexible in all but the most exceptional of situations

(Van Deusen et al. 1980), and it is seldom considered mandatory to do a particular thing at a precise moment. From the medical point of view, the tight scheduling of the hospital could not accommodate an unpredictable arrival time whose repercussions would be felt throughout the day in other rescheduling adjustments.

Second Emergency, Hospital B

As long as Mr. L. remained stable and free of outwardly visible symptoms, there remained no conviction on the part of his family members that an underlying or ongoing liver disease was actually present. He simply did not appear to be sick. His apparent general good health, the culturally shaped sense of time flexibility, and his personal dread of the endoscopic procedures all combined to lead Mr. L. to miss a number of scheduled sclerotherapy appointments. In addition, he discontinued his prescription medications, as they were expensive and (from his point of view) not obviously necessary. Some four or five months after the initial crisis, Mr. L. suffered a second critical bleeding episode. In the small hours of the morning he again began to vomit blood; he immediately awoke his nephew and asked him to drive him to the emergency room at Hospital B.

Mr. L. was admitted to the Medical Intensive Care Unit, where he required considerable effort, attention, and transfusion over the course of several days, to become stabilized. Once released from intensive care, Mr. L. was transferred to a surgical floor of the hospital, a floor unfamiliar to him from any of the overnight stays associated with his sclerotherapy. In these new surroundings, he found himself facing a team of physicians whom he had never met. These strangers strongly recommended that he undergo surgery for the placement of a venous shunt, a device designed to decrease the likelihood of rebleeding of the esophageal varices. (By physically rearranging the circulatory mechanism involved, the shunt reduces the localized blood pressure through deflection of a certain volume of the blood from the liver.) In effect the proposal represented a surgical solution to problems attributed to Mr. L.'s discontinuation of his medical routine of sclerotherapy and medications. The proposal, by providing for an internal mechanism to control Mr. L.'s bleeding varices, addressed the physicians' concern that this "uncooperative patient" might again fail to adhere to his medical therapeutic regimen, with dangerous (and possibly fatal) results.

For a second time, Mr. L. was presented with consent forms and pressured to make a decision. From the surgeons' point of view, the decision in favor of the shunt had already been made; the scheduling of the surgery and its preliminary procedures (including an angiogram, terrifying to Mr. L. in its own right) waited only for the patient to "catch up" to the decision. Though Hmong patterns of decision making were by this time a part of Mr. L.'s medical record, and the medical and nursing staff made genuine efforts to respect them, his care givers were frustrated by the conflict with their own deeply felt sense of time requirements. The nursing staff requested a patient-care conference focusing on cultural issues, and were extremely accommodating of Mr. L.'s special needs. Nurses gave him detailed explanations of all procedures proposed, illustrating their explanations with photographs and diagrams from anatomy books. They arranged for the hospital kitchen to prepare rice-water for him, as his regimen once again restricted him to clear liquids, and this generous step helped to relieve one genuine source of suffering: being forbidden to eat rice. Mr. L. was appreciative of these efforts, but remained resistant to the pressure he felt was attempting to coerce him to reach a conforming decision about the proposed surgery. His bleeding had again been controlled, and he was not in any imminent danger. However, there remained the sense of urgency to action that characterizes both the problem-orientation of conventional medicine and the administrative concerns of a hospital that beds not be "needlessly" occupied or time "wasted."

The conventional division of hospital labor into specialized services with wholly separate staffs and separate locations in the hospital can be baffling to anyone not familiar with the institutional structure. In Mr. L.'s case it raised an additional culturally based issue. Mr. L. became insistent that he see his hepatologist (i.e., his "own" physician), and urgently requested a conference to deal with this new crisis and the decisions it would entail. He was firm in his position that unless he could talk to Dr. O. first, he would refuse to consider the surgery at all (B. L., interview, November 1989). When Dr. O. came to confer, Mr. L. explained that he had dismissed the other physicians' advice and suggestions out of respect for him. He had been extremely careful not to insult or anger Dr. O. by suddenly switching his allegiances or behaving as if the opinions of strangers might carry equal weight with Dr. O.'s own judgments. Mr. L.'s insistence on confirmation of everything by his own physician had been an annoyance and an inconvenience in the hospital system, where it was interpreted as a slow-down technique and a form of noncompliance. From Mr. L.'s point of view, however, it was an essential enactment of his respect for and obligation to a man to whom he owed an immeasurable debt of gratitude—perhaps to whom he even owed his life.

Mr. L.'s eldest brother (the head of his household and of the extended family) and the president of the Philadelphia Hmong community also attended the conference with Dr. O., and I was there as a cultural interpreter. In this meeting, Dr. O. presented Mr. L. with the four alternatives open to him, from the biomedical point of view, in dealing with his type of chronic liver disease. These were: (1) do nothing, with the 90 percent chance of rebleeding, each episode carrying about a 20 percent risk of bleeding to death; (2) continue the sclerotherapy, at the rate of about once a month (intervals possibly longer, depending on progress of the treatments), with the requirement for follow-through in taking medications and keeping appointments; (3) undergo the shunt surgery (which would remove the necessity for additional sclerotherapy but would carry its own cumulative aftereffects); and (4) have a liver transplant. He took pains to explain each alternative to Mr. L.'s advocates, and to answer all of their questions regarding medical understanding of how the disease worked and what would and would not affect it. He attempted at once to be considerate of the cultural differences and needs, and to be firm about his own position and the medical considerations he felt were paramount.

As a result of his second crisis (which occurred at roughly the time the physicians in Hospital A had predicted he might die), Mr. L.'s advocates became convinced that something indeed must be wrong with his liver. They felt that Dr. O., in his careful explanations, and in reviewing some laboratory results for them, had "proved" the existence of the liver disease called hepatitis—though this conviction has, even up to the present, provided them with no clear conception of what this entity might be. Mr. L. acknowledged, during this conference, that he had played a part in his most recent crisis by missing his treatment appointments. The recurrence of severe esophageal bleeding convinced him that the prescribed treatments might have preventive value. The decision reached by Mr. L. and his family and community elders favored resumption of his previous therapeutic regimen, with the stated understanding that Mr. L. had specific responsibilities to the treatment and that he would carry them out. Shunt surgery was ruled out as firmly, and with as much relief, as transplant initially had been. The shunt surgery necessarily entails certain disconnections of the liver from the rest of the person, and a consequent decrease in the liver's access to vital fluids (blood). This suggestion was as frightening, as cognitively dissonant, and very nearly as fraught with spiritual risk as the prospect of the transplant itself. In conventional medical terms the shunt surgery procedure is categorically different from transplant, being many times more common and much less risky. In the Hmong conception of all that they entail, the two courses of action are not nearly so distinct.

At this stage, *all* parties to Mr. L.'s treatment were convinced that the option of liver transplant was out of the question. The Hmong participants had quickly and early on evaluated the situation and ruled out transplant. Mr. L. was accepting of, indeed preferred this course of action, observing, "If I am going to die, I want to die with my [own] liver." From the medical point of view, by the time of his second emergency admission Mr. L. was no longer considered a good candidate for transplant. Physicians and surgeons had serious doubts about his prospects for compliance with the complex (and perpetual) postoperative regimen. This raised economic and ethical issues within the medical framework: livers are a scarce commodity, not to be misallocated to those who will not or cannot be committed to their subsequent care. The agreement to rule out transplant greatly reduced the tension of the medical encounters for everyone. It is most significant in this case that although all parties felt satisfied with this decision and the agreement was mutual, *none of the reasons for rejecting this option was held in common* by the two groups involved in Mr. L.'s care.

Epilogue

At this writing, Mr. L. has dramatically outlived the three- to four-month survival prediction he received at his first emergency hospitalization. Six years after the initial crisis, Mr. L. is stable and well, and has experienced no further acute or critical episodes. He has completed an associate's degree in mental health technology, has married and had a child, and is employed as a social worker in human services for poor families. He requires no ongoing medications and returns to the hepatologist for a checkup about once every two years. He continues simultaneously to observe traditional Hmong religious practices and herbal medications as preventive health measures and as integral parts of everyday life. He follows a health-promoting diet that includes specific traditional foods, food combinations, and food restrictions (by his own and his family's choice), and largely excludes salt and caffeine (in response to medical recommendations).

Within three years of his initial crisis, Mr. L. had become quite acculturated to the American hospital subculture (Dr. O., personal communication), changing his responses to time considerations and to the procedures themselves. He had become confident in going unaccompanied to his appointments, which after the first year began to be handled on an outpatient basis. Mr. L. views his now infrequent checkups as important and reliable ways of tracking his status, and of screening for potential problems before they become critical. He accepts much, though not all, of what conventional medicine offers by way of both explanation and treatment. Biomedical opinions modify rather than replace his traditional views, and are modified by them in turn.

Mr. L.'s composite health care strategy exemplifies the commonly found circumstance of use of a vernacular health care system together with conventional medicine, with each system addressing specific aspects of the health problem.

Mr. L. continues to feel that there is a very real problem in the American medical system's lack of understanding of Hmong culture, and he disagrees strongly with certain specific beliefs and practices of biomedicine. He views physicians as people who possess important special skills and knowledge, but who are also ordinary and fallible human beings. He finds it crucial to take both of these considerations into account. At the same time, he believes it is important for people with serious health problems to go to the Western doctor, and he encourages and assists other members of the Hmong community to do so. He envisions a future of necessary cooperation between these two cultural systems, trying "to reach both side[s] to understand one another. We [are] not going to take any blame or blame anything to someone else" (B. L., interview, November 1989). He expects there will have to be flexibility on both sides.

Conclusion

The kind and extent of differences which can exist between conventional medicine and a vernacular health belief system are well illustrated in this case history. Such differences in beliefs, goals, and values are by no means confined to recent immigrants or to ethnic minorities. In cases such as this one, the differences in belief are made highly visible by the cultural distance and ethnic differences between physicians and patient. In the chapter that follows it becomes clear that—though not perhaps so dramatically visible—equally significant differences between conventional medical and vernacular health beliefs are also found in patient populations *not* culturally, ethnically, linguistically, educationally, or economically distant from their physicians.

Notes

1. For thorough histories of the Hmong see Young 1962; Geddes 1976; Mottin 1980.

2. "Brother" in the Hmong usage includes "brothers from the same mother and father" (i.e., full siblings, a usage equivalent to that of Western societies) and "brothers from the same grandfather," a usage referring to males in a patrilineal descent line traceable to a single grandfather, a kinship relation emphasized in Hmong society. Mr. L. had three male-sibling brothers, of whom two are still living, in Laos. As he has no siblings in the United States, the uses of the terms "brother" and "sister" in the remainder of this chapter refer to the broader, clanal meaning of the terms.

3. Survival estimates based upon aggregate statistics are frequently given to patients. These may be given as or interpreted as individual odds, and individual patients frequently outlive them. Many patients take such occurrences as evidence that physicians are less knowledgeable than they claim to be; are too quick to "give up on them"; are too limited in their knowledge of other therapies that might extend survival; or are using frightening statistics to manipulate them into compliance with medical recommendations about which patients may have misgivings. When the interaction takes place across quite divergent health belief frameworks, outcomes that vary significantly from medical predictions may help to create or reinforce distrust of medical motives and add to the body of experiential evidence that supports the vernacular belief system. This has been a frequent occurrence for Hmong patients in the United States (Xoua Thao, personal communication).

4. Indigenous Hmong strategies for controlling bleeding include herbal medicines and verbal spells, both of which are considered effective, but neither of which works extremely quickly (BL. interview, November 1989).

5. In the disease/illness model (Eisenberg 1977), such a cultural interpretation offers an example of the possibility of a person's having a disease (organic pathology or dysfunction) without an accompanying illness, even in the presence of some physical manifestations that biomedicine classes as symptoms.

6. Such a step is not absolutely impossible but would so fly in the face of profound cultural values that it could be taken only at very high social and personal cost. Few would choose such a course.

7. Women belong to the family and clan of their fathers until they marry, at which time they become members of their husband's lineage. The new lineage membership replaces their former lineage membership, though married women still retain some filial obligations to their parents, especially as the parents age and when they die.

8. In Laos this person would be the headman of the village. In their resettlement, the Hmong choose heads of their communities within their host cities or regions. For a fuller description of the village headman's position and responsibilities, see Geddes 1976.

9. There are risks of spiritual death, as well as risks of physical death, in Hmong culture (Xoua Thao, personal communication).

10. In the summer of 1989 a Hmong man who had returned to Thailand after living in the United States and Canada, and after having had a lengthy hospitalization and subsequent iatrogenic complications, was advising Hmong in Ban Vinai refugee camp not to go to the United States. He warned that American doctors take the organs of sick or dead people and sell them for food (Sally Peterson, personal communication).

11. The Hmong have suffered discrimination and various forms of persecution in their host countries for hundreds of years. They have, as a consequence, a lengthy historical basis for a sense of themselves as "outsiders" and for a general wariness of the motives of non-Hmong who are in a position to cause potential harm. It should also be noted in this connection that many other groups feel the same distrust of the motives of physicians, and the same fear of being used for experimentation or for nonmedical ends. For a distressing number of groups it may be said that these fears are founded at least in part on actual historical events, such as the Tuskegee syphilis study and sterilization practices carried out among some Native American and Latino groups.

12. Chao Song, personal communication, regarding description of stones as resembling grains of rice, and the use of red cloth or thread by sorcerers. See

also Bliatout (1986) regarding bones and nails, and Thao (1986), who calls the intruded stones "egg stones" (translation).

13. For this reason, at least some subset of traditional Hmong religious views remain a part of Hmong culture even in countries of resettlement where Hmong refugees have adopted other religions. Conversion to Christianity began in Laos in the 1950s, under the influence of missionaries. Other Hmong were converted to Christianity in the 1970s in the refugee camps in Thailand, or as a part of their resettlement under the sponsorship of Christian organizations. Some have discontinued many or most of their traditional religious practices and identify themselves as Christian; others are only nominally Christian; and still others combine both systems. Mr. L. and his family are among this last group, and do not experience conflicts in practicing within both religious frameworks.

14. I include here only the briefest summary of relevant aspects of Hmong religious belief, as they bear particularly on the medical case under discussion. For a richly detailed ethnography of the Hmong religious system, see Chindarsi 1976.

15. "Broken liver" is a near equivalent to the Anglo-European "broken heart," with the main symptoms being grief, worry, loneliness, and feelings of loss and insecurity and the primary causes being loss of family members, quarrels between family members, or a break in family unity (Bliatout 1982b).

16. There is considerable variation on this point in the written sources, perhaps attributable in part to varying interpretations of what is meant by the term "soul" (note that Bliatout refers to three "major" souls, implying that there may yet be other, minor souls), or perhaps a reflection of the well-documented clanal variations in the details of religious belief and practice. Mottin (1984) observes that "[t]he Hmong believe that every human being possesses several souls, but they do not quite agree on their number." Thao (1986) refers to only one soul, Bliatout (1986) to three, Lemoine (1986) to five, and Chindarsi (1976) to seven—though after locating the seven he also adds that "Hmong say their shadow is a soul which is outside the body" and take great care not to injure it. (Chindarsi 1976:31). Chindarsi also cites Young (1962) as reporting three souls, while Mottin (1984:102) says that the number of souls identified may be "two, [. . .] three, seven, nine, twelve or even thirty-two," depending on "which number a particular person might see as the perfect number." The different numbers of souls also have different corresponding anatomical locations, or parts of the body which they animate (Mottin 1984). Mr. L. claims that the greatest number of souls would be 120, and reports soul-calling ceremonies in which all 120 are called to return. He also feels that there are twelve major souls, and that of these the single most important "stay[s] in our head somewhere" (B. L., interview, November 1989). Chindarsi sums up: "it can be seen that the question of souls is not a straightforward one—different informants give different numbers and locations of the souls. The main concern of the Hmong is not so much in the numbers or natures of souls, as in their well-being, which affects the body and life itself" (Chindarsi 1976:30).

17. I refer to karma in a broad sense here, to indicate the general accumulation of ethical credits and debits that derive from a person's actions during life, and whose consequences shape future destiny in existences to come. A form of this concept enters into the Hmong reincarnation complex. Bliatout (1986:351) says that the soul that leaves the body at death to go to the afterworld may

"eventually be reborn (either as a human or [as] something else)." Chindarsi describes the reincarnation cycle as repeating "twelve times as a human, then twelve times as an animal, and twelve times as a human again, in an endless cycle," and also reports that when a Hmong dies "his soul goes to the sky world, where it comes before the gods for judgment. If a man has lived a good life his soul can be reincarnated straight away according to the stage he has reached in the cycle of reincarnation. If he lived a bad life then the soul is sent to pound rice and do menial jobs for the people in the sky. When he has served as much punishment as he has merited, his soul is released to choose a license and be reincarnated" (Chindarsi 1976:30). VanDeusen et al. (1980) do attribute to the Hmong a "belief in the theory of karma," though the word is not used by Hmong, and the authors do not elaborate on the theory. Chindarsi's description of the soul's judgment and its effect on reincarnation sounds somewhat akin to the Buddhist and Hindu concepts of karma, though in the Hmong variant the soul does not pay for misdeeds in one life by living a subsequent life (or lives) of punishment or burden but rather fulfills such sentences in the sky world before being permitted the next earthly incarnation.

18. Untimely death, such as by murder, war, or accident, may unnaturally cut short the term of a soul's charter for a given lifetime. It is this interruption of a life in full vigor that makes it difficult for the spirit to move on to the afterworld, as it is "not ready to leave yet," and "the part of [stay is] stronger than the part of go." Death during, or as a result of, surgery falls into this category for Mr. L., who illustrated his explanation of untimely death to me with the example, "if you die by accident or by operation" (B. L. interview, November 1989).

19. Hmong culture does not in general regard dream content as fictive, or as derived from one's own psychological processes. Certain classes of dreams are communicative, and these provide another primary means by which ancestors can make their needs known to their living family members.

20. In Hmong culture quite a number of denizens of the unseen world respond as well to ceremonies that are routinely performed by any male head of household and that do not require a specialist. These include cyclical ceremonies to honor ancestral and household protective spirits and to chase away troublemaking spirits, as well as smaller-scale healing practices such as routine soul-calling ceremonies that may be undertaken before it appears necessary to enlist a shaman for a sick person's aid (Chindarsi 1976; Geddes 1976; Bliatout 1982a).

21. Bliatout (1982a) translates the Hmong name not as the academic category name "shaman" but more literally as "person with a 'neng.'" ("Neng" is an English phonetic rendering of *neeb*, itself a romanized rendering of the name for the helping spirit which assists the shaman in his interactions with the spirit world. Hmong is not a written language, and possesses no indigenous script, so written renderings reflect Western alphabetical and phonetic structures.) For descriptions of shamanic ceremonies, see Bliatout (1982a), Moréchand (1968; 1984), and P. Thao (1986). Lemoine (1986) gives additional details, as does Chindarsi (1976).

22. The sick person is not held responsible for such events, and sickness is seen not as a punishment but as a means of communication for ancestral spirits who have no other voices with which to call attention to their needs (Bliatout 1986). Lemoine (1986:348) points out that the sick person "is always represented as a victim of an assault from outside powers or of an accidental

separation from one part of his self. When this situation has been identified and overcome by the shaman, health is recovered. At no point has there been a feeling of guilt associated with the suffering." He adds, in a footnote to this observation, that "[e]ven when illness is provoked by angry ancestors to whom the patient did not offer proper rituals, he is not made to feel that he is 'bad,' only that he has made a mistake that can be corrected" (p. 348).

23. For detailed descriptions of the categories of spirits, entities, and spiritual hazards included in the indigenous Hmong cosmology, and of types of ameliorative and propitiatory ceremonies, see Bliatout 1982 (the first chapter includes a description of shamanism and its religious context), and Chindarsi 1976.

24. This attitude reflects in part the general Western tendency to regard the magico-religious healing practitioner as not doing anything "real."

Chapter 4
Vernacular Health Care Responses to HIV and AIDS

Sicknesses that do not respond well to conventional medical care, or for which few conventional treatment options exist, frequently motivate people to develop purposive self-care routines and to explore a range of forms of potential treatment. Serious illnesses with poor prognoses may especially quickly lead people to expand their health care strategies beyond the bounds of conventional medicine, in an effort to multiply their therapeutic options. Such actions may be undertaken regardless of prior knowledge of or exposure to other treatment systems (Hufford 1988a), and indeed often include periods of research and concerted inquiry aimed at discovering options of which the interested parties had previously been unaware. These self-designed health care regimens may be quite complex, incorporating information and practices from widely diverse sources. The more serious the health threat and the more refractory to treatment, the greater is the number of additional therapeutic measures likely to be brought to bear.

As a devastating disease with a poor long-term prognosis, and often with minimal response to a medical armamentarium that is still quite limited, HIV/AIDS[1] is exemplary of the kind of health crisis that promotes the widest possible range of vernacular treatment responses. This chapter reviews the HIV/AIDS alternative and complementary therapies movement which is centered in the organized gay male community in the United States. This movement encompasses the broadest spectrum of nonconventional therapeutic measures used in all stages of HIV infection, and provides a detailed example of the use of vernacular healing methods by a population whose socioeconomic profile is that of a "mainstream" patient group: middle-class, well-educated, and familiar with conventional medicine.[2]

The Gay and PWA Communities

The gay male community is large, amorphous, and widely distributed geographically. Its size, distribution, and diversity sustain several well-defined subcultural groups, as well as a macroculture characterized by generally shared bodies of tradition, custom, lore and language, and a clear and articulated sense of group identity among members. Members refer to themselves collectively as a community and a culture, both informally and in their printed media. The principal criteria for membership are self-identity as a homosexual or bisexual male, and self-selection for affiliation.[3] Though gay men are of course represented in all races and ethnicities, social classes, and geographical regions, members of the organized gay male community tend to be white, well-educated, middle-class, and urban (Altman 1986; Ellerman 1988; Gevisser 1988; Peterson and Marin 1988). Characteristically, these are professional men with well-developed problem-solving skills, accustomed to a good measure of autonomy, strongly motivated to take social and political action on their own behalf, and having excellent social and historical reasons for being skeptical of established authority. Given the very recent history of the medicalization of homosexuality—only removed in 1973 from the psychiatric canon of treatable disorders—members of the gay community have reason to resist medical authority in particular. In view of the nature and pace of governmental and medical responses to the HIV epidemic, particularly in its early years, they are also amply motivated to insist on taking an active role in the management of their own health care.

A subset of the gay community are also members of the "PWA (people with AIDS) community," whose sole criterion of membership is HIV seropositive status.[4] As of early 1993, an estimated 44 percent of HIV/AIDS cases are outside the gay community (Centers for Disease Control and Prevention 1993), and this percentage is growing as the rate of infection has been dramatically slowed among (especially white) gay men. The designation "PWA" was coined in the gay AIDS activist movement (Altman 1986) and is still most common in that speech community, though its referent is any and all persons with HIV disease, regardless of gender, identity, or affiliation. In this discussion I focus on the intersection of the gay community and the PWA population, because it is this group primarily who have mounted a deliberate, informed, and well-organized grass-roots response to the HIV/AIDS epidemic that includes an enormous variety of vernacular treatments. Their efforts have resulted in the establishment of a nationwide network of conventional and alternative/complementary treatment information and evaluation, lay referral networks and supply lines, systematic data gathering, and extensive empirical testing (often involving intergroup coordination). The organized gay male community has produced a radical shift in the relationship between HIV-positive patients and health care providers, medical researchers, and government funding and regulatory bodies. It is also (for the time being, at least) members of this community, more than other PWAs, who have the greatest access to, and derive the greatest benefit from, this purposeful and well-coordinated response.[5]

HIV/AIDS and the Gay Rights Movement

The disease now known as AIDS, or more broadly by the recent medical coinage "HIV disease," was initially identified in gay men at the turn of the decade of the 1980s. In its early history in the United States, the syndrome was thought to be largely or entirely confined to the gay male population and was initially referred to in medicine as GRID, an acronym for "gay-related immune disorder" (Altman 1986). The disease very quickly became politicized—in part because of its challenge to existing medical knowledge and technology, and in part because its early identification with gay men brought about a social construction of the disease not as a public health threat but as a contained problem affecting a bounded group stigmatized by the wider society. Medical science had nothing to offer but palliation. The early response of the federal government was that the problem would have to be handled locally.[6] The Reagan administration's disinterest in AIDS was quickly perceived within the gay population as an expression of a deeper antipathy to supportive actions where "unpopular minorities" were involved (Altman 1986). At the local level, it was the gay communities themselves that responded, having gotten a clear sense from "official" sources that no one else would properly look after their needs.

In the 1970s, the decade preceding the appearance of AIDS, there was in the United States an escalating and widely disseminated popular distrust of government and other authorities, coupled with a growing climate of self-determination, pride of identity (based on ethnicity, region, national origin, gender, sexual preference, and other identity factors), and agitation for the rights of individuals and identity groups. Consumer activism increased, along with its concomitant, an insistence on accountability on the part of providers of goods and services; these social actions were extended into the arena of health care (Levin, Katz, and Holst 1979). Feminism included in its social critique a hard look at, and ultimately a rejection of, the paternalism and authoritarianism of conventional medicine. The women's health movement constructed a popular and professional health care sector responsive to the specific needs, interests, and values of women,[7] bolstered by a strong rhetoric of self-determination and practical training in self-care. These included such radical provisions as the de-medicalization and de-hospitalization of childbirth, assertiveness training for the medical encounter, and training in lay- or self-provision of such procedures as vaginal and pelvic examinations, menstrual extractions, and midwifery services. The feminist health movement became one of the models for the early health care organizing of the gay community (Altman 1986).

The gay rights movement rejected the medicalization and social stigmatization of homosexuality and reclaimed a public identity for homosexuals. Gay activists began a program of organization building parallel to that of the women's movement, resulting in numerous local advocacy and activity groups, as well as such national political organizations as the National Gay Task Force and the National Gay Rights Advocates. Recognition of specific gay health concerns (not the least of which were the assumptions and attitudes of many health care providers) made health care rights an organizing issue. By the mid-seventies the National Gay Health Coalition had been founded, and in 1978 the annual National Gay Health Conferences began. Increasingly, gay men and women publicly declared their sexual orientation, enlarging the community of support for others to follow suit. Scores of gay health care professionals, lawyers, politicians, and others in professions enjoying high social status openly declared their sexual identities; many chose to devote their professional talents to the movement. In 1973 the Gay Nurses Alliance was formed, and in the mid-seventies a gay caucus was initiated within the American Medical Students' Association. In 1977 the Bay Area Physicians for Human Rights Association (BAPHRA) was founded in San Francisco by gay physicians, specifically to address gay health care and human rights issues (Altman 1986).

AIDS made its appearance just at the end of this decade of reduction of confidence in medical authority, creation of interest group–oriented health care movements, and intensive organization in the gay community. Nearly all major American cities by then had become home to a significant array of gay organizations including both general and special interest associations (Altman 1986). A nationwide infrastructure, assembled over the previous decade, permitted very rapid and far-reaching mobilization of forces and dissemination of information. The rapid responses of the gay community to the AIDS epidemic were accomplished through activation of existing organizations and networks, and appeal to the ideology and rhetoric of gay pride and gay community solidarity, which were by then well established (Altman 1986; Shilts 1987).[8] San Francisco was (and remains) a major hub of gay rights activity and throughout the HIV epidemic has been on the leading edge of the gay community's response to the AIDS crisis. Homosexual and bisexual men make up a not inconsiderable constituency in the city's population.[9] They are on the whole affluent, well organized as a community, and have local political clout. Predating AIDS, gay groups also had significant political presences in a number of other major U.S. cities, among them Los Angeles, Washington, Houston, Boston, Minneapolis, Chicago, Philadelphia, and New York. The Gay Men's Health Crisis in New York was founded in 1981, one of the first and largest organizations created within gay communities directly in response to HIV/AIDS.

An additional factor spurring the ongoing response of the gay community is that conventional medicine has had relatively little to offer for treatment of the new disease; and understanding of HIV disease processes and their implications, while it has increased exponentially in the past decade, remains fraught with gaps and speculation. HIV/AIDS represents "a contravention of the general trend in modern medicine. It is an anachronism. In a society and a medical profession grown accustomed to the idea that the fight against disease is being progressively won, the appearance of a virulent new disease is an astonishment" (Gong 1987:122). The epidemic has pressed medical science and practice to the limits of their capabilities. The discovery of retroviruses to which humans were susceptible had just barely preceded, at the end of the 1970s, the first reported cases of AIDS (Altman 1986). The discovery of a retroviral agent for HIV/AIDS was made in 1983/1984;[10] antibody testing to confirm infection with HIV was licensed by the Food and Drug Administration (FDA) for public use in early 1985. In the first decade of the epidemic only one drug, azidothymidine (AZT), was approved for use against the HIV virus, and that not until 1987. Because of toxicities, astronomical costs, and diminishing therapeutic returns it is still not available to all PWAs. In the past two years two additional antiviral drugs (ddI and ddC) have been approved, and over the last decade a number of drugs have been added to the list for use against the opportunistic infections to which immunocompromise makes PWAs susceptible. Though research efforts have increased geometrically over the course of the epidemic, the standard process leading to FDA approval for new drugs takes as long as ten to twelve years, which may be as much as two or three times the remaining life expectancy of a person with HIV disease (Gevisser 1988). Even the new "fast-track" approval process, inaugurated in 1989, takes three to four years to bring a drug from initial testing to approval. These circumstances clearly move PWAs and the gay community to take matters of treatment and experimentation into their own hands with a particular seriousness of purpose.

Characteristics of the Vernacular Therapies

Like their conventional medical therapeutics, the vernacular healing practices used by people with HIV/AIDS are intended to produce antiviral action, immune system enhancement, and prophylaxis and control of opportunistic infections. In addition, many therapies are undertaken for pain relief and other symptom control; for control of adverse side effects of conventional chemotherapeutic agents; and for promotion of mental, emotional, or spiritual well-being and the general enhancement of health that is believed to accompany the improvement of these states. (See Table 3 for PWA classification of alternative therapies by putative effects.) Some vernacular practices have more than a single projected outcome. For example, some activities whose immediate goal is pain control or symptom relief also have as a longer-range goal the improvement of immune function resulting from the removal of pain and other symptoms as significant stressors. Improvement in immune function should, in turn, have preventive value against opportunistic infection.

Many PWAs are using a multi-pronged approach to managing their illness, combining some degree of participation in conventional medicine with several vernacular modalities. A sample clinical practice survey in Philadelphia showed a 40 percent rate of use of alternative and complementary therapies (Anderson et al. 1993). There is continual active discussion and debate about therapeutic substances and practices among PWAs. Not surprisingly for a community as numerous and diverse as this one, many points of view are represented, and frequently there are conflicting opinions of the utility or safety of particular treatments as well as differing interpretations of their mechanisms of action. While many of the therapies are harmonious with one another, others are mutually exclusive. In general, the gay PWA community's approach to HIV/AIDS therapies combines a strong self-determination in use of conventional pharmaceuticals (including foreign drugs not approved for use in the United States) and alternative modalities, with the concerns for holism, nutrition, low toxicity, and interest in new applications of traditional knowledge that typify the more general New Age and health foods movements (see Hufford 1971a; Levin and Coreil 1986). The goal is improved *quality* of life, not merely increased *quantity* (Jonathan Lax, personal communication).

The vernacular health care strategies of PWAs are variously referred to within the community as "alternative" therapies (meaning alternatives to the conventional medical modalities, generally with alternative modes of supply) and, increasingly, as "complementary" therapies—stressing the use of nonconventional approaches as adjuncts or com-

TABLE 3. Alternative Therapies Classed According to Putative Effects.

IMMUNOMODULATORS (implies stimulant/strengthening effect)

Botanicals

Echinacea (purple coneflower)
Astragalus (tragacanth)
Shiitake mushrooms or Lentinan extract pills
Ginseng (*Panax schin-seng* and *Panax quinquefolius*) "rejuvenator" vs. chronic fatigue, stimulant to thymus and pituitary glands, central nervous system stimulant (extensive use recommended under knowledgeable supervision only)
Traditional Chinese herbs (used with or without acupuncture in a comprehensive program aimed at a broad range of responses in addition to immune system stimulation)
Aloe vera oral gel
Mistletoe extract pills

Nutritional Supplements

NAC (N-acetylcysteine; to promote glutathione production in cells; antioxidant)
Thymus extracts (to stimulate T-cell production; dosages restricted to avoid overstimulation of immune system)
L-Lysine (amino acid)
Blue-green algae (spirulina; "Blue-Green Manna")
Commercial supplement tablets combining several herbs: "Astra-8," "Immunecomp," "Maximum Defense," "Vita-Mune"
Zinc (caution: low threshold of toxicity)
Selenium (caution: low threshold of toxicity)
Vitamins A, B, C, E

Prescription Pharmaceuticals (off-label uses)

Disulfiram (Antabuse®)
Cimetidine (Tagamet®), Ranitidine (Zantac®)
Low-dose alpha-interferon
Pentoxyfylline (Trental®)
Levamisole
Proleukin®

Foreign Pharmaceuticals and Products

Imuthiol/DTC
Ribavirin
Isoprinosine

Physical Therapies

Shiatsu or acupressure massage (believed to improve overall health and immune function by removing significant energy blockages)
Chiropractic

TABLE 3. *(Continued)*

Metaphysical Therapies

Prayer
"Psychoimmunity"; Louise Hay books and videotapes

ANTIVIRALS

Botanicals

Echinacea (purple coneflower)
Shiitake mushrooms or Lentinan extract pills
Hypericum (St. John's wort); (specifically identified as antiretroviral. Cautions: photosensitivity, hepatotoxicity; contraindicated when liver enzymes are elevated, or in the presence of subjective signs of impaired liver function. May be taken instead in synthesized form, hypericin)
Traditional Chinese herbs
Pau d'arco (also Tajibo/Taheebo; *Tabebuia impetiginosa*)

Nutritional Supplements

L-Lysine (against herpesviruses)
BHT (commercial antioxidant; to eliminate "atmosphere of oxidation" conducive to viral replication)
NAC (N-acetylcysteine; to promote glutathione production in cells; antioxidant)
Vitamin C

Foreign Pharmaceuticals

Dextran sulfate (specifically identified as antiretroviral; now controversial)
Compound Q (toxicity warning)
AL-721 (specifically identified as antiretroviral; now largely out of favor)

ANTI-FUNGAL AND ANTI-YEAST AGENTS

Botanicals

Pau d'arco (also Tajibo/Taheebo; *Tabebuia impetiginosa*)
Garlic (odorless tablet forms available; therapeutic and prophylactic use)
Traditional Chinese herbs
Ligustrum (privet; as mouthwash for candidiasis)
"Candida Cleanse" (commercial herbal formula; contains echinacea and astragalus)
Chaparral tea

ANTIBIOTICS

Garlic (odorless tablet forms available; therapeutic and prophylactic use)
Traditional Chinese herbs

ANTITUMOR AGENTS

Botanicals

Echinacea (purple coneflower)
Astragalus (tragacanth)

TABLE 3. (*Continued*)

Shiitake mushrooms or Lentinan extract pills
Pau d'Arco (also Tajibo/Taheebo; *Tabebuia impetiginosa*)
Spirulina (blue-green algae)

Other Natural Substances

Shark cartilage

Nutritional Supplements

Vitamin C

FOR KAPOSI'S SARCOMA SKIN LESIONS SPECIFICALLY

Homeopathic remedies

Mistletoe
Phytolacca (poke root)
Periwinkle (vinca)

Botanicals

Aloe vera (topical)
Mistletoe extract pills

SYMPTOM CONTROL

Traditional Chinese medicine: herbs and/or acupuncture (symptom abatement follows resolution of imbalances). A printed handout distributed at a monthly alternative therapies discussion group asserts that "100% of long-term survivors are using some form of Chinese Medicine weekly."
Aloe vera (Egyptian burn plant): topical, for skin lesions and ulcerations; oral gel, anti-inflammatory
Ligustrum (privet): internal, for diarrhea; as mouthwash for candidiasis; topical, for skin problems
Chiropractic

FOR SIDE EFFECTS OF CONVENTIONAL MEDICAL THERAPY

Iron: to overcome anemias and reduce fatigue resulting from AZT, chemotherapy
"Blue-green Manna" (a blue-green algae): to combat liver toxicity of AZT, pentamidine
Marijuana tea: for nausea secondary to chemotherapy
L-Arginine (amino acid): to combat liver toxicity (contraindicated in presence of herpesvirus infections or their prodromal signs)
Traditional Chinese herbs
Acupuncture
Visualization; guided imagery
Chiropractic

plements to conventional therapeutics, and eliminating the suggestion perhaps implied by the term "alternative" that these therapies ought to be used *instead of* biomedical treatments. Usage varies within the community and its media, and the terms are frequently used either in conjunction or interchangeably. Many of the practices and substances in the repertoire of the HIV alternative therapies movement are also used as unconventional cancer therapies—several with long histories in this connection—and many are in wide general use in the health foods and holistic health movements, though they may also have HIV-specific modifications or applications.

No listing of alternative and complementary approaches to HIV could ever conceivably be comprehensive. Because of the intense experimental and theoretical research activity surrounding HIV/AIDS, both in the official research echelons and at the grass-roots level, the proliferation of new information and hypotheses is swift, and staggering in volume. Treatment possibilities and strategies change constantly in response to new discoveries of apparent beneficial and deleterious effects of scores of substances and a virtual infinity of permutations in their possible combinations. So rapid are the changes that PWAs refer to particularly popular new treatments as the "cure of the week" or the "treatment *du jour*," anticipating with irony born of past experience that they may yet fade from the scene (Lax, personal communication). What follows is a description of several of the strategies most commonly reported between 1987 and 1993, culled from medical and nursing literature, health foods and HIV alternative therapies advocacy literature, the AIDS alternative therapies information network, and ethnographic fieldwork (interviews, participant observation in PWA alternative therapies discussion groups) in the Philadelphia PWA community between 1990 and 1993. It cannot be overstressed that these descriptions represent only a limited and specific moment in the complex and rapidly changing environment of the PWA community's responses to HIV/AIDS.

Nutritional Approaches

People with HIV seropositive status report a heightened consciousness of the importance of nutrition to their health. This concern is actively promoted throughout the PWA community and is supported by physicians. The understanding of what constitutes good nutrition may differ radically between PWAs and medical professionals, however, with standards generally being more complex and defined minimum requirements higher in the nonmedical model. PWAs often share with members of other vernacular health belief systems a conviction that physicians' training in and understanding of nutrition and diet is incomplete, inadequate, or even incorrect (see O'Connor 1993). All PWAs I have spoken with have adopted some form of special diet and/or nutritional supplementation to promote optimal health and functioning. The most common form of supplementation is vitamin and mineral megadosing. Vitamin and mineral supplementation is generally aimed at boosting immune function, based on an awareness that certain immune deficits are associated with vitamin or mineral deficiencies (Rakower and Galvin 1989), and the concomitant assumption that megadose intake will help to repair deficits and promote higher-level functioning. In general, vitamin and mineral therapy is aimed at restoring cell-mediated immunity by increasing T-cell (CD-4)[11] counts and T-cell activity (Meisenhelder and LaCharite 1989), though particular constituents may have other specific functions. Vitamin C, for example, is frequently taken to increase the infection-fighting activity of phagocytes, white blood cells that consume foreign matter in the body. Most frequently used are vitamins A, B_1 (thiamine), B_6 (pyridoxine), B_{12} (cobalamin), C, D, and E; mineral supplements are generally zinc and selenium (see Table 4).

Vitamins A and C have reputations as free radical scavengers, promoting a healthy immune system both by preventing free radical formation within the body and by stabilizing existing free radicals. In addition, vitamin A is credited with repair of damaged nerve cells and enhancement of vision, considerations of importance to PWAs affected by or concerned about HIV-related neuropathies or cytomegalovirus (CMV) retinitis. The B vitamins are regarded as stress reducers, and as correctors of metabolic irregularities brought on by stress. Pantothenic acid, a constituent of the B vitamin family, is additionally thought to increase assimilability of vitamin C. Vitamin C, among its other properties, is believed by many to strengthen the body's general resistance to viruses (from the rhinoviruses of the common cold to HIV) and to stimulate eliminative processes (Serinus 1987). The latter quality is significant to those who hold a theory of disease based upon the build-up of toxins in the body, since all eliminative functions have a role in the removal of such toxic matter. Vitamin E is taken to promote wound healing and cell and tissue regeneration, zinc to rebuild and stimulate the immune system, and selenium to strengthen cell membranes (Serinus 1987), as well as to boost immune responses. Iron may also be taken as a supplement, though there are sharp differences of opinion as to its safety. Some feel that iron supplements enrich the blood and help to prevent or overcome anemia (a frequent side effect of AZT and other chemotherapies) and to reduce fatigue and improve energy levels. Others consider it to be toxic or to promote certain opportunis-

TABLE 4. Vitamin and Mineral Supplements.

Vitamins	
A	Free radical scavenger; promote repair of damaged nerve cells, enhancement of vision (cf. HIV neuropathies, CMV retinitis).
B complex	Stress reduction; correct stress-induced metabolic irregularities; increase assimilability of vitamin C.
C	Strengthen resistance to viral infection; stimulate eliminative processes (explanatory model attributes disease to accumulation of toxins in the body).
E	Promote wound healing, cell and tissue regeneration.

Minerals	
Selenium	Elevate immune function, strengthen cell walls.
Zinc	Restore and stimulate immune system.
Iron	Prevent/overcome anemia; reduce fatigue/improve energy levels. (Controversial: many PWAs feel iron intake promotes opportunistic infection by providing beneficial growth environment for infectious agents.)

Note: Vitamin and mineral supplements may be used in moderate or very high doses. Theory of megadosing is based on association of vitamin and mineral deficiencies with certain immune deficits. Consequent belief is that high intake of these substances will help to repair deficits and promote higher-level immune functioning.

tic infections by providing an iron-rich growth environment that benefits infectious agents. One couple participating in a group discussion of alternative therapies strongly discouraged any supplemental iron intake, noting that they even avoid brands of multivitamin tablets that contain any iron whatsoever (WTP[12] alternative therapies discussion group, March 1990).

There is widespread awareness in the PWA community of contraindications for certain supplements, and warnings are part of the information network. For example, while the amino acid L-Arginine is widely used by health foods enthusiasts as a stimulant to the immune system and as a liver regenerator, it is contraindicated for those who are troubled with infections caused by viruses of the herpes family, for which it is also recognized as a stimulant (Serinus 1987:123–124; WTP alternative therapies discussion group, March 1990). Even arginine-rich foods, such as citrus fruits, chocolate, peanuts, and almonds (Serinus 1987) may be eliminated from the diet when herpesvirus infections are a persistent problem. Supplemental intake of zinc and selenium are also singled out for careful control, since both have low thresholds of toxicity (WTP alternative therapies discussion group, March 1990).

Two forms of blue-green algae, Spirulina and Blue-Green Manna,[13] are taken as drops or in tablet form to stimulate the immune system, to provide essential amino acids and micronutrients, and to enhance trace mineral absorption. The algae preparations are sold as food items (not medications) in health food stores and through private distributors. Both are valued as protein-rich supplements. Spirulina has the additional reputation of having anticancer properties, while Blue-Green Manna is thought especially to act on the thymus gland (thereby promoting T-cell production) and to detoxify the liver (Strawn 1989). This quality is of interest to PWAs, since liver toxicity is a side effect of Bactrim® and of pentamidine, the drugs most frequently used against the opportunistic infection *Pneumocystis carinii* pneumonia (PCP).

In addition to vitamins and minerals, a number of items sold as foods or food supplements are used medicinally. NAC (N-acetylcysteine), an amino acid derivative, is taken as an antioxidant and as a stimulant to cellular production of glutathione, which is commonly deficient in T-helper and other blood cells of HIV-positive people (*AIDS Treatment News* #152, 5 June 1992; hereafter cited as *ATN*). Antioxidants are promoted on the theory that HIV virus reproduction requires an environment of oxidation, which can be significantly restricted through taking antioxidants (WTP alternative therapies discussion group, March 1990). There is additional speculation among both PWAs and researchers (e.g., Roerderer et al. 1992) that NAC may have antiviral activity as well, though there is as yet little agreement on effective dosage. The amino acid L-Lysine is a standard antiviral treatment and a preventive measure against outbreaks of herpes, within the health food movement. Some PWAs also use BHT (butylated hydroxytoluene, an antioxidant used commercially as a food additive to retard spoilage) for herpes control, though most who recommend BHT use it as an HIV antiviral on the basis of some research claims that it breaks down the protective coating of HIV and other retroviruses (Dwyer et al. 1988; Serinus 1987). Soy and/or egg lecithin are used to create the homemade version of AL-721, an experimental antiviral drug first synthesized and tested in Israel. AL-721 was not approved for use or testing in the United States for a number of years after its Israeli developers reported that it inhibited HIV viral replication in vitro, but word quickly spread that the substance was fairly easy to replicate or closely approximate at home. AL-721 home formulations continue to be used by some PWAs, although the drug is generally considered ineffective and "passé" in most circles (printed handout, WTP alternative therapies discussion group, March 1990). Organically bound iodine (found in seaweeds), chlorophyll, barley greens or their extracts, and wheat grass juice are reputed to stimulate the thymus gland (Badgley 1987; Serinus 1987) and may therefore be consumed as immune-boosting dietary supplements. Thymus extracts, derived from animal glands, are likewise popular as potential immunomodulators (Serinus 1987; WTP alternative therapies discussion group, March 1990). For "routine immune stimulation," commercial supplement-combination capsules such as brandnames Immunecomp, Maximum Defense, or Astra-8 are taken. These are generally taken in restricted dosages, to avoid overworking the immune system and producing adverse, rather than beneficial, effects (printed handout, WTP alternative therapies discussion groups, March 1990, April 1990). Bovine colostrum is sold as a supplemental source of protein and "natural antibodies," and is taken by some PWAs for its reputed antibiotic properties (Serinus 1987; Danielson, Stewart, and Lippert 1988).

Complete dietary regimens most often followed are macrobiotics, the anti-yeast diet, and adaptations of a system published as the Immune Power Diet (Berger 1985) (see Table 5). Of Japanese origin, the macrobiotic diet is based on the principle of balance and harmony between yin and yang forces in the body, and its restoration and maintenance through the yin and yang properties of foods, together with the practice of meditation.[14] Proper balance promotes harmony and health, and diseases result from imbalances between these polar—but interconnected—qualities. The modern American macrobiotic diet specifically addresses diseases such as cancer and AIDS as the results of long-term imbalances. The basic diet consists of 50 to 60 percent whole grains, 20 to 30 percent vegetables, 5 to 10 percent legumes and seaweeds (or "sea vegetables"), and 5 percent soups based on miso, a fermented soybean paste (Meisenhelder and LaCharite 1989; Rakower and Galvin 1989). Fish is permitted only occasionally, and liquid intake is generally restricted. Meats and fowl, all refined sugars, wheat products, and eggs are proscribed because they are too yin or too yang (Rakower and Galvin 1989). Those who support the macrobiotic approach to health feel that this diet and its attendant lifestyle can restore balance and harmony, promote optimal health, remove the underlying cause of HIV/AIDS, or render the virus inactive or incapable of producing immune system deficits. Some simply observe that "macrobiotics live longer" (WTP alternative therapies discussion group, April 1990). Other PWAs have strong negative feelings about this very restrictive diet, based on the conviction that it is insufficient in caloric and protein intake for seropositive or actively symptomatic people, who need to maintain a good body weight and ample nutrient intake (A., personal communication; WTP alternative therapies discussion group, April 1990).

The Yeast-Free Diet is primarily aimed at preventing opportunistic

TABLE 5. Special Diets.

Macrobiotics

Aim: To achieve and maintain a balance between yin and yang energies in the
 body
Underlying theory: Disease results from long-term imbalances.
Practice: Promotes whole grains, raw or lightly cooked vegetables, sea vegetables, soy products; restricts liquid intake, fish; proscribes meats and fowl, all
 refined sugars, wheat products, eggs
 (Controversial: many PWAs feel protein intake and total calorie consumption
 are dangerously inadequate)

Anti-yeast diet

Aim: To prevent yeast and fungal infections
Underlying theory: Yeast-containing or yeast-promoting foods create a yeast-
 favorable environment in the body.
Practice: No yeast-containing or fermented foods or beverages, and none that
 may incidentally contain yeast or be likely to promote yeast growth (e.g.,
 packaged foods, refined and raw sugars, cheeses, fruit juices in any form,
 "leftovers"); also proscribes coffee and tea

Immune Power Diet (Berger 1985; not formulated by author with reference to
HIV/AIDS)

Aim: To achieve and maintain maximum immunocompetence
Underlying theory: Food sensitivities or allergies, often undetected, provoke
 continual immune responses, which over time tax and ultimately deplete the
 immune system.
Practice: Eliminate "immuno-toxic" foods, especially cow's milk, wheat, yeast,
 eggs, corn, soy, cane sugar, and all products derived from or containing these
 ingredients; identify and eliminate individual sensitivities (especially suspect
 are foods which are usual centerpieces of the personal diet, and those for
 which one experiences cravings). Simultaneous vitamin and mineral supplementation are essential (recommended dosages exceed U.S. RDAs, but fall
 below megadose amounts).

yeast infections (candidiasis, or thrush), a frequent problem for people
with HIV/AIDS. This diet excludes all yeast-containing or fermented
foods and beverages, including all yeasted breads, as well as any foods
that may incidentally contain yeast or be likely to promote yeast growth,
such as packaged "ready-to-eat" foods, refined and raw sugars, maple
syrup, honey, cheeses, fruit juices in any form, and all "leftovers"
(Rakower and Galvin 1989). Also eliminated are coffee and tea (Meisenhelder and LaCharite 1989). The theoretical principle of the yeast-free
diet is that the ingestion of yeast-containing or yeast-promoting foods
will create a yeast-favorable environment in the body, thereby increasing susceptibility to *Candida* infections, which then further weaken the
immune system. The purpose of the diet is preventive, and it is specific

to a fairly narrow range of problems. (Note that yeast-free and mac-robiotic diets are incompatible with one another, since such fundamen-tal constituents of macrobiotics as miso [a product of fermentation] and whole-grain wheat are proscribed by the yeast-free diet.)

The Immune Power Diet (not originally developed with reference to HIV/AIDS, but rather as a general health-promoting diet) is based on the theory that most people have at least some undetected food sen-sitivities or outright food allergies that provoke immune responses. Over time, continued consumption of these foods will, through over-stimulation, tax and ultimately deplete the immune system, leaving the individual vulnerable to illnesses. Certain foods are felt to be directly "immuno-toxic," causing lymphocytes and other critical components of the cellular immune system to self-destruct, thereby weakening general immunity through depletion of available immune system cells (Berger 1985). Though the spectrum of food sensitivities is unique to each individual, the foods most often implicated are cow's milk, wheat, yeasts, eggs, corn, soy, and cane sugar, as well as all products made from or containing these ingredients. The individual constellation of specific sensitivities is discovered through an initial dietary phase of elimination of all the above-named items, followed by the gradual reintroduction of a single food at a time coupled with observation of any adverse reactions. Signals of food sensitivities include such symp-toms as nausea, headache, fatigue, rashes and other skin conditions, weight control problems, moodiness, frequent infections or minor illnesses, joint pain, and so forth. Other foods implicated are any which an individual especially craves, or consumes very frequently (ibid.:29). Additional problem foods and food additives may be detected directly by "cytotoxic testing" (offered by the creator of the system, an M.D.), in which blood cells are exposed to food extracts and observed micro-scopically for adverse reactions (ibid.:39).

Within this framework, the ideal diet for any individual excludes all foods to which sensitivities are discovered, and is always supplemented with vitamins, minerals, and essential amino acids. Ideally, supplement combinations are individually distinctive, though general programs may also be determined using the published guidelines (ibid.:242–249). Supplements are consumed in quantities larger than the usual "recommended dietary allowances" (RDAs) but smaller than typical megadoses; emphasis is placed on keeping supplement dosages within a proper therapeutic range. The usual supplements are vitamins A, B complex, C, D, E, and K; zinc, iron, selenium, and copper; and selec-tions from a spectrum of twenty-two amino acids. Benefits to health are described in terms of strengthening the thymus gland, increasing numbers of T-cells and macrophages, boosting antibody responses, and strengthening the responses of immune system cells. The dietary regimen is intended to rebuild depleted immune systems as well as to provide "preventive immune nutrition" (ibid.:261). Though the development of this nutritional system had nothing to do with responding to HIV/AIDS, its focus on restoration of damaged immune function and its explicit emphasis on the health of the thymus gland and increases in T-cell counts make it relevant to the health concerns of PWAs, with only minor modifications.

Herbal and Related Therapies

A number of herbal or herb-derivative remedies are used to control HIV/AIDS and its related infections, as well as to boost the immune system and to directly combat the HIV virus. Most have been used medicinally for centuries and are found in a number of herbal traditions with a variety of theoretical bases. Some PWAs are using herbs under the direction of a naturopath or other formally schooled herbalist (including both ethnic Chinese and non-Chinese practitioners of traditional Chinese herbalism). Others design their herbal regimen on their own, with the aid of reference books[15] or in consultation with friends or other PWAs who are part of the alternative treatment information network. There are as many personal preferences and uses for herbs as there are personal variations in health and response to medications; those mentioned here are only the herbs that appear to have the widest general currency in treating the causes and effects of HIV/AIDS.

Most widely recommended by naturopaths is echinacea, commonly known as purple coneflower. Its rootstock has long been used to make a tea or tincture used to treat skin eruptions that are believed indicative or expressive of contaminants in the blood (Lust 1974), as well as sexually transmitted diseases and cancer, also interpreted as expressions of impurities in the blood (Grieve 1982). Its traditional uses and associations with cancers, contaminated blood, and sexually transmitted diseases make echinacea an obvious candidate for use in HIV/ AIDS. Within the HIV alternative therapy network, echinacea is considered "the herb of choice for treating immune deficiency" (Serinus 1987:33) and has a reputation for both antiviral and immunomodulating action (see also Tyler, Brady, and Robbers 1988:470–471). Use of echinacea is typically intermittent, with the herb being taken for some number of consecutive days, followed by a respite period of twice or three times that number of days: a typical schedule, for example, might be ten days "on" and twenty or thirty days "off." Other PWAs take echinacea only symptomatically, for example, in response to early cold or flu symptoms, increase in fatigue, or decrease in sense of overall energy or vitality. Though some people do use echinacea as part of a constant regimen, cautions circulate regarding risk of overuse with resultant hyperstimulation of the immune system. This in turn is thought to contribute to further compromise of immune function, and possibly to promote development of autoimmune responses.

Astragalus (tragacanth), traditionally used as a demulcent to soothe irritated mucous membranes (Grieve 1982:821), is used in HIV/AIDS treatment to improve lymphocyte and macrophage function (Steinberg 1990:185), thereby enhancing immune response. Some attribute antitumor effects as well to the use of astragalus (Martin 1988:43). Also used as immunomodulators are ginseng, and shiitake mushrooms or their extracts. Shiitake mushrooms, native to Japan but now readily available in health and specialty foods stores in this country, are felt to increase macrophage and lymphocyte function (Steinberg 1990). They are also considered to have antiviral properties, which are not diminished by cooking (Serinus 1987:216–217). Lentinan, a derivative of the mushrooms, is used in Japan in the treatment of some cancers (*ATN* #19, 5 December 1986). Those who advocate the use of shiitake mushrooms recommend frequent, even daily, consumption (WTP alternative therapies discussion group, March 1990).

In Chinese herbalism, ginseng has been revered for thousands of years as a general panacea and "considered especially valuable for feverish and inflammatory diseases, for hemorrhage, and for blood diseases" (Lust 1974:206). In Western herbal traditions, it has a reputation as a "rejuvenator," restoring energy and combating fatigue, and as a stimulant to the central nervous system. Its reputation in tradition gives ginseng a natural affinity for HIV/AIDS. In this context it is taken as a restorative in chronic fatigue (WTP alternative therapies discussion group, April 1990), as a general immune system booster, and as a specific stimulant to the thymus and pituitary glands (Serinus 1987: 216). Different varieties of ginseng are recognized to have different modes of action, and the species as a whole is regarded as extraordinarily powerful. For these reasons it is commonly recommended that it be used with the oversight and consultation of a knowledgeable herbalist. If it is being taken within a yin/yang therapeutic framework, it is thought best that consultation be specifically with a practitioner of traditional Chinese medicine.

Long in traditional use (in many parts of the world) as a natural antibiotic, garlic is used prophylactically in HIV infection as both an antibacterial and antiviral agent. Ideally, it is consumed raw, and in substantial quantity: five to fifteen cloves daily (Serinus 1987:122). It is very widely used by PWAs, though many joke that either they or their lovers cannot tolerate the smell (WTP discussion group, March 1990). When "garlic breath" and related garlic odors (such as garlic-scented perspiration, when consumption is very high) are considered problematic or when consumption of fresh garlic is inconvenient or impossible (for example, during hospitalizations), an odorless tablet form is substituted. These tablets are readily available in health food stores and from private suppliers.

A more recent import to herbalism in the United States is Pau d'arco (also known as Tajibo, or by its anglicized spelling, Taheebo), the inner bark of a tree native to the South American Andes (*Tabebuia impetiginosa*). Because of its reported antifungal properties, some people take a daily prophylactic dose against opportunistic yeast and fungal infections (Steinberg 1990:185). The herb has a reputation as an anticancer substance, and is believed by some within the HIV alternative treatment network to have antiviral properties as well (Serinus 1987: 216). It is taken in tablet form, or as a tea.

St. John's wort (*hypericum*) has been used historically for its tranquilizing and antidepressant effects (Lust 1987:344), as well as in pulmonary and urinary disorders (Grieve 1982:708). Its primary interest to PWAs stems from the discovery reported in 1989 that two of its active principles, hypericin and pseudohypericin, have been shown to have antiretroviral action in vitro (Steinberg 1990:185). PWAs taking St. John's wort are aware of its potential liver toxicity, as well as its potential for producing skin photosensitivity (Lust 1987:396; WTP alternative therapies discussion group, March 1990). They recommend taking the photosensitivity in stride and avoiding prolonged exposure to the sun, but caution that anyone with a history of hepatitis or other liver disease avoid St. John's wort or use it with vigilance and medical monitoring, discontinuing the herb if liver enzyme levels become elevated or if familiar liver-related symptoms appear (WTP alternative therapies discussion group, March 1990). More recent opinion suggests that the herb form, in any feasibly consumable quantity, does not deliver sufficient amounts of active principle, and that PWAs wishing to use it would do better to seek access to the drug forms, now available in some official clinical trials.

Certain herbs find their main uses treating the symptoms of the opportunistic infections to which PWAs are susceptible. Aloe vera is used topically, in accordance with its time-honored traditional uses, to promote healing of both skin ulcerations and the lesions of Kaposi's sarcoma (KS). Aloe vera gel or capsules may also be taken internally for immune system stimulation or as an anti-inflammatory. Because of its astringent properties, an infusion or decoction of ligustrum (privet) is taken internally to combat diarrhea. It is also used as a mouthwash or gargle (e.g., for oral candidiasis, or thrush), and applied topically as a soothing and therapeutic wash for skin problems (Lust 1987; Martin 1988). Chaparral tea is used against candida, and a tea of marijuana to combat nausea, especially the nausea produced by conventional chemotherapy (Serinus 1987:137–138, 143). Dwyer and colleagues (1988) report the use of injections of mistletoe extract to inhibit tumor growth, and some people also take it in pill form to control KS (printed handout, WTP alternative therapies discussion group, March 1990).[16] Two popular commercial herbal tincture formulas intended specifically for use in HIV/AIDS are "Vita-mune" and "Candida Cleanse." Both contain the widely used herbs echinacea and astragalus, along with other herbal ingredients selected for their immunomodulating, antiviral, or antibacterial reputations.

Special Preparations of Herbs

Flower Essences

A common New Age use of herbs is in the form of flower essences, first developed by Dr. Edward Bach, a British physician and homeopath, in the 1930s (Cate 1986). Bach's pharmacopeia included thirty-eight essences. More recent flower essence practitioners and user associations both in Britain and the United States have expanded this list, which is now considered to be open-ended. New essences are added on the basis of experimentation and reports from users.[17] Flower essences are infinitesimal dilutions of various flowering plants which are selected not for their pharmacological properties, but rather for innate spiritual or metaphysical qualities which they are intended to impart to those who use the distillates. Indeed, presence or absence of pharmacological activity in the plant species selected is a moot issue for production and use of the essences.

Flower essences are prepared in a manner intended to capture and enhance the inherent "life energy" of the plant through proper harvesting and preparation techniques; these include a positive mental attitude on the part of the harvester, and steeping of flowers in clear water by exposure to direct sunlight.[18] They are commercially manufactured but may also be self-prepared by anyone with access to the appropriate plants in ecologically desirable growing conditions (e.g., free from man-made environmental pollutants). Only the flowering parts of the plant are used. Because the flowers are usually found at the top of the plant, "closer to the heavens," they correspond to the "higher planes" of individuals (Michael DiPalma, N. D., personal communication). Unlike homeopathic remedies, which they resemble in their infinitesimal dilutions, flower essences aim specifically to "help balance the mental, emotional, physical, and spiritual aspects of the individual," on theoretical grounds that "the basis of disease is found in disharmony between the spiritual and mental aspects of a human being" (Strawn 1989:189).

Flower essences are usually taken orally (sublingually) in microdoses, but they may also be used in baths and applied topically. Doses of flower essences are typically accompanied by silent recitation of prescribed "affirmations," or statements designed to promote optimistic thinking and positive mental states, since it is believed that negative thoughts encourage disease and a positive mental outlook promotes health at all levels. Within this system, it is believed that physical healing proceeds from prior establishment of mental, emotional, and spiritual well-being and balance. In the context of HIV/AIDS, the use of flower essences is intended to help establish and maintain the necessary conditions for optimal health in HIV-positive persons.

Homeopathy

Homeopathy represents a specialized use of herbs, minerals, and animal materials, which form the basis of its pharmacopeia.[19] Homeopathy is used by PWAs both to prevent and control opportunistic infections and in an effort to eradicate HIV/AIDS through addressing underlying conditions that allowed the HIV virus to become established in the body in the first place. According to homeopathic theory the "terrain," or inherited constitutional predisposition, makes individuals especially susceptible to certain classes of sickness. Among the predisposing hereditary factors are "miasms," or traces of specific prior serious diseases in one's family heritage. Especially significant in the homeopathic construction of sexually transmitted disease states are the syphilitic miasm and the sycotic miasm, or residuum of familial gonorrhea. These are typically treated by homeopathic practitioners with syphilinum, mercurius vivus, or aurum in the case of syphilitic miasm; and with medorrhinum, lycopodium, or thuja in the case of gonorrheic (sycotic) miasm (Serinus 1987:147–148). It is believed that the successful treatment of these underlying constitutional predispositions will establish conditions supportive of eradication of subsequent sexually transmitted diseases, including venereal herpes (a frequent complication of HIV infection), active syphilis or gonorrhea, and nonspecific urethritis.

The basis of selection of homeopathic pharmaceuticals is the principle that "like cures like"—that is, a substance (or remedy) that will produce in a healthy person a certain set of symptoms, or "symptom picture," is therapeutically indicated for sick persons who present with the same symptom set. New substances can always be added to the pharmacopeia on the basis of new empirical testing procedures (called "provings"), following this general principle. It is important to a grasp of homeopathic theory to recognize that remedies are not posited to work according to pharmacological principles, but rather to act energetically to stimulate the body's own healing response or vital energy. Some homeopaths, noting a similarity between the symptoms of AIDS and those of penicillin overdose, have speculated that a homeopathic preparation of penicillin might be effective against AIDS (Ullman and Cummings 1984). By the same reasoning cyclosporine, a drug used in biomedicine to induce immunosuppression following organ transplant (to minimize risk of rejection of the new organ by the host's immune defenses), is considered by some to be a candidate for homeopathic use against HIV/AIDS. A holistic health study group based in California has suggested that a homeopathic preparation of cytomegalovirus (CMV) would be effective against CMV infection, herpes (a related virus), and as a treatment for and a preventive measure against HIV/AIDS itself (Serinus 1987:124, 146). Some homeopathic practitioners also recommend homeopathically prepared dilutions of a PWA's own blood as a preventive against progression of HIV infection (Jonathan Lax, Julian Winston, personal communications). It should be noted that these last-named items are theoretically consistent with homeopathic principles, but I do not know them actually to have been used by PWAs.

Specific symptomatic episodes prompt PWAs interested in homeopathy to seek the remedy that corresponds to their constellation of symptoms at a given time. Since homeopathic treatment is individualized to match specific symptom complexes, rather than to address disease entities, it is impossible to create a listing of "most common" remedies for complications of HIV/AIDS. There are differences, however, in the ways in which homeopathic practitioners conceptualize and respond to the presenting problems of PWA patients (completely individualized), and the ways in which PWAs treat themselves with self-selected homeopathic remedies. Certain commonly recurrent problems have in fact become associated with particular remedies, especially in the realm of self-care where theoretical consistency is not usually an issue. For example, the skin lesions of KS are frequently treated with homeopathic preparations of mistletoe, phytolacca (poke root), and vinca (periwinkle) (Serinus 1987:139).[20] PWAs may also self-treat symptomatically with such remedies as arnica for musculoskeletal aches and pains, and nux vomica for extreme nausea. In so doing, they are typically applying homeopathic solutions to specific and especially troubling symptoms, an approach which in many ways more closely resembles allopathic than homeopathic prescription practices. This illustrates the common vernacular practice of adapting available healing resources (including biomedical ones) to personal needs and interpretations—not on the basis of theoretical principles, but on the pragmatic basis of "what works."

Traditional Chinese Medicine

PWAs who have acquired some understanding of traditional Chinese medicine (usually through workshops and seminars, or as a result of their own research) may favor its treatment program, incorporating both acupuncture and Chinese herbs.[21] This system views sickness as the product of imbalances or disharmonies within the body, and their relationship to disturbances in the flow of vital energy throughout the body. Pathogens are recognized as being among the immediate agents of disease states, and their eradication may be a part of the treatment process. The emphasis of treatment, however, is on the restoration of the sick person to a state of balance and harmony, partly through redirecting blocked or misplaced energy within the body. Treatment is individualized to each person and to the presenting stage and character of the illness. Diagnostic techniques may include reading of a series of pulses (different from the pulses known to Western medicine), and visual inspection of the tongue for a variety of indications. Practitioners may also make a variety of other observations, including careful observation of a patient's demeanor and self-presentation, and attentive listening for cues during a detailed interview and review of bodily systems and functions. Diagnostic techniques typically precede each treatment to help determine the course the treatment should follow.

Central to this system is the concept of *qi* (also anglicized as *ki* or *chi*), the vital force or life energy, and its subtypes. Qi moves through the body via pathways called meridians and its flow and distribution can become blocked, causing localized deficiencies or excesses that lead to pathological states. Pathology can also occur as a result of deficiencies of qi or other vital substances that may be systemic rather than localized. Pathological states or their predisposing conditions may be constitutional (i.e., inborn), or may have developed over a long period of time, owing to other imbalances (Randi Freedman, R.Ac., personal communication). The traditional Chinese medical conception of physiological function differs substantially from that of conventional Western medicine. Organs are related to each other in systems whose interconnections are based upon their mutually influential meridian(s), the relationship of the individual organs to the five basic elements (wood, fire, earth, metal, and water), the properties of yin and yang and their distribution by organs, and specific interrelated organ functions.

"According to [traditional Chinese medicine], HIV illness represents a severe depletion of qi and thus [of] organ system function, particularly the lung, kidney, and spleen" (Sanders 1989:40). The Kidney system is regarded as the source of qi, and the Lung system as "ruling" the qi. The lungs are most vulnerable to external pathogens, because they directly exchange internal and external elements. Underlying imbalances disrupt the flow and function of qi, making the lungs susceptible to infection; this in turn affects the function of qi in other systems of the body. The nosology of traditional Chinese medicine conceptualizes disease in ways that dovetail with common symptom patterns in HIV disease and its opportunistic infections. A major symptom of deficient qi in the Kidney system is chronic fatigue, while repeated respiratory diseases (such as the pneumonias that plague PWAs) indicate deficient qi in the Lung system. "Other symptoms, such as chronic cough, reflect a disruption of interaction between the Kidney and Lung systems" (Sanders 1989:41) which disturbs the distribution and regulation of the element of water within the body. The lungs are paired with the large intestine as eliminative organs, and disruption of qi along their shared meridians can result in serious intestinal symptomatology, another problem with which PWAs are frequently plagued. The lungs also control the protective qi (*wei qi*), which resides chiefly at the surface of the body. Resistance to infection or illness is indicated by the strength of one's wei qi (Sanders 1989). Deficits in wei qi may include symptoms such as spontaneous sweats, frequent chills, and decreased resistance to illnesses such as colds and flus (Randi Freedman, R.Ac., personal communication).

Symptom patterns reveal particular kinds of systemic disturbances and deficiencies of qi. Treatment combines herbal medications with acupuncture stimulation of indicated points and meridians. It is intended to address the organ dysfunction indicated by the symptoms, rather than directly to correct the symptoms themselves. Melioration of underlying causes will in turn lead to symptom control. Herbal teas or soups address imbalances in inner states (excess/deficiency), and essential qualities (heat/cold, wet/dry) and elements within the body, while acupuncture treatments "'unblock the qi' and assist the organ system to perform its function, which is followed by relief of the symptoms" (Sanders 1989:40). Traditional Chinese medicine is very highly regarded within the PWA community, perhaps especially in large urban centers, where practitioners are most readily accessible. A printed handout distributed at a monthly discussion group on alternative therapies in Philadelphia asserts that "100 percent of Long Term Survivors are using some form of Chinese Medicine weekly" (WTP alternative therapies discussion group, March 1990). Most PWAs using traditional Chinese medicine see it as a complement to conventional Western medicine,[22] enhancing vitality and immune response while helping to control symptoms and reduce the side effects of chemotherapy, radiation, and HIV-related drugs.

Many asymptomatic PWAs use traditional Chinese medicine as a health maintenance program at stages in their HIV infection in which no drugs are medically indicated and their interactions with physicians are restricted to periodic monitoring visits. PWAs whom I have interviewed repeatedly observe that biomedicine does nothing for those who are asymptomatic and have not yet reached laboratory thresholds used as markers for initiating drug therapy. Many begin traditional Chinese medical therapy as their first intervention, feeling that it is foolish to do nothing but "wait to get sick" between discovery of HIV-positive status and the time that symptoms appear or CD-4 counts drop. There are also those who prefer to avoid for as long as possible the toxicities of conventional Western therapeutics and rely primarily on the Chinese system even after they have reached threshold CD-4 counts at which medical therapy is recommended. The Quan Yin Acupuncture and Herb Center in San Francisco has a program specifically for PWAs, based on a belief in the antiviral and immune balancing effects of acupuncture and Chinese herbs. In general, the center discourages (but does not forbid) the concomitant use of drugs, especially cancer chemotherapeutic agents; however, they were early supporters of the prophylactic use of aerosolized pentamidine for PCP (Martin 1988).

New Age and Holistic Approaches, Touch and Energy Therapies

Holistic approaches to AIDS and HIV infection address physical, mental, emotional, and spiritual aspects of the person and the disease. Most often mentioned by PWAs are those therapies discussed above, and others which have broad currency in the New Age healing movement generally and which center on practices, actions, and states of mind. These are used to enhance overall health as well as specifically to combat HIV/AIDS. Visualization and Guided Imagery are popular techniques that use focus of concentration on the generation of mental images, sometimes following the suggestions of a facilitator, to create a positive state of mind, induce relaxation, and help bring about behavior changes that will have beneficial effects and (in some interpretations) will directly stimulate healing.[23] All types of meditative practice have some following within the PWA community. These are used by individuals primarily to promote relaxation and reduce stress and fatigue. In conjunction with personal meditation, various forms of yoga may be practiced, using stretching exercises, deep or patterned breathing, and specific series of body postures "to achieve a sense of awakening, balance, and stamina" (Strawn 1989:187). Some group meditations are aimed at providing benefit to others, or even at attempting to positively alter the global conditions for control of HIV/AIDS.

A number of massage and other bodywork therapies seek to promote well-being at all levels of health, in addition to directly addressing physical symptoms. Shiatsu and Acupressure are Asian massage techniques that stimulate critical points on the meridians through which life energy flows (see the discussion of traditional Chinese medicine, above). Restoration of unobstructed vital energy flow is aimed at correcting organ dysfunction, providing symptom relief, increasing immunity, and reducing stress. The most far-reaching interpretations include the possibility of eliminating disease, provided pathology has not progressed too far by the time treatment is initiated. A few Philadelphia shiatsu practitioners offer their services free of charge to PWAs in weekly sessions at local, grass-roots PWA organizations; most of those taking advantage of this service are using the therapy for relaxation and for relief of stress and specific symptoms, including fatigue and pain. Chiropractic theory sees the potential for ameliorating HIV/AIDS, like any other disease state, through restoring and maintaining proper flow of the Innate Intelligence through the body. Chiropractic intervention is aimed at underlying conditions that produce symptoms and leave the body susceptible to pathogens. Some even see the possibility of rendering the virus dormant or incapable of generating progressive disease, assuming one begins treatment soon enough. Those PWAs with whom I have spoken who see a chiropractor regularly all reported doing so only for symptom relief or to enhance overall wellness.

Nurses who practice Therapeutic Touch (TT) have reported finding this modality beneficial for treating symptoms and effects of HIV-related conditions (Newshan 1989; Strawn 1989).[24] In the theoretical framework of TT, symptoms are interpreted as expressions of blockages or disruptions in the human "energy field" (Krieger 1975; Newshan 1989), susceptible of melioration through an "intentional transfer of energy through the nurse to the client" (Newshan 1989:46). "[T]he client sits or lies comfortably while the practitioner works in a meditative state" (Strawn 1989:189); critical to the success of Therapeutic Touch is the practitioner's conscious intention, during the procedure, to help or heal. Newshan (1989) reports that this healing technique has been found to be very effective for pain control and anxiety reduction, and that the respiratory distress associated with PCP and other AIDS-related pulmonary complications responds quickly to TT interventions. Gastrointestinal symptoms are reported to respond more slowly, as are fevers, whose intensity can nevertheless be reduced by this means (Newshan 1989:47–48). PWAs have found Therapeutic Touch beneficial both in hospitals and in informal healing sessions in other settings.

Other forms of "energy healing" favored by PWAs include Qi Gong (or chi gong), a learned ability to move and adjust qi within the body through concentration, which may be a form of self-care or may be sought from a practitioner; psychic healings of various types; and laying-on of hands by healers in a number of belief contexts. A variety of touch and energy transfer therapies may be used concurrently, as exemplified by R., whom I met at an alternative healing techniques workshop for PWAs. He is a registered nurse with an active interest in incorporating alternative therapies into his own and his patients' treatment regimens. He regularly sees a chiropractor, has an occasional shiatsu massage, and uses self-administered crystal healing techniques. In addition he has at least twice gone for treatment to Gregorio, a Filipino psychic surgeon who now resides in the United States and conducts healing sessions around the country (R., personal communication).[25] Philadelphia's grass-roots PWA advocacy and self-help organizations schedule regular sessions in which a variety of alternative practitioners are available to work with interested members. Some practice multiple modalities: for example, one offers several distinct massage styles, as well as polarity therapy; another is primarily identified as a Reiki healer, but also practices psychic and spiritual healing and Therapeutic Touch.

The Japanese system of Reiki is another frequently used method of energy transfer or laying-on of hands for healing (Strawn 1989). The Reiki healer is understood to be a channel for the energy of the Universal Life Force, which passes from the universe, through the healer's hands, and into the client (WTP alternative healing methods workshop, March 1990). In Reiki, as in most vernacular health belief systems, a clear distinction is made between healing and curing. Healing includes many aspects of enhancement of well-being, but it will not necessarily cure disease, nor will it keep people from dying of HIV/AIDS. One practitioner explains, "Reiki is not a weapon in the battle against death—that outcome is completely out of the channel's hands.

Physical pain associated with disease in its advanced state can be lessened by Reiki, for a more peaceful transition" (Printed handout provided by Bill Tomaszewski, Certified Reiki Channel, WTP alternative healing methods workshop, March 1990).

Though Reiki practitioners differ in their methods, a typical Reiki treatment includes balancing "the seven major *chakras*, or energy centers" of the body (Strawn 1989:188). One of these, the heart chakra, is located anatomically in the area of the thymus gland, with which some PWAs believe it to be associated (Bamforth 1987; Serinus 1987). Since this gland figures so prominently in HIV/AIDS because of its role in the production of T-cells, energy-based treatments directed to this area of the body (either as gland, chakra, or meridianal points connected to organ systems) are used by many PWAs, including those who do not profess to believe in the healing system as a whole.

Crystals, especially the different varieties of quartz crystals, are used by interested PWAs in ways that parallel their general use in the New Age healing movement. Crystal healing enthusiasts claim that the piezoelectric properties of crystals that are the basis of their scientific uses also function to make them conductors and modifiers of other energies (Strawn 1989:187). This is especially claimed for quartz crystals, though by extension it is believed to be true for other crystalline minerals and gemstones as well. Color is also often incorporated into crystal therapeutics, with particular colors (and thus particular minerals) selected for specific effects, association with particular chakras, or association with specific desired qualities (spirituality, intuition, energy, etc.) (Chocron 1983). Crystals may be prescribed and applied by practitioners, or personally selected and used in self-care. They may be worn as amulets to absorb negative energies or enhance personal growth, worn or carried as energy transmitters to help the body properly use nutrients, centered over the forehead (the Third Eye chakra) to focus meditative thoughts or intensify psychic vision, or applied to any of the seven chakras to focus healing energy there (Biltz, unpublished manuscript). Crystals are also used as adjuncts to other healing techniques (including conventional drugs for HIV and its associated opportunistic infections) "to potentiate the energy of the healing source that is being directed into the client" (Strawn 1989:187), improving its depth of penetration or rate of absorption in a manner analogous to the synergistic augmentation of the action of one drug by another.

Psychological and Metaphysical Approaches

Psychological and metaphysical healing methods have an enormous following among PWAs taking a holistic approach to treating HIV/

AIDS. Within these types of healing strategies claims have been made of the possibility of "healing AIDS" or of being "totally healed of AIDS" (Serinus 1987:8). Though this usage of the terms sounds as if it means "curing" and "cured," the same sources also report the deaths of individuals who have previously made claims of "total" healing (Serinus 1987:8). The emphasis, when further explanation is made, is on the sense that these people had "healed their lives," thus enabling them to live fully for the balance of their lifetimes and to die without "unfinished business" (though some also interpret physical death not as a terminal event but as a metaphysical or spiritual "stage" or "crossing point"). The central concept of several alternative psychological/metaphysical approaches is "psychoimmunity" (Serinus 1987), a system-specific interpretation of the principles of psychosomatic illness that places special emphasis on "psychospiritual" aspects of disease. The concept of psychoimmunity rests on the theory that disease (usually written as "dis-ease") is the product of "negative thought forms," which both create the conditions for disease and are themselves physically manifested as diseases. (The concept of psychoimmunity is sometimes supported by reference to the emerging and still controversial medical field of psychoneuroimmunology, with which it shares some common principles, but with which it is by no means identical.)

Jason Serinus is a principal proponent of this philosophy, outlined in his book *Psychoimmunity and the Healing Process: A Holistic Approach to Immunity and AIDS*. It is his theory that HIV/AIDS has essentially been created by self-hatred among gay men and by rejection and social isolation of gay and other affected populations. Noting the connection between "the collapse of the thymus gland" (Serinus 1987:82) and AIDS, and the location of the thymus in the heart chakra, Serinus observes, "AIDS is not a sexual disease at all; it's really a disease of the heart. . . . It's essential to recognize that it manifests among members of culturally disenfranchised minorities to whom we have turned off our hearts, and who sometimes turn their hearts off to themselves" (Jacobs and Serinus 1987:35). "It is this isolation, often internalized as self-hatred or lack of acceptance, which allows the AIDS virus to incubate once it has entered the system" (Serinus 1987:82).

The very different pattern of HIV/AIDS in Africa, where it primarily affects the heterosexual population and is a disease of families, is explained within this theory as owing to the general oppression of undeveloped countries by the predominantly white global political powers, as well as to the specific oppression of blacks within Africa by whites within Africa. (Given the current demographics, this theory would probably be expandable to the heterosexual spread of HIV in the United States and to most instances of vertical transmission from mothers to children *in utero*. Serinus offered no explanation for exposure through transfusion, nor for the infection of people with hemophilia through their conventional medical therapies.)

The road to prevention and healing through psychoimmunity requires complete commitment and a dramatic reorientation of one's life and habits of mind, to achieve a genuine and lasting change in attitude. Infected and susceptible people must consciously embrace positive thinking and avoid the damaging influence of their own and others' "negative thought forms." A holistic regimen of healthful foods, herbs, and other alternative therapeutic actions is recommended as a complement to psychospiritual healing efforts. Though proponents of psychoimmunity do not advocate leaving conventional medical care, they stress the need to work only with positive-thinking, and preferably holistically oriented, physicians. Conventional medicine is full of "negative thought forms," including stigmatization of homosexuality, care givers' projected frustrations at their own limitations in being able to help PWAs, and the tendency to treat a diagnosis of HIV/AIDS as a "death sentence." These attitudes are to be avoided as overtly hazardous to one's health. Likewise, gay and PWA support groups that focus too heavily on problems associated with HIV disease, or on issues connected with death and dying, are felt to be disease-reinforcing in their "negative energy." Workshops and training sessions in developing optimism and positive attitudes are recommended for starting and keeping oneself on the healing path; personal responsibility for making the changes and embracing healing is stressed.

Perhaps most acclaimed among such inspirational training courses are those of Louise Hay, who maintains a schedule of nationwide speaking and workshop engagements and is a favorite featured participant in seminars and conferences on coping with HIV/AIDS.[26] Hay is described in one New Age publication as a "unique blend of spiritual evangelist and transformative therapist," whose insight derives from the personal experience of having healed herself of cancer (Jacobs and Serinus 1987:34). She professes the beliefs that "all physical illness is a result of negative thought patterns that allow disease to flourish" and that changing thoughts can literally change reality (Jacobs and Serinus 1987:34). In the late 1980s, her weekly healing meetings for PWAs, held in West Hollywood's Plummer Park, reportedly attracted an average attendance of close to four hundred people (Jacobs and Serinus 1987). Hay teaches affirmations for changing thought patterns, believing that "positive thoughts that encourage self-esteem, self-worth, and self-love" can physically strengthen the immune system; she feels it is possible to render the HIV virus dormant by psychospiritual means. Louise Hay's books, audiotapes, and videotapes are best-selling items in the PWA community.

Though there is a strong emphasis on spiritual development and spiritual aspects of health and illness, there is little discussion in the gay PWA alternative healing network of specifically religious approaches to healing. This may be attributable to the tension that exists between many religious institutions and the gay community over the issue of homosexuality.[27] A 1988 survey of Philadelphia PWAs revealed that only one-third of respondents listed any religious affiliation; of those, just over one-third felt that their religion was a significant source of support in coping with AIDS (Ellerman 1988). It should be noted, however, that the survey question addressed formal institutional religion; information about individual religious actions and sentiments was not sought, and many religious healing actions fall into this category. Some members of Philadelphia PWA discussion and healing groups mentioned that they pray both directly for the improvement of their health and for the ability to accept their situation with grace and equanimity (which will improve their spiritual health, and possibly therefore their physical health as a secondary outcome). One group member said that he regularly consults the scriptures for guidance and understanding in his daily life and applies his interpretations of scriptural counsel to his HIV disease for spiritual healing purposes (H., personal communication). In a 1990 clinical practice survey of PWAs' use of alternative and complementary therapies, 39 percent indicated that they used religious healing means, including prayer, as therapeutic measures to deal with their HIV disease (Anderson et al. 1993). St. Luke's Episcopal Church in Philadelphia holds a weekly healing service that is advertised in PWA newsletters and specified as "open to people with AIDS and HIV disease and their families, friends and lovers" (*Critical Path* 1[7]:17; hereafter cited as *CP*), and the local chapter of Dignity sponsors a weekly AIDS Prayer Group.

Conventional Pharmaceuticals and Underground Drugs

Vernacular health care practices are not confined solely to activities and substances not embraced by conventional medicine. For all groups of people (not only PWAs), such practices typically also include uses of pharmaceuticals in ways for which they were not "officially" intended. Such adaptations are well documented in the literature dealing with self-care and folk/popular health beliefs and practices, and have a number of variations. These include such measures as (1) use of prescription medications only in response to presence or intensity of symptoms (irrespective of professional directions for their use); (2) personal modification of dosages for reasons of convenience, lifestyle necessity, perceived optimal efficacy, avoidance or moderation of side effects, and so forth; (3) use of medications according to the dictates of a vernacular explanatory model (for example, the hot/cold system operative in many Latino populations [see Harwood 1971, 1981]); (4) prescription-sharing with a neighbor or family member with similar symptoms; and (5) self-medication with "leftover" prescription drugs when new symptoms appear.

In the PWA community, self-regulation and self-determination in use of prescription drugs and other pharmaceuticals take place on a much larger scale than has been documented for other groups, and encompass several activities that are relatively rare in other illness contexts. These include (1) use of foreign drugs not approved for sale or clinical use in the United States; (2) use of drugs having experimental status in FDA-approved clinical trials, but obtained through underground sources and used privately; (3) "off-label" uses of FDA-approved prescription drugs; (4) prescription sharing, including sharing of drugs obtained through participation in clinical trials (Jonathan Lax, personal communication); and (5) black market and other underground purchases of prescription drugs. All of these practices allow for self-control of certain aspects of the treatment program. In addition they provide access to treatments that would otherwise be unavailable to the PWA, or which might compromise anonymity—an important concern for many PWAs who wish to avoid the stigmatization and discrimination that frequently accompany disclosure or discovery of HIV-positive status.

Since use of AZT is now synonymous with HIV seropositivity, black market purchase of the drug is a method adopted to protect anonymity. AZT (and other drugs) can be purchased from prescription holders who do not use their full dosage or supply (Kolata 1988; Kwitny 1992). Willing sellers advertise in the gay and AIDS-specific press, by bulletin-board notices, or by word of mouth. Prescription sharing between close friends or lovers is not uncommon and may involve any prescription drug to which one partner has access but from which the other is excluded by his physician. Exclusion may be a matter of a physician's personal preferences in restriction of particular drugs or may follow general medical treatment guidelines such as the established CD-4 threshold for prophylactic use of aerosolized pentamidine. PWAs who exceed the threshold CD-4 counts, but who disagree with the medical consensus that they do not yet need PCP prophylaxis, may accompany a friend or lover to his monthly pentamidine treatment and "share a couple [of] puffs" for their own benefit (WTP alternative therapies discussion group, April 1990).

"Off-label" uses of prescription drugs are uses for purposes in which the drug appears effective, but for which it was not officially designed or intended and is not specifically marketed. Common examples include use of disulfiram (Antabuse), marketed for control of alcoholism, and of the ulcer drugs cimetidine (Tagamet) and ranitidine (Zantac), for their immunomodulating side-effects (WTP alternative therapies discussion group, April 1990). Pentoxyfylline (Trental) is recommended to counteract wasting syndromes and for possible antiviral action, and veterinary levamisole (a puppy-wormer) for "immunopotentiating effects" (*CP* 3[9], Winter 1993). Such uses require either the cooperation or acquiescence of prescribing physicians, or access to alternative sources of supply: for example, drugs with both human and veterinary applications may be acquired through friends or relatives who are veterinarians (WTP alternative therapies discussion group, April 1990); several are also available through buyers clubs.

Drugs that are in various stages of FDA-approved clinical trials are vigorously sought through foreign or underground sources. The official clinical trials typically give access to a very limited number of people, sometimes as few as ten to twelve subjects. Even in larger studies, admission criteria in terms of permissible health status, definable disease stage markers, or restrictions on uses of other therapeutic agents disqualify many PWAs and act as a deterrent to still others who may technically qualify. In addition to foreign and underground purchase, some experimental drugs (such as AL-721, now largely out of favor) can be made in home versions, or obtained through alternate supply. The French experimental drug DTC (Imuthiol), for example, obtainable through the underground, is also a common "reagent-grade chemical, not prepared for human use," which can be purchased very cheaply and then analyzed for purity and safety for human consumption (*ATN* #29, 10 April 1987). It is "quite easy to make in a laboratory; an organized community can easily get around a [possible] ban" (*ATN* #29, 10 April 1987).

Most of the underground drugs are used under the supervision of peers and sympathetic health professionals, sometimes in the context of "guerrilla clinics" (*ATN* passim; Gross 1987; Kolata 1988). Originally organized to oversee PWAs' use of DNCB (dinitrochlorobenzene, marketed as a photographic chemical, and used topically both to control KS and for general immunomodulating effects), the guerrilla clinics are underground alternative health care sites that oversee the administration of certain nonapproved drugs and monitor patients throughout these treatment regimes. PWAs attending guerrilla clinics procure their own drugs and bring them to the clinics; there are no fees for services, and no drugs or other therapeutic products or services are sold. However, detailed records of results are kept, so that treatment methods can be evaluated across a population and through time. Eighteen months after the inception of guerrilla clinics, for example, *AIDS Treatment News* was able to report that DNCB still had "thousands" of users, and that "instructions for use have changed . . . as the 'guerrilla clinic' movement gains experience" (*ATN* #14, 26 September 1986. Quotes are from an update added in April 1988 for a bound volume of prior *ATN* issues.)

In addition to these special clinic sites, there are also PWA-organized "treatment study groups" (*ATN* #60, 1 July 1988), in which members systematically test, record, compare, and discuss results of specific treatments and treatment combinations. Private physicians sympathetic to the alternative therapies and treatment activist movements also agree to monitor PWAs acquiring and taking underground drugs on their own (Booth 1988). A formal underground clinical trial, organized and administered by San Francisco's Project Inform and involving physicians and patients in four cities, was carried out on the Chinese drug Compound Q (trichosanthin) in 1989 (Thompson 1989; Arno and Feiden 1992; Kwitny 1992); participating PWAs purchased and supplied their own drug (see also Hamilton 1989; Wyss 1989; *ATN* #77 and #78, 21 April and 5 May 1989). The underground trial was initiated during the time when reports were circulating that trichosanthin showed promise, but FDA approval for official trials of the experimental drug was still pending (for a detailed description, see Kwitny 1992).

Some PWAs have enrolled in treatment programs in foreign countries, using drugs not available in the United States. Many went to Paris, for example, for treatment with the experimental French drug HPA-23 following publication of actor Rock Hudson's Parisian treatment (Clark 1985). More frequently, though, PWAs have traveled (and sent emissaries) to purchase foreign drugs to import for use at home. Significant examples include the massive purchases of ribavirin and isoprinosine in Mexico (Kolata 1988; Arno and Feiden 1992; Kwitny 1992), AL-721 in Israel (Kolata 1988), dextran sulfate in Canada and Japan (Booth 1988; Gevisser 1988; Arno and Feiden 1992; Kwitny 1992), and Compound Q in China (Wyss 1989; Kwitny 1992). Many of these drugs are available over the counter in the countries where they are purchased, though others have required much more complex negotiations (see Kwitny 1992). In response to pressures from the PWA community and treatment activists, FDA regulations were changed in mid-1988 to grant official sanction to importation of foreign pharmaceuticals in three-month supplies intended for personal use (i.e., not for resale) (Booth 1988; Arno and Feiden 1992; Kwitny 1992).[28]

Buyers Clubs

In the mid-1980s, West Coast AIDS treatment activists formed the first buyers clubs, primarily to facilitate large-scale purchases of specific foreign pharmaceuticals for redistribution to their membership (see *ATN* #30, 24 April 1987). By facilitating import of larger quantities, buyers clubs reduced the cost of the drugs to members and eliminated the expense and the fatigue of travel for individual PWAs. Buyers clubs were soon to proliferate nationwide.[29] There are now upwards of a dozen large-scale clubs located in populous cities, and numerous smaller local clubs in other areas. The larger clubs are generally open to national membership, and a few are incorporated as nonprofit corporations (*ATN* #43, 23 October 1987). The buyers clubs conduct worldwide searches for drugs, attempting to find any products that may be efficacious in treating any and all aspects of HIV disease, and to find them at the lowest prices. The demand for their services is significant: one of the founding members of a New York buyers club estimated in 1988 that their weekly business ran to about $60,000 (Kolata 1988); another cited annual business figures of some $625,000 in 1991 (DeBlasio 1992) and close to $827,000 in 1993 (Huppert 1993). The clubs typically charge a membership fee, and individual orders are pooled to facilitate bulk purchases and price negotiation. Clubs may stock, or broker the supply of, vitamins and dietary supplements, over-the-counter products, alternative therapeutic agents, and domestic and foreign pharmaceuticals and their available knock-offs or "bootleg" versions (such as bootleg ddC, produced by independent chemists and widely available before, and on a reduced scale following, FDA approval of ddC for HIV therapy).

Some of the larger clubs retain lawyers to serve as legal consultants, as well as to represent the club in the event of a legal challenge (Booth 1988). Clubs with sufficient resources contract commercial laboratories to test any products about which they have questions, to assure product identity, quality, and safety (*ATN* #43, 123 October 1987; Healing Alternatives Foundation brochure, n.d.). Larger buyers clubs publish regular inventory and price lists; names, addresses, and price lists of suppliers from whom members can order vitamins and nutritional supplements directly; fact sheets on specific substances; and sometimes treatment information newsletters. Some clubs will supply information on the availability of black market AZT and other prescription drugs; and some will supply certain drugs only if the buyer has a prescription or can supply a physician's affadavit or monitoring agreement (*CP* 3[9], 1993).

The Information Network

The extent, sophistication, and success of the grass-roots treatment network are possible because members of the gay community are, generally speaking, a savvy middle-class group with a wealth of skills and experience, access to and familiarity with modern information management technology, and often the discretionary income to pay for alternative treatments and for the travel they sometimes require. The professional cross section of the gay and PWA communities is a microcosm of the professional variety of American society at large. It includes, for example, physicians and nurses, holistic and alternative health practitioners, analysts, microbiologists and other scientific researchers, writers and investigative journalists, pharmacists, chemists, lawyers, politicians, strategic planning and organizational development consultants, computer information specialists. Members of this population, taken in the aggregate, have a considerable range of abilities to bring to bear on PWA issues: they are familiar with research methods, accustomed to synthesis and analysis of data, well rehearsed in a range of organizational and communications skills, and practiced in the formulation of sound argument. They are explicitly aware of the concept of the cultural construction of reality, and they employ it themselves in articulating constructions that differ in salient points from those of the medical, scientific, and regulatory establishments. They read the (international) medical and scientific press (as well as publications of the alternative health care movement), carry out empirical studies on themselves, maintain records and establish databases, and report to others on their findings.

The community expresses a commitment to the idea that PWAs must "do as much of their own research as possible" (*ATN* #64, 9 September 1988), and should persist both in asking questions and in demanding and exercising the right to contribute to the definition of what kinds of questions ought properly to be asked: "Why not simply trust the experts who have the information, and the recommendations and policies they publish? Because no one familiar with how AIDS has been handled could reasonably trust the authorities with his or her life" (*ATN* #15, 10 October 1986). Activists encourage PWAs to take the initiative not only in doing their own treatment research but also in "researching the researchers" and their protocols. Their goals are both to be as informed as possible and to exert influence on the course of the "official" research (see also Skloot 1993). Observing that "[k]nowledge is our key to fighting the HIV epidemic and the HIV beaureaucracy," Critical Path AIDS Project in Philadelphia urges:

Adopt a principal investigator. [. . .] Read their papers. Read their protocols. Discuss their research with them and their staff. Their staff is often more candid. Find out what they researched before AIDS. Find out their consultancy arrangements.

Reading is fundamental. Get hold of the latest scientific journals. Start a science club to discuss important articles and share what you learn. Attend scientific meetings in your community and represent your point of view. (*CP* 1[9/10]:25)

The gay PWA community has developed an efficient, effective, and high-tech communications system that operates on an international scale to relay up-to-the-moment treatment information among numerous and often distant locations. One member stressed "how rapid information dissemination can be," explaining, "We used to be promiscuous with our bodies; now we are with treatment data—and *frequently with the same far flung partners*. London hears from New York, Montreal talks to Seattle, and Philadelphia keeps up with Redondo Beach" (Jonathan Lax, personal letter; emphasis in original). When dextran sulfate came to the attention of PWAs through its mention in a letter to the editor of a medical journal, both the news of its potential as a treatment and information on how and where to obtain it moved rapidly throughout the PWA community. Within weeks, trips to Tokyo to buy dextran sulfate "became so routine that detailed subway maps to certain pharmacies in Tokyo began to circulate around New York City, San Francisco, and Los Angeles" (Booth 1988:1280).[30]

In addition to word-of-mouth channels (broadly construed to include a range of technological intermediaries, including telephone, electronic mail, and fax), the gay community has instituted and supported a formal information exchange network. Among its resources are several treatment newsletters, some with national circulations of fifteen thousand and upward. Primary among these resources are *AIDS Treatment News* (published biweekly since April 1986), *Treatment Issues*, Project Inform's *PI Perspectives*, *Critical Path*, *Body Positive*, and *BETA (Bulletin of Experimental Treatments for AIDS)*. Innumerable local newsletters with smaller circulations also exist. The major newsletters report on new and speculative findings culled from the medical and scientific research literature; on results of community-based research efforts; and on anecdotal information reported by PWAs based on their individual and collective personal experiences with both conventional and alternative or complementary treatments. Newsletter editors have on occasion conducted reader surveys to gather information on particular alternative therapies—mailing out survey questionnaires with the newsletter, including reminders in subsequent issues, and publishing the tabulated results upon completion of the survey (e.g., *ATN* #33, 5 June 1987; #39, 28 August 1987; #63, 26 August 1988; #64, 9 September 1988; #69, 18 November 1988; #91, 17 November 1989).

Bibliographic citations accompany many articles and topical bibliographies are also available. Some of these are intended specifically for physician use and information, pulling together diverse sources that practicing physicians are unlikely to have the time to search out for themselves. In one instance, information on potential benefits of combining two experimental drugs for HIV therapy was garnered from a Japanese newspaper by a man who worked professionally as a Japanese translator and had a personal interest in HIV/AIDS issues. He passed the information on to *ATN*, where it made its first English-language appearance (*ATN* #32, 22 May 1987). *ATN* subsequently offered to broker correspondence between interested American physicians and the Japanese researcher, using the volunteered services of the professional translator. Several of the major information newsletters are also available on-line through computer networks accessible by modem from home computers. Some electronic bulletin board services allow for real-time exchange of information between participants. Most accept anonymous log-ons (one accepts the password "AIDS" from all users), and many of the services allow for downloading of files for personal use. Publishers and operators of these information resources can in many instances be queried through toll-free nationwide telephone hotlines, electronic mail, and fax.

This AIDS-specific grass-roots press publishes, in addition to conventional and unconventional treatment information, detailed warnings and advisories about treatments considered dangerous or fraudulent; lists of contraindications for specific therapeutic interventions (conventional and complementary); information on locations and enrollment criteria of approved clinical trials; and articles addressing issues such as access to treatments, ethics of treatment research and experimental drug trials, and other matters of private and public policy. Guides to "official" AIDS information databases and alternative on-line services are published, as are regularly updated lists of major buyers clubs and their addresses, and subscription information for other newsletters. Topics covered include "best" and "worst" treatment survey results (both conventional and unconventional); lists of substances for which the PWA community urges formal trials; calls for volunteers interested in participating in alternative treatment protocols; guidelines for evaluating (conventional and unconventional) therapies; preventive health education matters for health professionals, and so forth. Many of these publications are designed to be useful to health care professionals, as well as to members of the gay and PWA communities, and most of them

explicitly state the value the community places on working in partnership with conventional medicine.

The "Multiple Choice" Strategy

Vernacular treatment strategies for HIV disease are generally intended to supplement rather than to supplant conventional medical
care. This was not always the accepted popular wisdom, however, and
the community has been divided on this issue in the past. "When the
epidemic really began to take off, there was the thought that you would
either 'heal naturally' or you were 'into drugs'" (Jonathan Lax, personal letter). The PWA ethos now emphasizes that, whatever else one
does to deal with AIDS, one must not forgo conventional medical
treatment or (for those who still prefer to avoid drugs and "go natural")
at least consistent medical supervision and monitoring. A handout
entitled "HIV Alternative Medicine and Adjuncts," composed and
distributed in Philadelphia, is headed by the proclamation "!!SEE
YOUR DOCTOR WHO IS YOUR ALLY IN ALL MEDICAL MAT-
TERS!!" (WTP alternative therapies discussion group, March 1990).
Alternative or nonconventional treatments are increasingly referred to
simply as "complementary therapies," the term both emphasizing and
incorporating the presumption that they are to be used in conjunction
with conventional medicine.

A good physician is considered essential to HIV care, and augmentation of the medical routine with self-care actions is often considered to
be of equal importance. As one respected HIV/AIDS self-care manual
puts it:

The first step is to see a doctor. Even if you decide to pursue an alternative
therapy, there is no substitute for consulting with a doctor who can monitor
your vital signs, blood work, etc. Any alternative practitioner who tells you to
stay away from physicians should make you immediately suspicious. If your
medical doctor advises you not to try anything alternative, you should question
that advice as well. (Moffat et al. 1987:119)

Disclosure of treatment actions to *all* practitioners is advocated:

It is important for different care-givers to communicate with each other so they
do not do things that will contradict each other. Your doctor and your herbalist
may be giving you medications that can react with each other and put you in
danger. If each knows what the other is doing, dangerous situations can be
avoided. (ibid.: 119)

PWAs whose physicians are not receptive to their nonconventional
adjunct treatments are urged, if at all possible, to change physicians.

Responsibility and authority are identified as matters for open negotiation between PWA and physician.[31] PWA activists assert that maximum authority in the health care program belongs with the person
whose life is on the line: one man observed that his physician "'doesn't
have a vote, he has an opinion' in treatment decisions" (Gross 1988:
182). Treatment activists in Philadelphia created and distributed an
"HIV Standard of Care" in the spring of 1992 (Act Up/Philadelphia,
Science and Medicine Committee 1992). These photocopied docu-
ments were intended to serve a dual purpose: to inform PWAs, and to
be given by PWAs to their physicians both as a guideline and as a
minimum acceptable standard of care upon which PWAs are entitled to
insist.[32] These recommendations, and the philosophical and political
positions they embody, receive attention well beyond their community
of origin: five thousand copies were distributed at the Eighth International Conference on AIDS in Amsterdam in June 1992 by members of
the Philadelphia PWA community who attended this global scientific
conference as registered delegates. Updated versions of the "Standard" that incorporate new information, as well as the latest thinking
on long-familiar problems, are circulated locally at intervals. A 1993
revision was published in *Critical Path* under the front page headline,
"A Standard of Care *by Which to Measure Your Doctor*" (*CP* 3[9], 1993;
emphasis added). Such realignments of authority between PWAs and
their physicians assign the PWA-as-patient a role of competence, and in
a sense place the timeworn shoe of (non)compliance upon the other
foot: it is the physician who is now expected to come into line with
treatment recommendations. Should a physician be unwilling or unable to provide the outlined standard of care, the PWA patient is urged
to press for an explanation of the reasons for this shortcoming. If the
situation cannot be remediated, the PWA should, if possible, change
doctors.

A dozen years into the HIV/AIDS epidemic there is as yet a limited
understanding of HIV disease, and notwithstanding several recent
advances, a still more limited range of medical therapies. The formal
channels for development of new treatments are cumbersome and
bureaucratically slow, and PWAs tend to share a conviction that new
treatment research is driven by profit and politics rather than motivated by concern for patient benefit or public health (see also Shilts
1987). In this climate, PWAs not surprisingly feel it is critical personally
and actively to explore additional therapeutic modalities. Incidence of
use of alternative and complementary therapies has been reported
variously as ranging from 29 percent (Greenblatt et al. 1991) to 40
percent (Anderson et al. 1993) of surveyed PWAs.[33] Within this segment of the gay PWA community, standard therapeutic strategy now

includes the combined use of conventional medical and complementary therapies, selecting some experimental and some relatively well-established treatments from each domain. Treatment options (of both kinds) are pursued for as long as they appear fruitful, discarded or replaced as they appear to fail or reach a point of diminishing returns, or as more promising options become available. This eclectic and malleable approach has taken shape especially during the past five to seven years. One community member characterizes it as a sort of "cafeteria approach":

taking AZT from allopathic medicine, acupuncture, eating better (but still not "well" in the macrobiotic sense), trying the underground drug *du jour*, etc. Almost a rotation diet of medical self-empowerment. What's changed? First, a greater recognition that the allopath [conventional medicine] increasingly does have something to offer. Second, the consumers have reported (by word of mouth) that the natural/Chinese approaches make one feel better. (Jonathan Lax, personal letter; emphasis in original)

It is definitive of a "good AIDS doc" that s/he be receptive both to the use of complementary therapies and to active participation of the PWA in designing and evaluating the total treatment regimen. Local level "doctor report card" networks, both word-of-mouth and in loose-leaf reference manuals housed at local AIDS advocacy and information organizations, pass along critiques of physicians that include state-of-the-art evaluations of their medical knowledge and treatment regimens and descriptions of their receptiveness to alternative therapies and patient partnership in case management. The same sources provide evaluations of a variety of alternative practitioners, including whether they have any treatments specifically tailored to HIV/AIDS and whether they offer (as most do) reduced fees to HIV-positive clients. "Best" practitioners, both conventional and alternative, come well recommended and are usually in high demand.

Other PWAs: Communities of Color

Though the focus of this chapter is on the responses of the largely white and middle-class gay community, it is necessary to briefly treat responses of other specific population groups seriously affected by HIV/AIDS, because the contrast is so instructive. Currently, the fastest-growing rate of HIV disease is found among inner-city, poor black and Hispanic people (Drake 1988; Colbruno 1990).[34] Though homosexual transmission accounts for some percentage of HIV/AIDS in black and Hispanic populations, needle sharing in injection drug use plays a major role in HIV transmission in these communities: "[u]nlike

AIDS cases among Whites, nearly half of the cases of AIDS among Blacks and Hispanics have occurred among heterosexual intravenous (IV) drug users or their sexual partners" (Peterson and Marin 1988: 871). Women and men who earn money by selling sex are at high risk for infection; if they have turned to prostitution to support an injection drug addiction, they multiply their risk. Increasing numbers of children are being born with HIV infection, acquired in utero. As of 1993, an estimated 74.4 percent of all women with AIDS were women of color (Centers for Disease Control and Prevention HIV/AIDS Surveillance Report 1993:8). By the late 1980s, "[o]f all children with HIV infection, 80%were black or hispanic. . . . It has been estimated that 73.1% of the babies diagnosed with AIDS (most of whom are black) have at least one parent who uses . . . IV drugs" (Lester and Saxxon 1988:564).

African American and Latin American cultures, like all cultural heritages closely associated with specific ethnic identity groups, have well-developed traditional vernacular health belief systems with long histories and continuing vitality. The flexibility and adaptability that characterize vernacular health belief systems virtually assure their continued relevance both to long-familiar and to newly emerging health problems. It should come as no surprise, therefore, that HIV/AIDS is addressed within the framework of these traditional healing systems; on the contrary, it would be remarkable indeed if such a pressing issue did *not* become incorporated into vernacular healing traditions in any cultural group.

HIV/AIDS and African American Traditional Health Beliefs

A California study conducted in 1989 (Flaskerud and Rush 1989) describes the assimilation of HIV/AIDS to the African American traditional health belief system and its associated practices. This study, based on interviews with twenty-two black women of two generations, demonstrates that in the context of this folk healing tradition, HIV/AIDS may be interpreted as having either "natural" or "unnatural" causes, depending on interpretations of the circumstances of infection in individual cases. Either category can include sickness brought about by supernatural agency: divine causes, in the "natural" category; and demonic or magical (witchcraft, sorcery) causes in the "unnatural" category.[35] All interviewees in the study reported being aware that "'you get AIDS from sex with the wrong people or from needles when you're using drugs,'" but only three of twenty-two felt that exposure was confined to these routes. It was additionally widely believed that one could get HIV/AIDS from "'impurities in the blood, the air and food,'" as well as from "lowered resistance due to impurities, poor health habits, exposure to cold, cyclical weaknesses (especially true for women and babies), and improper nutrition" (Flaskerud and Rush 1989:212). "Poor health habits" included such things as irregular bowel movements, poor diet, failure to treat other infections, and general lack of cleanliness. Some women felt that HIV/AIDS is contagious through being coughed at, especially when one's resistance is low to begin with.

All of these circumstances represent instances of "natural" illness. Though treatments recommended in these cases are not detailed in the study, it is reasonable to assume that they also follow the pattern of the tradition. Treatment would thus include—in addition to conventional medical care—avoidance of cold and chills, attention to cleanliness, dietary modulation, herbs, prayer, patent medicines (especially tonics and laxatives), and any positively evaluated prescription medications available from family and friends. Any or all of these measures could be used both preventively and remedially. Some bodily signs may not be construed as disease symptoms, but as the body's reaction to unclean or imbalanced states; for example, diarrhea and skin eruptions may be interpreted as "'the body's [way of] trying to clean itself out'" (ibid.: 213), and therefore as positive signs. Such manifestations may not be reinterpreted as symptoms to be treated unless they become chronic or debilitating.

Supernatural causation of AIDS within the "natural" category of diseases[36] is restricted to imposition of the disease by God, either as a test of faith or as punishment for sin. It is important to recognize that such a view does not imply disbelief in or lack of knowledge of the germ theory of disease, nor does it imply lack of awareness of a viral agent for HIV disease. Rather, this view *incorporates* such agents, and their effects on health and the body, as figuring among the ways in which God allows or causes sickness to take place as a test or as retribution. Fundamentalist Christian denominations, which usually view homosexuality as sinful, may believe that "AIDS is a punishment from God for the way homosexuals live" (Mays and Cochran 1987:229); such interpretations vary by specific religious context, however. Infant cases of HIV/AIDS tend to be seen as visitations on the young of the sins of their parents (Flaskerud and Rush 1989). Cases of HIV/AIDS acquired through transfusion are considered to be tests of faith. One woman observed that such cases have "'two purposes: to test your faith, and to show someone else that God can heal you'" (ibid.:213). Healing actions to be taken in the case of divinely imposed sickness lean heavily to expiation of sin, recitation of psalms and verses of scripture, and prayer (ibid.: 213). Prayer as an intervention takes many forms, including individual prayer both by sick persons themselves and on their behalf by other concerned individuals; group prayer in both institutional and private devotions; and submission of the names of persons in need of healing to an intercessory prayer chain in which participants "call [the sick person's] name to the Lord" and urge healing for him or her (Lula Mae Jones, personal communication).

Supernatural causes placing particular cases of HIV/AIDS in the "unnatural" disease category include actions of "evil spirits, demons, the Devil and witches" (ibid.: 213). Witchcraft (also known in African-American folk tradition as conjure, hoodoo, and "working roots") may be practiced by any person with malicious or punitive intent for another, or the services of a specialist may be engaged for the purpose (Snow 1974; 1983). "Remedies for attack from evil included reciting the 23rd Psalm, reading Scripture, prayer, studying God's Word, thinking positive thoughts, and reminding oneself of good times: 'Fret not yourself because of evil doers.' Other remedies mentioned were to ask for assistance from voodoo women or persons with [divinely conferred] powers of healing" (Flaskerud and Rush 1989:213). HIV/AIDS in homosexuals is not invariably interpreted as punishment for sin ("natural"); it may also be caused by the Devil or other evil spirits ("unnatural"). Some interviewees considered injection drug use and homosexuality to be unnatural (i.e., demonically motivated) behaviors, which caused people to become sick with HIV/AIDS: "'You're being controlled by evil spirits; evil spirits cause you to live this life'" (ibid.: 213).

Some view the AIDS epidemic as a fulfillment of the prophesy of plagues in the Book of Revelations, which "involves both punishment for sin and the work of the Devil" (ibid.:213). It is considered by those sharing this interpretation—which, it should be pointed out, is by no means confined to African-American religious contexts—to be one of many current signs of the approaching apocalypse. Irrespective of specific denominational affiliation, the majority of participants in the California study emphasized the importance of prayer for people with HIV/AIDS. Though ordained ministers can provide spiritual healing, considered to be very important, individual prayer was considered the most important healing activity once a diagnosis of HIV/AIDS is received. In the treatment of HIV/AIDS, as in any disease for which there are no medical cures (and for some individuals, in any disease whatsoever), it is considered that "'[d]octors can doctor, but only God can heal'" (ibid.:214).

HIV/AIDS and Some Latino Healing Resources

Traditional theories of health and illness in Latino cultures have also assimilated HIV/AIDS to their explanatory models and healing practices. Exposure to cold and dampness, and to both external and internal impurities, may either cause or predispose to illness. Excretory matter, blood, and other bodily fluids may be felt to be inherently impure or to contain impurities and exposure to these substances to pose a danger of contagion. Exposure to cold and to dampness, lack of moderation (of any sort), improper diet or being too thin, states of weakness (including menstruation and the postpartum period for women), and cosmic or planetary cycles may lower resistance and predispose to infection, or may directly cause illnesses (see Harwood 1981b; Trotter and Chavira 1981; Flaskerud and Calvillo 1991). Several aspects of these traditional etiological models are readily syncretized with medical explanations of exposure to HIV; examples include concerns with blood and body fluids, lowered resistance (cf. immunodeficiency), and immoderate behavior (such as intravenous drug use, homosexual sex, or high-risk sexual practices in either homosexual or heterosexual contexts). Illnesses can also have supernatural causes, including hexing, witchcraft or *mal puesto*, effects of evil spirits or of the Devil, and divine punishment for sin. HIV/AIDS may be assimilated to these explanatory categories as well (Flaskerud and Calvillo 1991).

Vernacular healing resources indigenous to Latino populations in the United States include use of medicaments and foods according to principles of hot/cold balance (see Harwood 1971), herbalism, dietary modifications, use of tonics and vitamins (including injectable vitamins—see Marin 1990; Marin and Marin 1990),[37] a range of physical therapies, curanderismo (see Trotter and Chavira 1981), and a variety of religious and spiritual practices. Healing practices likely to be in most common use vary by region of the country and by the specific Latino cultures and countries of origin represented. HIV and other very serious diseases often call for spiritual or supernatural healing interventions (Flaskerud and Calvillo 1991). Among these are included prayers and blessings; protective and healing amulets and talismans worn or carried on the person; herbs taken internally or applied topically for medicinal purposes; consultations with ritual specialists of various types; and ritual baths and cleansing sweepings of both persons and places, with specific herbs selected for their symbolic or spiritual qualities and for their associations with spiritual figures and with well-known healers both living and deceased. Herbs and related supplies are sold in *botánicas*, the botanical and religious goods shops that are well patronized and common features of many Hispanic neighbor-hoods. Herbs selected may be used for specific medicinal actions, but also for innate qualities or spiritual potencies that make them effective against negative influences, ill fortune, evil spirits, and malevolent human agency. Specific combinations of herbs may also be used to make a sacred liquid that is both used externally for protective bless-ings and taken internally for spiritual and healing purposes. Shop-keepers of botánicas, like pharmacists in drugstores, serve as commu-nity consultants on health and related issues. Because of the salience of these consultative functions, community AIDS education activists in New York have recently engaged keepers of botánicas in several His-panic neighborhoods, as well as spiritualists and other religious fig-ures, as community AIDS educators and promoters of safe sex and other preventive measures (Derr et al. 1992; Rivera 1992).

The Two-Tier Vernacular Health Resource System

There is no parallel in communities of color to the organized gay community's HIV treatment, support, and information network, and PWAs of color do not participate in significant numbers in the gay PWA community or its network. Men of color who have sex with men fre-quently do not affiliate with the organized gay community, and this is especially true if they are also in the lower income strata (Altman 1986; Mays and Cochran 1987; Lester and Saxxon 1988; Peterson and Marin 1988). Reasons for this division include the gay movement's and the commercial gay world's mirroring of the segregation patterns of the general society (Altman 1986:100); social class differences affecting both attitudes to care and financial access to resources and support systems; and the strong cultural prohibitions in many communities of color against adopting or being assigned a homosexual identity (Alt-man 1986; Peterson and Marin 1988). Heterosexual men and women of color are even less likely to be associated with the gay PWA move-ment (if they are aware of it in the first place). In the early 1990s it remains true that the great majority of HIV/AIDS "forums, confer-ences and organizations involve an extraordinary overrepresentation of whites [and men] and a real failure to involve others" (Altman 1986:100). Attendees at special programs are typically white, middle-class, and middle-aged, and so do not represent a proportional cross section of the population at risk (Altman 1986). This is as true of conferences dealing with alternative and complementary therapies as it is of academic and scientific conferences focusing on more conven-tional topics.[38]

Although the public image of HIV/AIDS as a "gay white disease" is changing, this image has been so firmly entrenched for so long that culture-specific educational efforts have had to be designed to dispel it. Culturally specific and ethnic interest-group organizations, such as the National Minority AIDS Council, the Haitian Coalition on AIDS (New York City), and BEBASHI (Blacks Educating Blacks About Sexual Health Issues, a Philadelphia advocacy and education group) have been formed to meet the challenge of providing culturally relevant treatment, prevention information, and support services. Posters and leaflets proclaim a crucial message: "You don't have to be white or gay to get AIDS." Local level culture-specific organizations, however, "unlike a group such as the Gay Men's Health Crisis, . . . cannot call on an affluent and politically sophisticated community for assistance" (Altman 1986:73). It is not their inner-city constituents who subscribe to alternative treatment newsletters, fax their drug and supplement orders, which they pay by credit card, to buyers clubs, peruse the medical and scientific journals, negotiate with physicians, reach on-line treatment information services by modem from their home computers, and draw upon their discretionary income to pay for foreign pharmaceuticals and other complementary therapies.[39]

The principal purpose of sketching these comparative vernacular treatment responses to HIV disease is not to point out culture-specific differences in the explanatory models or in the particular treatments used by the mostly white gay community and the black and Hispanic communities from which examples are drawn (although that is significant and useful information). It is rather to illustrate the social class–specific differences in quantity and range of available information and treatment options for people living with HIV disease. The gay PWA community has been spurred to action by the sentiment, "we have to look after our own, because no one else will."

For gay men this is not an impossible burden. For the [economically] marginal victims of AIDS, for black and hispanic drug users, for poor women forced into prostitution, this becomes cruel piety. (Altman 1986:28. See also Gross 1988; Gevisser 1988.)

In the context of HIV and AIDS, the stereotypes of "marginality" so long associated with use of unconventional health care practices carry a special irony: it is precisely the groups of people to whom these stereotypes are typically applied who make the *smallest* use of vernacular treatment strategies. "The majority of the persons who have supported complementary therapies are middle- and upper-class white men. Unless these therapies are modified to be available and sensitive to the needs of people of various cultural, ethnic, or socioeconomic backgrounds, complementary therapies will probably remain a luxury item for an elite segment of those infected" (Strawn 1989:193). In vernacular health care options, just as in conventional medical care, a two-tier system exists. It is the "mainstream" people with HIV/AIDS, the members of more privileged social classes, who have greater access to both conventional *and* alternative healing resources—just as they have access to more of *all* social resources than do the minority poor.

Summary

HIV/AIDS is widely addressed by both innovative and traditional vernacular healing strategies, and this should occasion no surprise. Anyone who receives a devastating diagnosis is quite likely to begin to search for all available resources for coping with the situation (Hufford 1984, 1988a), and to reason about which treatment prospects to try, why they might be beneficial, and how to gain access to them. This is a general fact of the human response to pressing problems, both individual and collective, and needs to be recognized as a matter of fact in health care. The gay PWA community has responded to the AIDS epidemic with an extraordinarily vigorous elaboration of vernacular treatment strategies to augment conventional medicine. What is unique about their particular response is its enormous extent and purposeful organization: the collection and dissemination of alternative treatment information; the establishment of an underground consumer-regulated supply network; the radically new ways in which the community has extended the uses of vernacular strategies; the overt challenges to and successful negotiations with regulatory and research bodies; and the assertion of personal authority in care. A 1989 Safe Sex poster proclaimed: "Cultures are known not only by their art and architecture but also by the way they respond in a time of crisis. History will define gay men's response to AIDS as nothing less than extraordinary" (San Francisco AIDS Foundation 1989). It is a response unprecedented in the history of the relationship of vernacular and conventional health care, and one whose social and political ramifications reach far beyond the realm of HIV and AIDS.

Notes

1. Following one of many current usages, I use the term "HIV/AIDS" to designate the full spectrum of HIV disease from asymptomatic seropositive status to the fully developed immune deficiency syndrome.

2. I continue to use "mainstream" here as it was operationally defined in Chapter 1, i.e., having English-language fluency, a minimum of a high school education, and familiarity with the conventional medical system; obviously this

term has certain ironies when used to refer to gay men, who have long been stigmatized by, and therefore in many senses forced out of, the mainstream of U.S. society. Note also that the term "patient group" represents only a clinical point of view: people are only "patients" when they are in, or being viewed from within, medical settings.

3. The issue of identity is central to affiliation: many men who have sex with men do not self-identify as homosexual or bisexual and may therefore avoid membership in the gay community and its organizations and functions.

4. The term PWA, meaning "person(s) with AIDS," reflects a deliberate social and political insistence on identification of those who are HIV infected as *persons*, rather than patients—a conscious and emphatic demedicalization of their public (and private) image. This term has a range of differing usages, as well as a number of competitors in various segments of the HIV-positive population. Some restrict PWA to persons with AIDS only, while a much larger segment use it as a shorthand for *all* persons in all stages of HIV disease. Some have chosen PLWA (person living with AIDS) to stress not only the person-vs.-patient aspect of identity, but also a focus on *living* meant to counteract the public (and private) perception of HIV-positive status as a "death sentence." Some have now modified the terms to PHIV or PLHIV as more explicitly encompassing the full spectrum of HIV disease, rather than focusing upon its manifestation only in the diagnostic category, AIDS.

Because it allows for linguistic consistency and follows the usage still most widely found in the community of reference and throughout its media and its organizational acronyms, I use PWA as my shorthand term. I intend it in its broadest application, as a term of reference to the full spectrum of HIV disease and its manifestations (which corresponds as well to the range of applicability of the health care practices discussed in this chapter).

5. For detailed treatment of the political action aspects of the HIV alternative therapies movement, and for treatment activism generally, see Gamson 1989, Arno and Feiden 1992, and Kwitny 1992.

6. Once an infectious agent had been identified, many members of the gay PWA community continued to feel that the government's only overt concern was insuring the safety of the blood supply, i.e., not attention to the care of those infected but to the preservation of those uninfected (Jonathan Lax, personal communication).

7. The definitive work on the subject is Sheryl Burt Ruzek, *The Women's Health Movement: Feminist Alternatives to Medical Control* (New York: Praeger, 1978). In retrospect it must be recognized that the "values of women" enshrined in the women's health movement were often the values of middle-class white women, which did not necessarily apply to women of other social classes or to women of color who frequently had different sets of concerns and different possibilities for action. In the current decade there are several women's health contingents, including local and national culture-, ethnicity-, or class-specific groups.

8. This is not to suggest that there was unanimity of opinion in the national gay community, or even in its regional and local subsets. For a thorough discussion of the community's internecine political struggles in coping with AIDS, see Shilts 1987.

9. Estimates of the percentage of the San Francisco gay population vary wildly, and it is difficult even to average them in any meaningful way. For example, a 1984 estimate placed the figure at roughly 10 percent (Bethell

1988); a 1986 estimate at 20 percent (Gong 1986); and a 1992 San Francisco Department of Public Welfare estimate at 8.01 percent.

10. French and American scientists both claimed the discovery, as a result of separate research; the dual claim accounts for the two dates given. See Shilts (1987) for detailed documentation of the international competition for credit for the discovery.

11. Throughout this chapter, I follow the common parlance usage of the PWA community in referring to CD4 lymphocytes generically or interchangeably as "T-cells."

12. WTP is used throughout this chapter as the abbreviation for a grassroots PWA support and advocacy organization in Philadelphia, whose full name is We the People Living with AIDS/HIV of the Delaware Valley, Inc. Members refer to the organization conversationally as "We the People," and in written shorthand as "WTP."

13. Blue-Green Manna is a brand name for a specific subspecies of blue-green algae found in Klamath Lake, Oregon; this species is also available under other brand names. "Blue green manna" may be used as a generic name in the common parlance, in much the same way as the brand name Kleenex is used to refer to facial tissues generally.

14. For detailed descriptions of the theory and practice of macrobiotics, see George Ohsawa, *Zen Macrobiotics* (Los Angeles: Ohsawa Foundation, 1965) and Michio Kushi, *The Book of Macrobiotics* (Tokyo: Japan Publications, 1977). Specifically addressing the use of macrobiotics in AIDS is Tom Monte, *The Way of Hope: Michio Kushi's Anti-AIDS Program* (New York: Warner Books, 1989).

15. One popular self-help reference work is Christopher Hobbs, *Superimmunity: Herbs and Other Natural Remedies for a Healthy Immune System* (Botanica Press, 1985), a primer specifically devoted to the use of herbs in the context of HIV infection and other immune disorders. Others include John Lust, *The Herb Book* (New York: Bantam Books, 1974) and Jethro Kloss, *Back to Eden* (Back to Eden's Book Publishing Company, 1992; originally published 1939).

16. Chaparral tea, marijuana, and mistletoe are also widely used as vernacular treatments for cancer (U.S. Congress, Office of Technology Assessment 1990).

17. The Flower Essence Society (California) prints and distributes a standardized form for collection of practitioner and user data on new essences, as well as on new uses of familiar essences. The form requests information as to diagnoses, types of essences selected and method of selection, dosage and frequency of use, simultaneous recommendations or modalities used, and changes experienced during treatment cycle. A waiver on the form, if signed, permits use of the information for research and its anonymous publication in the Members' Newsletter.

18. For a fuller description of the underlying theory and the details of preparation, refer to literature from the Flower Essence Society (available in New Age bookstores and health food stores).

19. I have arbitrarily selected these grounds for discussing homeopathy under the broader rubric of herbalism and related therapies. Most homeopaths and their clients, given the classificatory categories I use in this chapter, would probably place it under the heading of energy therapies, which would be consonant with current homeopathic theory about mechanism of action of homeopathic remedies. For full explanations of homeopathy, see Harris Coulter, *Homeopathic Medicine* (St. Louis: Formur, Inc., 1975) and Dana Ullman,

Homeopathy: Medicine for the Twenty-First Century (Berkeley: North Atlantic Books, 1988).

20. The conventional chemotherapeutic agent for KS, vinblastine, is also derived from a species of vinca, the Madagascar periwinkle.

21. For a detailed treatment of traditional Chinese medicine and its complex theoretical and philosophical foundation, see Ted Kaptchuk, *The Web That Has No Weaver: Understanding Chinese Medicine* (New York: Congdon and Weed, 1983). For detailed interpretation of HIV/AIDS and traditional Chinese medicine, see Qingcai Zhang and Hon-yen Hsu, *AIDS and Chinese Medicine: Applications of the Oldest Medicine to the Newest Disease* (Long Beach: Oriental Healing Arts Institute, 1990).

22. Certain aspects of traditional Chinese medicine have even been incorporated into the therapeutic program available in San Francisco General Hospital's Alternative Therapy Unit, started specifically in response to the needs of AIDS patients (Gong 1986).

23. See, for example, Jeanne Achterberg, *Imagery in Healing* (Boston: Shambhala, 1985) or Bernie Siegel, *Love, Medicine and Miracles* (New York: Harper and Row, 1986). Siegel has quite a following among PWAs, as well as among cancer patients.

24. For a thorough explanation of Therapeutic Touch and its introduction into nursing practice, see Dolores Krieger's books, *The Therapeutic Touch: How to Use Your Hands to Help or Heal* (Englewood Cliffs, NJ: Prentice-Hall, 1979) and *Foundations of Holistic Health Nursing Practices: The Renaissance Nurse* (Philadelphia: J. B. Lippincott, 1981).

25. Gregorio's practice is illegal in the United States and this client reports that the healer is watched and harassed by the FBI. Nevertheless, the healer has a large and loyal following of clients who are advised of his scheduled visits to their area through a lay referral network (word-of-mouth and printed flyers) and who are willing to risk harassment themselves to keep their appointments with him.

26. Other major figures, especially on the conference circuit, are physicians Elisabeth Kübler-Ross (who rose to prominence with her studies of death and dying in the 1970s) and Bernie Siegel. Each has also recently written a book on the subject of AIDS, with a metaphysical/psychospiritual point of view.

27. There are a number of gay-identified religious groups, however, such as the international nondenominational Metropolitan Community Church (Altman 1986), Bet Mishpachah (Jewish; Washington, D.C., area), Affirmation (a Methodist and a Mormon chapter), Integrity (Episcopalian), the Lifeline Baptist Caucus, Lutherans Concerned, the Brethren/Mennonite Council, and the Catholic organization Dignity (Van Ness 1988).

28. The radical effects of this decision are not restricted to people with AIDS, but apply to any person suffering from any ailment, thus extending the public policy influence of the PWA and AIDS treatment activist movements into a much wider sector.

29. The alternative cancer therapies movement also spawned buyers clubs, but not nearly on the scale nor with the degree of organization of the current PWA buyers clubs.

30. By the time the FDA ruling on private importation of foreign pharmaceuticals was changed in July 1988, dextran sulfate was in formal FDA-approved clinical trials, though enrollment in these was very restricted. Project Inform of San Francisco estimated as many as 2,500 people were using the drug regularly before the new FDA ruling (Booth 1988).

31. This insistence on forging new authority relationships extends to the research and regulatory agencies as well. In October 1988 for example, a group of 1,000 AIDS activists demonstrated outside FDA headquarters, shouting, "We're the experts; Let us in!" (Gevisser 1988).

32. The document has recently been translated into Spanish and is distributed in both languages, as well as having been published in both English and Spanish versions in *Critical Path* 3[9], 1993.

33. Members of the Philadelphia gay PWA community estimate even the highest of these findings to underrepresent actual rates of use (personal communications).

34. Terms identifying race and ethnicity have the following referents in this chapter: "white" refers to whites not of Hispanic heritage; "black" refers to blacks not of Hispanic heritage. "Hispanic" denotes those self-identified as of Spanish or Latin American cultural or ancestral heritage, regardless of race (see also Peterson and Marin 1988:871). It is acknowledged that all of these referents for racial or ethnic identity are problematic.

35. For a complete explanation of the construction of these two broad classificatory categories and how they affect healing strategies, see Snow 1974, 1983.

36. Flaskerud and Rush, citing Snow (1974), explain the "natural"/"unnatural" division as part of the introductory material in their article. However, for reasons which they do not elucidate, they then go on to reclassify the division as "natural"/"supernatural." I have re-sorted these authors' results into the categories originally used by Snow and cited by these authors in their introduction.

37. Marin and Marin (1990) have noted that home injection of vitamins and prescription medications is practiced by a small percentage of some Latino groups, and that this practice should be considered in light of its risk for HIV transmission (see also Marin 1990; Flaskerud and Calvillo 1991)

38. A two-day seminar in Philadelphia entitled "Fight Back Against AIDS" (April 1990) had an advance registration fee of $195/person and an on-site registration fee of $225/person. Much larger was the Second International Conference on the Traditional and Complementary Therapies in the Prevention and Treatment of AIDS (subtitled "Changing the Odds: Living Long and Living Well, an Idea Whose Time Has Come"), held in a major hotel in Washington, D.C., in February 1990. Advance registration for this conference was $250/person ($275 after the advance-registration deadline). In addition, special workshops had separate registration fees of $25 and $65 per person, and luncheons or dinners with the featured speakers could be joined for $30 and $100 per person. Videotapes of certain sessions could be purchased for $40 and audiotapes for prices ranging from $10 to $15; complete sets of audiotapes were available for $125 for the current conference, and $100 for the previous year's tape set. The fee structure and the demographics of HIV disease, taken together, determine a great deal about the probable makeup of the audience for such events.

39. One member of the gay PWA community, pointing out this disparity, queried a reporter: "Does an 18-year-old black kid know egg lecithin from a hole in the ground? . . . And if he knows, does he have $200 to pay for it?" (Gross 1988:183).

Chapter 5
Implications for the
Health Professions

The immediate message of the foregoing chapters is that nonbiomedical health belief systems are alive and well; that they are in very common use by all kinds of people; and that health professionals should
ask patients about them and expect to find them among their patients'
healing resources. The larger message this phenomenon evokes is that
patients are authoritative agents of their own health care,[1] and this
social fact needs to be recognized and taken seriously by health professionals. Patients evaluate health care options in a range often much
broader in scope than that of the conventional medical system. They
make decisions on the authority of their own knowledge and experience—which differ from the knowledge and experience of health
professionals—and they do so notwithstanding professional disagreement with many of their choices and conclusions. They pursue the
therapeutic goals most valued by themselves, whether or not these
coincide with the goals most valued by clinicians. Patients, in the end,
not health professionals, determine the actions they will take with
respect to health and illness, including when, how, and from whom
they seek care, and how they pursue the recommendations of their
various care providers. "Patient" is a small part of most people's identity, and not generally the one that supplies the main frame of reference within which important decisions about life are made.

Conventional medicine has reached a watershed in the confluence of
many streams of change: a rising public disaffection with conventional
medicine and its practitioners (related to much deeper social currents;
see Freidson 1987; Levin, Katz and Holst 1979); public demands for a
broadening range of participatory rights in the clinical relationship;
legal recognition of patients' rights to self-determination in acceptance
or rejection of medically recommended treatments; the changed profile of health problems in the population at large; rapid technological

innovation and its attendant ethical dilemmas; the recent and burgeoning corporatization of health care; and the increasing ethnic diversity and multiculturalism in American society, to name but a few of
the most obvious considerations. All of these elements have contributed both to shifts in and accentuation of the patient's perspective in
relationships with the official health care system. Health professionals
and patients alike will benefit, and the quality of care improve, by a
reframing of the customary provider-patient relationship to recognize
patients' authoritative agency and engage it as a resource in identifying
and working toward common goals.

Health Care Pluralism

The multiplicity of vernacular healing systems to which people of every
ethnicity, cultural background, educational exposure, and social class
have recourse create de facto health care pluralism in the United States
(as in other complex societies). Recent estimates suggest that at least one
in every three Americans uses alternative healing resources at some
time (Eisenberg et al. 1993), and these resources show no signs of diminishing in popularity. The reactions of health professionals to vernacular
healing systems range from irritation and reflex condemnation, to
general uneasiness, to reasoned and informed selective disagreement,
to cautious and selective endorsement, to active participation both as
referring practitioners and as clients. Whatever the preferences and
responses of health professionals, however, the existence and popularity of vernacular health belief systems is a fact of modern life that
needs to be recognized as a relevant factor in health care, and one with
bearing upon clinical concerns.

It is useful to bear in mind a few summary facts about this phenomenon. In general, patients' use of vernacular healing modalities is the
result of reasoned choices and an effort to multiply therapeutic options
to obtain optimal care for their felt needs. Conventional medicine does
not and cannot provide everything that people need in order to cope
with all aspects of the experience of illness (Hufford 1988a), or to meet
their desires to achieve or maintain optimal health. It ought therefore
to be expected that people will seek elsewhere to attain desired health-
related ends for which medicine does not provide. To the extent that
they find them helpful, patients generally feel committed to and satisfied with their vernacular healing systems (as with the conventional
system). This holds true irrespective of health professionals' opinions
of the systems, and regardless of whether or not health professionals
agree with their attribution of causal relations between the therapeutic
practices and changes in health status. Simple argument invoking

medical or scientific authority is unlikely to be successful in persuading participants in vernacular health belief systems to change their minds or their behavior.

Users of vernacular healing resources are frequently of the stated opinion that biomedicine does not know all there is to know about a variety of health issues and treatment possibilities. This may be considered a critique, or simply an artifact of the way in which medicine has historically delimited its territory. Most do not expect physicians and other conventional practitioners to be knowledgeable about alternative healing modalities, and so may be unmoved by health professionals' assertions that such-and-such a technique or substance "is not known to have any real effect." (Quite commonly in my fieldwork experiences, interviewees have made an observation to the effect that "they" [i.e., scientists, health professionals] may not know that this is effective, but *I* do.) The assertion that "there is no scientific evidence" that a substance or technique is efficacious seldom has a deterrent effect on people using vernacular healing techniques, in part because many of them are well aware that there has been little scientific investigation of most vernacular therapies, and hence little production of scientific evidence one way or the other.[2] Further, most have other evidential standards in addition to—indeed, often in preference to—the findings of scientific investigations. Anyone who obtains the desired effects from any healing effort (including biomedicine), especially if s/he obtains them repeatedly or obtains them after efforts with other strategies have failed, is likely to be convinced of the therapy's efficacy on the basis of personal experience. This constitutes empirical evidence and is typically considered both trustworthy and sufficient. People who know through experience that a given technique works (or works for them, at least) are unlikely to be perturbed by a lack of scientific evidence demonstrating efficacy: no such corroboration is needed, and its lack is a moot issue. Science is not necessarily discredited, but is simply regarded as only one possible source of valid information. Similarly, if a disagreement arises between this person and another (say, a health professional or an academic) who considers the system to be ineffective or its mechanism of action impossible on grounds of theory, personal experience will always hold the evidential and epistemological high ground for the experiencer.

Some "alternative" practices, such as acupuncture, have begun to be selectively incorporated into conventional medical settings. Many patients, however, prefer to seek outside the bounds of conventional medicine for their adjunctive therapies, because they are seeking a different cognitive framework, a different level of skill, and different interaction patterns as well as specific therapeutic interventions. A number of people whom I have interviewed in my fieldwork, for example, have emphatically stressed their preference for a licensed acupuncturist with full training and certification in traditional Chinese medicine (TCM) over a physician-acupuncturist. Two principal reasons are cited: (1) the physician receives "only about 100 hours" of training (P., personal communication), while the schooled practitioner of TCM pursues a four-year curriculum that includes double or triple that amount of direct clinical training and is therefore considered to have the superior background and skills; and (2) the physician typically reinterprets the application of acupuncture within the biomedical model, while the schooled practitioner of TCM views the health problem and treatment rationalization in an entirely different interpretive framework. Since problem definition constrains the range of solutions that suggest themselves, many people prefer a practitioner who will conceptualize the health problem in an entirely new way, opening up new possibilities and shedding new light on the matter. They are specifically seeking a new paradigm as well as a new range of treatment options. This is as likely to be true of people who are using conventional medicine and acupuncture simultaneously to manage a problem (i.e., approaching it from more than one angle) as it is for those who have found conventional medical approaches unsuccessful and moved to acupuncture as a next line of effort.[3]

The range of circumstances that can prompt people to use vernacular health care measures is as at least as numerous and diverse as those which prompt them to seek conventional medical care. Indeed, it is probably broader, as alternative systems address an even wider range of problems. Some of the circumstances most likely to prompt use of vernacular healing resources are summarized in Table 6. With or without the health professional's blessing or permission, people will continue to make decisions for themselves about their health needs and about which therapeutic options best address them. Patients have authoritative agency in self-determination, a position that is recognized and sustained in the principles of biomedical ethics, and in such aspects of the legal code as the federal Patient Self-Determination Act. Ethically, patients "are free to choose alternatives that physicians may think ill-advised, so long as the rights of others are not abridged" (Cross and Churchill 1982:110); legally, they are entitled to make such choices and pursue them wherever the therapeutic options themselves are legal.[4]

Vernacular health belief systems are an active component of American health care resources and are as unlikely to fade away as is conventional medicine itself. A large and growing number of vernacular health belief and treatment systems draw adherents from every ethnicity, social class, and educational level. These systems address aspects

TABLE 6. Conditions Under Which Alternative Health Care Measures Are Most Likely To Be Used.

- Serious, chronic, debilitating, or terminal illness, especially when conventional medicine has limited success in controlling symptoms or disease processes. (Examples: HIV disease, chronic fatigue syndrome [CFS], multiple sclerosis [MS], autoimmune disorders, cancers)
- Acute or chronic conditions for which conventional medicine has little or nothing curative to offer. (Examples: headache, persistent back pain, various skin conditions, colds, allergies, fatigue, weight control, asthma, rheumatic diseases, pain syndromes)
- Conditions for which a person prefers nondrug, noninvasive approaches, and which have popular reputations for nonmedical management success. (Examples: insomnia, allergies, colitis and other disorders of the digestive system, pregnancy and childbirth, asthma, headache, back pain, arthritis)
- Desire to replace recommended medical therapies that are offensive or impair quality of life, or with which a person disagrees. (Examples: invasive therapies, drugs with significant toxicity, disfiguring treatments, drugs with mood-altering or sense-altering side effects, extended or lifelong regimens)
- Need to control side effects of conventional medical therapies (while not wishing to discontinue the therapies).
- Dissatisfaction with treatments, outcomes, or personnel and attitudes of conventional medicine.
- Failure of conventional therapy.
- Inability of physicians to arrive at a diagnosis, especially after lengthy efforts or exhaustive testing.
- Diagnoses that are too vague, that are offensive to the patient, or with which the patient disagrees. (Examples: persistent "fever of unknown origin" [FUO]; illnesses in which mental illness or psychosomatic processes are considered to be sole or contributing factors)
- Illnesses that conventional medicine does not recognize as diagnostic categories. (Examples: folk illnesses; new diseases, e.g., CFS)
- Instances in which conventional medicine is considered to be addressing symptoms, but not underlying causes. (Examples: allergies, digestive disorders; illnesses in which spiritual or supernatural causal factors are implicated, from the patient's point of view)
- Instances in which conventional medicine is felt inadequate to address a person's health concerns. (Examples: nutrition, prevention, health maintenance or promotion of "wellness," preference for natural rather than synthetic medicaments, preference for high patient involvement in determination of therapeutic course)
- Whenever a particular health belief system is part of a person's cultural heritage or identity-group culture, or part of a consciously chosen lifestyle.

of health care ranging from disease prevention and maintenance of wellness; through all manner of minor and grave acute ailments and injuries; to chronic, degenerative, and terminal illness and death. They encompass both conditions recognized and conditions differently interpreted or unrecognized by conventional medicine. The majority of people using vernacular healing strategies also use conventional medical care, either sequentially or simultaneously. They may use each system to which they have recourse for a variety of purposes. Some of those purposes may cut across systems as well, while others are specific to one particular system. Clearly, this vigorous and complex sphere of alternative and complementary vernacular health belief and practice has significant implications for conventional medicine and health care. These implications are likely to become more salient in the foreseeable future, given their interactions with a number of other social and cultural factors affecting health care in this country.

The Social Context of Medical Practice and Health Care Delivery

The current social context of professional medical practice in the United States—as in contemporary Western societies generally—poses problems whose complexity increasingly requires recognition and incorporation of nonmedical input from a variety of sources, from the management consultant to the ethicist to the social scientist to the patient. For the past two decades public opinion has been increasingly critical of medicine, in spite of acknowledging its many advances. Criticism has been leveled at the official health care system for several publicly identified reasons: for the exponential growth of technological interventions, blamed for both an increase in iatrogenesis and a drastic drop in humanism (read: genuine interpersonal concern and responsiveness) in medical practice (Wexler 1976); for rapidly and perpetually increasing costs; for the shamefully uneven quality of care for poor and for better-off patients; for the general lack of preventive and health-promoting care; for the arrogance, inaccessibility, and authoritarianism of many physicians; for the dehumanization and inflexibility of hospital care; and innumerable other dissatisfactions. These criticisms have come from every socioeconomic stratum of society, each with its particular grievances based in values, desires, needs, and experience. Dissatisfied citizens call for serious revisions in health care practice, including changes in the clinician-patient relationship. The called-for changes are expected to reflect shifts in authority relations between providers—especially physicians—and patients. These in turn will require recognition of incongruent, even competing, systems of values and goals that patients and providers bring to the therapeutic relationship.

Patient Expectations

Patient expectations of medical care have changed dramatically over the past fifteen to twenty years. Increasingly, all sorts of patients seek a relationship with health professionals that engages *their* questions and *their* values and does not merely consign them to roles of supplication and obedience (see Reynolds and Carson, 1976). Patient populations of every description seek greater responsiveness and attention to their health needs *as they themselves define them*. Middle-class patients especially constitute an increasingly knowledgeable group who tend consciously and overtly to value their own intellects and autonomy, and to dismiss pronouncements and arguments based in physicians' customary cultural authority rather than in solid and accessible explanations.[5] It is they who have founded and continually increased the popularity of the holistic health movement; they who actively seek and advocate the widest variety of alternative healing modalities for purposes ranging from prevention to active treatment, and for conditions ranging from the medically (but not necessarily personally) minor to the chronic and life-threatening; they who most firmly expect—even require—clinicians to be accessible and accountable to them in new ways.

Changes in the structure of the health care system itself, such as the extraordinary proliferation and regulatory influence of systems of third-party payment and the increasing corporatization of medicine, have contributed to public charges of loss of humanism in health care. Many patients, of all socioeconomic classes, believe or worry that concern for profit outweighs concern for people as a physician's primary motive nowadays, that the health care business is designed "so that the business rather than the patient may prosper" (Loewy 1989:12). The corporatization of health care has increased many patients' dissatisfaction with the system and heightened their sense of alienation and neglect of *their* concerns. Increasing managerial demands of the business of medicine require physicians to balance patient care against the requirements of the system, to the frequent detriment of the patient-physician relationship. Patients must navigate a maze of rules and bureaucratic obstacles in their efforts to secure appointments with those whose expertise and counsel they seek. System-centered "managerial determinations of appropriate medical care . . . are potentially in conflict with . . . patient-centered care" (Bosk 1987:472; see also Aiken and Mechanic 1987; Loewy 1989). *Procedures* are billable but *care*, or time spent with a patient, is not (see Stoeckle 1979). Reimbursement arrangements too often drive the clinical encounter, discounting the fact that *care* is a social and interpersonal, as well as medical, phenomenon (see Lowenberg 1989).

The shift in perspective from medicine-as-service to medicine-as-business transforms patients into "consumers" of health care. The business model embodies a fundamental change in moral view (Loewy 1989): while the classical patient-physician relationship was based on an ethic of trust and service, the consumer-provider relationship is based on savvy, skepticism, self-protection (on both sides), and the directives of the "bottom line." Ironically, it has also placed patients in a relatively more powerful position ideologically with respect to the system, for it has heightened their sense of their right to choose. Consumerism is based on choice. Consumers compare and critique, and they bring their own standards and preferences to bear in evaluating their purchasing options. They continue to patronize (and help to advertise) only those providers of goods and services who satisfy their needs within the framework of an adequate cost-to-quality ratio. Consumers decide both what they perceive their needs to be and how well they feel those needs are met by specific products and services.

There is widespread sentiment that patients should "shop around" until they find what they need in a physician or hospital, and that they can and should be forthright in questioning physicians, in expressing their own opinions, and in making clear what they need from the particular encounter or from the longer association. As previous chapters have shown, this is one of the fundamental political principles of the PWA, gay and lesbian health, women's health, and holistic health movements, and it is an approach likewise advocated by members of the generally disgruntled public. Central to this approach is a reconceptualization of the relationship and apportionment of authority between patients and physicians. Some consider the physician to be an expert consultant, whose advice is recognized as knowledgeable and important but whose recommendations may, like those of any consultant, be adopted in whole or in part or in some modified form of which the client is the final arbiter. More radically, some view the physician as a skilled contractor whom they "hire" and "fire" according to the skill, knowledge, and personal qualities that bear on how well s/he does the job. This relationship is seen as inherently asymmetrical, but inverts the classical asymmetry which has heretofore characterized the physician-patient relationship: "[the patient] is the administrator and they work for *you*" (H. C., personal communication).

The capacity to act on these sentiments varies with people's means to pursue their preferences: access to a variety of health care services by virtue of ability to pay or of comprehensive or flexible third-party coverage, access to transportation, and so forth. Even for poorer patients with restricted means and access, doctor switching (defined from the professional perspective as an "inappropriate" use of the system) is common and may reflect deliberate choices based on dissatisfaction with prior care and relationships, or on circulating information about who are the best physicians and which are the best hospitals for specific types of problems (see Salloway 1973). People who are able to do so may go to very great lengths to find the caliber of care and type of therapeutic relationship they feel best responds to their needs and values. For example, a professional couple in their forties, upon receiving a serious diagnosis for one of them, spent several weeks interviewing physicians (as well as other types of healers) before finding one who fit their requirements. These included a solid grounding in her own subspecialty; openness to innovative therapies and new explanatory possibilities; a concern with sound nutrition congruent with a health foods orientation; a willingness to engage both patient and spouse as partners in defining the care relationship; accessibility for ad hoc consultation as questions or issues might arise; and a personable, respectful, and interested manner. Though the illness was expected to require ongoing care for an extended period, the couple were willing to travel the two hours (one way) that separated their home from the physician whom they eventually engaged in order to secure the kind of care and therapeutic relationship they desired (Tony and Margaret Dale Barrand, personal communication).

Epidemiological Changes

Changes in the epidemiology of American health and disease alter the significance of the patient side of the patient-provider equation. The general aging of the American population and medicine's historical successes in controlling acute infectious diseases have shifted much of the demand for medical care to chronic conditions and long-term care strategies. Long-term illnesses require long-term involvements between patients and health professionals. Self-care becomes a critical resource in this context, and health professionals make efforts to promote and encourage it (see Levin 1976; Levin, Katz, and Holst 1979; Dean 1981, 1989c). Social, cultural, and behavioral factors contributing to health and illness are critical to the outcomes of these efforts, in which responsibility and authority will be negotiated between health professionals and patients and their families. The current epidemiological pattern increases the need for health professionals to be equipped to "understand the patient's motives and attitudes, as well as the family [cultural] and societal influences that will shape the way the patient treats himself or herself" (Banks 1979:281).

American Cultural Diversity

The population of the United States represents an enormously diverse range of cultural heritages, including hundreds which are indigenous to the continent. Diversity of cultural heritage has been the rule throughout the country's history of voluntary and involuntary in-migration of peoples, and American rhetoric has depicted the country as a melting pot. Though this image was adopted and celebrated as an ostensibly positive one connoting access for all, its underlying assumption was essentially that newcomers and indigenous peoples whose cultural origins and values were not those of the dominant class (that is, Anglo-European) could, and should, somehow be stirred in, melted down, and recast in the dominant mold—at least in a generation or two. In this way, they would mix in and "become American." In reality, this meltdown has not happened much of the time, for a complex variety of social and political reasons that lie far beyond the scope of this commentary. Instead, various groups have influenced and borrowed from one another; become acculturated to the dominant model to varying degrees; selectively maintained much of their native cultural heritage through several generations; consciously generated significant aspects of their own group culture; or actively restored and revitalized cultural identities and repertoires that had, through various circumstances, become dormant or been reduced or eviscerated.

There is a strong tendency within the health professions to think of culture as an "issue," or of cultural difference as a consideration, largely in terms of strongly ethnically identified populations, or those identified by health professionals as "ethnics."[6] While certain features of cultural identity, worldview, and expression are closely associated with specific ethnic groups, it is inaccurate to equate culture and ethnicity. All people reflect cultural shaping, regardless of their ethnicity, and all ethnicities encompass a range of cultural possibilities. Cultural features are also associated with many other aspects of identity and life circumstances including religion, social class, gender, sexual preference, geographic region, occupation, and so forth. Any individual can have multiple cultural memberships and influences, and any cultural group encompasses a great range of individual diversity. Cultures may be conceptualized as consisting of interpretive and expressive repertoires, upon which individuals draw selectively and in an infinite range of possible combinations, all of which are subject to personal modification. Thus, while it is possible to describe the ingredients in a cultural repertoire associated with any given group, it is *not* possible to predict on that basis how any individual member may believe or behave.

Multiculturalism, or cultural pluralism, is a fact of American life and therefore of American health care. Increasing cultural diversity will exert escalating pressure on the official health care system to broaden its perspectives and develop capabilities to be responsive to the needs of patients of all manner of backgrounds and beliefs. This will require recognition of the fact that conventional medicine is itself both a culture (and a diverse one at that) and a culturally shaped institution, reflecting the values and worldview of the historically and currently dominant segment of American society. Recognition of the importance of cultural issues in health care is already under way in medical settings, but has heretofore been narrowly focused on national origin or ethnicity (presumptively defined as nondominant cultural group identity). This gradually growing recognition has not yet encompassed the realization that many of the cultural issues are contributed by medicine itself: they do not just come through the door with patients. The "issues" are rooted in cultural differences, and "difference," by definition, requires at least two reference points. Differences are not within one, but between them both (or all). The differences are *relational*; that is, "different compared to what?"

Patients who strongly identify with a cultural heritage different from that represented by the values of conventional medicine may be expected to reject medical opinions and recommendations that violate deeply held values or that imply or openly declare their own cultural systems to be invalid, outmoded, or substandard. Mr. L., for example (Chapter 3), observed to me matter-of-factly that it was obviously impossible for anyone with common sense to accept the proposition that Hmong culture, which has served its people well for several thousand years, should suddenly be proved incorrect or insufficient (especially by members of a culture so historically young and inexperienced!). Yet this was the implication, if not the direct message, of many of his American physicians' efforts to persuade him to abandon his point of view in favor of their own. He had felt embarrassment for the sake of the physicians whose transparent ignorance had allowed them to make this absurd suggestion.[7] He had been shocked and offended at their summary dismissal of Hmong values and knowledge, and at their failure to show respect for even those Hmong adjudicators of the greatest wisdom and highest community status (for some, a status considerably higher than that of a physician in American society). Indeed, the physicians' lack of wisdom in these matters called into question for Mr. L and his family and community advocates the soundness and reliability of their medical judgments as well.

Cultural issues in health care include the values and goals of health professionals as much as those of patients (see Table 7). They include the special questions raised and considerations imposed by differences between the medical point of view and patients' beliefs and values, conceptions of health and illness, favored or required health care practices, decision-making patterns, dietary requirements or preferences, goals for treatment, "moral geographies" of the body that assign meaning to body parts (as clean, dirty, noble, base, etc.), conceptions of

Table 7. Cultural Issues in Health Care.

Cultural issues shape *providers'* attitudes and responses as much as those of *patients*. They include (but are not restricted to) such things as:

- definitions of what constitutes a problem, or stands in need of explanation or remediation;
- values and goals that determine what constitutes an appropriate response to problem situations;
- definitions of health, illness, and care;
- definitions of what constitutes a symptom, or of when a person is actually sick;
- conceptions of disease processes, their etiologies, and their interrelationships;
- constructions of the meanings of illness, both in general and regarding specific illnesses;
- "moral geographies" of the body, which affect how body parts are invested with meaning;
- expectations of the roles of sick people and of their care givers;
- religious or moral convictions that influence responses to health, illness, and treatment;
- behavioral rules for communication and for decision making;
- conceptions of necessary and of effective treatment for specific illnesses or aspects of illness;
- dietary patterns, and the ways in which foods are understood to relate to health and illness, as well as to other aspects of social life.

proper relationships between sick people and their various care givers, understanding of rights to contribute information, definitions of valid knowledge as a basis for action, and so on. All of us have a learned bias in favor of our own beliefs and values. This is as true of patients as it is of clinicians, of any one culture or worldview as of another. Cultural pluralism presents to the conventional health care system many epistemological and practical challenges, all of which require a framework of accommodation, or adaptive reconciliation, to bring about productive outcomes and good quality health care for all patients. It must be recognized that cultural diversity is not a problem to be solved (D. Hufford 1990; M. Hufford 1991) but a set of relationships to be negotiated. For the same reasons that lead us to cherish and protect biodiversity (the diversity of species), we ought to protect and cherish human cultural diversity. Because culture is the wellspring of all ideas and all possible solutions (Farley 1988b; Hufford 1990), cultural diversity provides us with "depth on the bench": a source of strength and adaptability, an enormous variety of ideas and resources, and a multiplicity of approaches to common human problems. In the arena of health care, it creates an expanded repertoire for discussion and implementation of health care options.

Taking Greater Account of the Patient's Point of View

The Issue of (and the Problem with) "Compliance"

There is enormous concern in the health professions with the issue of whether and to what extent patients accept and carry out medical advice in therapeutic and preventive regimens. This issue, called "compliance" (or, negatively, "noncompliance"), has essentially been conceptualized as a one-way street: the physician or other health professional determines and declares what is to be done; the patient is to do it. "Compliance" is a value-laden term, based on the assumption that the health professional is (and should be) in control of the therapeutic relationship (Stimson 1974; Conrad 1985; Trostle 1988). It suggests an image of the patient that "amount[s] to a moral prescription for patient behavior" (Stimson 1974:97) as malleable and obedient, a subordinate following the orders of a superior. A trip to the dictionary quickly outlines the foundations of the concept: to comply is "to conform or adapt one's actions to another's wishes"; compliance is "a disposition to yield to others;" and one who is compliant is "submissive" (Merriam-Webster's Collegiate Dictionary, Tenth Edition). In recent years there has been a move toward substitution of the term "adherence," based on recognition of the undesirable (to patients) qualities encoded in the relationship implied by "compliance" (see Sumartojo 1993). The shift, however, is almost always more semantic than substantive. To adhere is "to maintain loyalty," and adherence connotes "fidelity." While these terms at least do not *entail* fidelity or loyalty to a superior or to priorities established by someone else, their usage in the literature reveals them essentially to imply just that. The shift in terminology has not been accompanied by a real conceptual shift in defining the issue, which is still constructed from the sole point of view of the health professions and their goals. "Adherence" is, for all practical purposes, a euphemism for "compliance" and "nonadherence," though a newer usage, is still the same old "problem."

The unilateral model is conflict-based and focuses attention on a proliferation of efforts to successfully bring patients to heel. A critical flaw in this construction of the issue is its failure to take account of the real lives and circumstances, and of the active agency, of patients. This is especially ironic in that it omits from careful consideration the domain in which the action happens: that of the patient in his or her actual circumstances. It forecloses accurate description of the actual complexities of the interactions among health professionals and their goals, and patients and *their* goals in the real lived contexts in which they manage their health and their illnesses along with myriad other aspects of their lives. It reifies a false picture. Worse, it fosters pejorative images of patients and contributes an adversarial tone to provider-patient relations: the "noncompliant" patient is deviant, uncooperative, negligent, stubborn, ignorant, unreliable, or at the very least in default (Stimson 1974), a vexation to the health professional. His or her behavior is considered illegitimate. "Noncompliant" becomes an epithet (Trostle 1988), an adverse judgment of the presumed motives and character of the patient to whom it is applied. This view contributes to negative stereotyping and the damage that stereotyping always does, and tempts or allows health professionals to blame patients for not getting well.

The compliance/adherence model is formulated as if the patient were essentially a "blank sheet" (Donovan, Blake, and Fleming 1989; Donovan and Blake 1992), "not . . . able to make decisions of consequence regarding his illness or medication or . . . to evaluate the doctor's actions" and recommendations (Stimson 1974:100). It presumes "that the professional consultation signals an end to the patient's decision making about caring for the complaint," and "[denies] the legitimacy of behaviors that differ from the medical prescription" (Trostle 1988: 1305). But in fact, as we have seen throughout the foregoing chapters, patients do make evaluations, decisions, and choices about their health and its optimal care all the time. They derive their ideas from a variety of sources, among which conventional medical sources figure to varying degrees. People make treatment choices based on an enormous complex of interdependent variables: vernacular health beliefs (see also Donovan and Blake 1992:510) and the larger systems of values and ideologies in which they are embedded; personal experiences and the experiences of trusted others; competing social and economic demands (Trostle et al. 1983); the meaning they assign to specific illnesses and treatments (Conrad 1985); and what they themselves know about illnesses and about treatment options, both within and outside of the medical model.

Patients—people—*are* active agents in the course of their own health care (Trostle et al. 1983; Conrad 1985; Roberson 1983), and deliberately modify their medically recommended treatment regimens for all manner of reasons: they may be experimenting to see if they can get by with less; titrating their dosages according to their own theories or observations; attempting to avoid or reduce undesirable side effects; substituting a preferred "natural" product for a synthetically produced drug; altering a routine to bring it into congruence with the logistical realities of their working and social lives; or enacting a desire not to feel, be, or become drug-dependent (applicable to any category of drug; see Conrad 1985; Donovan and Blake 1992). One of the curious artifacts of the compliance/adherence model is that by constructing noncompliance as deviance, it portrays alterations from a clinically prescribed course as characteristics of *persons* rather than features of *situations* in which persons manage their health and treatment. Acceptance and following of a clinical prescription, however, "is not a personality trait, but a task-specific behavior" (Sumartojo 1993:1317) that can be affected by scores of circumstantial influences. Anyone (and any *sort* of one) may alter a prescribed regimen of one type but not of another; alter it under some sets of circumstances but not others.

To achieve a realistic picture of patients' behavior with respect to medications and treatments, we need to reconceptualize the issue. Conrad (1985) suggests reframing it as a study of patients' "medication practice[s]," though perhaps "therapeutic practices" would be more encompassing. Research needs to be expanded to include not just what patients have *not* done with reference to clinical prescriptions, but what they *have* done in addition or instead (Trostle 1988). It should not focus solely on the question, "why don't they do what I tell them to do (and how can I get them to do it)?" but cast a wider net to discover, for example, "what do they actually do?" "why are those the choices they make?" and "how can I incorporate this understanding into designing treatment plans?" The matter cannot rest only with increasing the measure of *responsibility* allocated to the patient to behave in certain ways, but must include recognition of the patient's *authority* to make reasoned choices as well—for patients are the only authorities on their own experiences of illness and its management in the context of their lives. Likewise, it cannot continue to place the burden of failures only on patients but must recognize the ways in which proposed treatment regimens have failed to match patients' understandings or meet patients' needs.

Significant numbers of people do not reorganize their lives so that they fall into line with a medical model or prescription, but rather the other way around: they "vary their medication practice on grounds connected to managing their everyday lives" (Conrad 1985:34). A realistic response to this truism calls for negotiating a working relationship between the providers' and the patients' perspectives on a given health care situation. This is not at all to suggest that the clinical and public health concerns of health professionals are not well founded, or that they do not propose an ideal course of action to achieve desired and important medical results. It is rather to observe that situations are seldom ideal, and that more players than the health professionals are involved as active managers of any health problem. Part of maintaining active participation in a pluralistic culture entails coming to recognize that one's own perspective is not the only one that exerts strong claims to being "right." Even when the professional position is right about the medical facts of the matter, there are many competing considerations, and the "medically correct" thing to do is not necessarily everyone's priority. An adaptive strategy calls for engagement of the patient's as well as the provider's points of view in negotiations that attempt to identify and increase common ground and work toward mutual solutions. It will take innovation on the part of health professionals to learn to construct multiple and flexible solutions, and will require some "modifications of services and changes in attitudes of personnel" (Curry 1968:1267; see also Roberson 1992) to bring about this shift in perspective and translate it into action. Perhaps one of the focal issues now should be "how medical staff can understand and participate in the decisions that patients already [make] about their medications" and other therapeutic and preventive routines (Donovan and Blake 1992:512).

Patient Education

Patient education (like "compliance," which it often aims to foster) also has been constructed as a one-way street: the health professional has knowledge to transmit; the patient is the receiver, whose job it is to "take it in." As with "compliance," the view is medicocentric and patients are essentially left out of the account except as objects of improvement. Whether its intended audience is individuals in the clinic, or whole communities in public health and outreach efforts, patient education is traditionally designed by health professionals on the basis of their own priorities and values, for which the patient education effort is an export vehicle. Intended beneficiaries are defined as "target" populations. A target is "something to be affected by an action or development": something to take action *at*, not *with*. These efforts are in the great majority sincere and well intended, motivated by genuine and deeply felt desires to help. Their primary goal is to promote important and real improvements in the health status of their intended audiences. Nevertheless, typical patient education efforts incorporate the same conceptual flaws as the "compliance" model: they are mostly unilateral designs founded on an assumption of professional dominance and authority, and incorporating a prescriptive view of an essentially subordinate and receptive role for patients. Patients are not recognized as having knowledge or as functioning as active agents themselves (see Reiser 1992).

Health professionals engaged in educational efforts intend to be agents of change (see Egeland 1978; Chambers 1989; Farley 1988a). One of the explicit goals of patient education efforts is to bring about change in beliefs and behavior patterns (both in individual patients and in patient populations), in particular to "penetrate the beliefs that thwart adoption of [medically] prescribed health behaviors" (Levin and Idler 1981:234). This is ordinarily conceptualized as "normalizing" (read: medicalizing) the views of the patient population, that is, bringing them into congruence with medical definitions of health needs and priorities and of the most appropriate means to meet them. Patients to be educated are often assumed to be "empty vessels" who, in the absence of medically accepted knowledge about health and illness, are assumed to have *no* knowledge about them as a basis for making choices or taking action (see Donovan, Blake, and Fleming 1989). The conception of patient education thus frequently operates on the basis of an extremely simplistic view of its mission: "communicate successfully with people so they will understand their health problems (usually as we, not they, define them) and they will want to change their behavior" (Foster and Anderson 1978:214). When the proposed changes do not occur, or when they come about very slowly, the cause is generally interpreted as "resistance to change" and defined as a "problem" which is located in the "target population" (Egeland 1978; Foster and Anderson 1978; Farley 1988a; Chambers 1989).[8]

As in the case of "compliance," a critical flaw in the unidirectional model of patient education is its equivalent omission of the actualities of patients: their circumstances, experiences, worldview, knowledge, values, self-perceived needs, and their agency in responding to these. The problem can be illustrated by a public health education example which follows a generic and familiar pattern. Health needs are identified in a community by medical and public health personnel, using "objective" (impersonal; outsiders') measures. Design of public health services to meet the identified needs is carried out exclusively by members of the professions, and is followed by large-scale "outreach" and education activities. The aim of these efforts is both to inform prospective patients about the availability of services and to "educate" them to the need for the services and so encourage their use. "Appropriate" use (defined from the professional perspective) should bring about the intended improvements in the health status of the population for whom the services are intended. Actual rates of utilization that are lower than the projected ideal will be classified as "under-use" of services (when they actually might indicate rejection of services as unnecessary, undesirable, or inappropriate by the community's standards; see Rempusheski 1989). Uses by patients in ways other than those intended by the designers will be classified as "misuse" of services (when they actually might be adaptive strategies employed by community members to shape the services to what they want and need). Here again, *situational* features are likely to be interpreted as characteristics of persons or of specific populations.

In efforts of this order, the actions and attitudes of health professionals often appear arrogant, misguided, superfluous, or absurd from the point of view of their intended beneficiaries. Members of "targeted" populations not infrequently see health professionals' efforts and exhortations as uninvited, even unwelcome, advances thrust upon them by outsiders self-appointed as competent to define their needs and to do their thinking for them. Efforts to bring patient groups "up" to the level of officially accepted health priorities and standards of knowledge or practice frequently engender resentment and rejection. This is especially likely to be the case when professional efforts are made across boundaries of race, ethnicity, cultural heritage, and social class—as public health efforts in particular very often are. As one community spokeswoman in Philadelphia put it: "The community *cannot* look at the medical profession as if they have *all* the answers, and the medical community must understand that they *don't* have all the answers" (Sheila Laney, President, Block Captains' Association of Southwest Germantown, address delivered at an internal symposium on prevention at the Medical College of Pennsylvania, 20 May 1993; manuscript; emphasis in original). The one-sidedness of the model contributes to the failure of many endeavors it engenders, very often making its hoped-for patient populations feel unconsidered and invaded: "The community is *not* a training ground for doctors because we are *more* than just an illness or a disease" (ibid.; emphasis in original).

The example of colonialism can help to illuminate this reaction. Historically, colonialists have imposed themselves on the indigenous populations of locations that they have selected for conquest, arriving uninvited and pursuing with implacable determination their own imported agendas. They have set about enforcing change with the "conviction and missionary zeal of a people who were certain that their way of life was vastly superior to that of the peoples who fell under their new-found dominion" (Chambers 1989:53). Colonialists have seldom acknowledged the validity of indigenous values and knowledge, their ethnocentrism leading them to assume instead that "their technological achievements . . . made self-evident their moral and intellectual superiority" (Foster and Anderson 1978:212). Health professionals, though clearly with less power and arguably with much more honorable intentions, have nevertheless operated from an analogous frame of reference. As a result they have often "found it difficult to believe that the 'obvious superiority' of their methods is not alone sufficient to win . . . acceptance" (Foster and Anderson 1978:225).

Health professionals' conviction of their epistemological and methodological superiority is not necessarily shared by patient populations, however. The fact that health professionals possess superior clinical knowledge and population-based health statistics does not translate into their possessing superior knowledge of every sort that is relevant to identifying, addressing, or resolving the health problems of a given group as its members themselves define and experience them. As the preceding chapters have shown, ordinary people have all manner of cultural and experiential knowledge about health and illness, and they constantly make decisions and take actions based on that knowledge. They continually evaluate the care they are offered and receive, discuss options with one another, learn from each other and from innumerable other sources. In addition, *they*—not the health professions— make the determination of where issues of health fit in among the competing concerns and priorities of their lives.

A solution to the colonial undercurrent of patient education and to the frequent failure of educational efforts to achieve their desired behavioral ends (whether in adoption of individual preventive actions, or in achievement of large-scale use of services such as prenatal care) must again entail a reformulation of the relationships involved. Communication, by definition, is not a one-way process. Effective education requires interchange. All parties to the issue—health professionals, patients, and participating community members—have a role in identifying and prioritizing health needs, framing the definition of the problems to be resolved, contributing to the design and delivery of the solutions, and serving as educators to each other and to the public. Adoption of a collaborative model will include a view of the issues "as they are experienced and defined by those persons who are otherwise most likely to be left out of the decision making processes" (Chambers 1989:xi). Intended beneficiaries need to be recognized not as "targets" of outsiders' actions, but as participating actors and contributors, with equal ownership of the effort and investment in its outcomes, right from the first. This will require a fundamental shift in orientation on the part of health professionals: from expecting "them" to become like "us" or to conform to professional goals and expectations (Farley 1988a), to a recognition that "we all" must be involved in moving toward mutually agreed upon goals in mutually acceptable ways. This view is equally applicable to public health and to individual patient educational interchanges. Its importance lies in commitment to making the effort, in willingness to initiate and sustain the dialogue—even when complete agreement on goals and means to their achievement is unlikely to be reached.

To bring about this change a new symmetry will have to be introduced into the relationships between health professionals and patients or patient populations. Health professionals will need to be able to see themselves as members of *a*—not *the*—value system; as coparticipants in, and not sole dictators of, health education and health services. The goal of modifying or changing attitudes and behaviors will have to expand to include modification of attitudes and behaviors of health professionals as well as of patients. Old questions and observations will have to be reformulated to be multidirectional. For example, it will not be sufficient to study how and why patient populations fail to understand or respond to health care initiatives and educational efforts without also seeking to understand how and why health care initiatives and educational efforts fail to prove interesting, meaningful, or engaging to patients. "It is clear that unless the members of a [particular] group come to share similar health priorities with the specialists who wish to help them, interest and cooperation in . . . projects will be difficult to achieve" (Foster and Anderson 1978:237). It should be equally clear that unless the specialists who wish to help any particular group come to share similar health priorities with the group members themselves, interest and cooperation in projects will be equally difficult to achieve. Mutual accommodation is required, incorporating both health professionals' and patients' perspectives.

Interactive patient education will necessarily entail provider education and is therefore more likely to promote mutual comprehension and appreciation. Each constituency can both teach and learn from the other. Understanding of cultural factors is essential to selection and promotion of particular health behaviors, since behavior is quintessentially culturally shaped (this is equally true for providers and for patients). Recognition of the existence, prevalence, and significance of vernacular health belief systems is critical for grasping their bearing on the ways in which people identify and define health and illness, and engage in treatment, prevention, and health promotion activities. All parties to the endeavor will have to grant legitimacy to each other's concerns, and recognize that *each* group (patients and health professionals) has significant and well-considered mandates to which its members must be responsive. A number of studies have demonstrated that interactive patient education efforts prove very successful in increasing patients' vested interest in adoption and pursuit of medically recommended therapies, in improvement of the overall patient-provider relationship, and in enhancement of long-term therapeutic outcomes (see, for example, Svarstad 1978; Anderson, Toledo, and Hazam 1982; Weidman 1982). Health professionals committed to their own beliefs about the important goals of medical care must surely find such outcomes desirable, warranting efforts to incorporate change. Accomplishment of the task—education for health promotion and improved health outcomes—must be given primacy over maintenance of established or emergent authority relations, and each constituency must be prepared to compromise to achieve mutually desirable ends. Collaboration and negotiation will not eliminate conflicts between belief systems, but they do make possible a degree of cooperation which—though perhaps not ideal from the point of view of either patients or providers—can be acceptable to and productive for both.

Medical Ethics

The activity of medical ethics (alternatively called bioethics or biomedical ethics) is not an effort to persuade or convince, but a process of moral inquiry aimed at negotiating conflicts among divergent but equally compelling mandates in medical action and decision making. This process entails the identification and comparative evaluation of all of the goals, and the means to their attainment, called forth by a particular set of medical and sociocultural circumstances. The eventual decision requires the establishment of moral priorities, in light of all of the actual circumstances and cherished ideals bearing on the case (Ackerman 1989). The field of biomedical ethics has been developed purposively and self-consciously as a secular philosophical enterprise with the goal of identifying and applying ethical principles that transcend the convictions of particular religions and the dictates of specific cultures (Engelhardt 1982). This goal embodies two fundamental concepts: (1) recognition of the plurality of systems of values in the world, which renders it impossible to establish by consensus a single vision of "the good life" or of proper action in all circumstances; and (2) a commitment to "framing an understanding of how a society will deport itself in conditions [in which] one view of the good life, or of the nature of man, will not be imposed by force" (Engelhardt 1982:65).

In the United States, primacy is culturally assigned to personal values and individual autonomy, in congruence with our cultural construction of personhood (see de Craemer 1983). Attentive respect for patient autonomy is considered a minimum operating condition for ethical medical decision making (Loewy 1989). In other words, in this enterprise the patient's point of view and authoritative agency are not only recognized, but are ideally weighed in the balance at least equally with the professional point of view. In many circumstances the patient's values and desires have primacy in determination of the highest order good and the path to its achievement. Cautioning that the health professionals are in a position to extend their "authority in technical matters over the patient's system of beliefs and values" (Pellegrino 1974:1290), bioethicists enshrine careful consideration of the values of the patient as one of the general operating rules of medical decision making. Some insist that good and ethical medical decisions cannot in fact be made "until the lay person supplies the value framework to be used" (Veatch 1985:3).[9]

Some form of ranking of "goods" is a requisite underpinning for the clinical ethical enterprise. Highest ranking and most compelling in the schema of many theorists is the patient's own chosen "good of last resort" or ultimate personal good: for example, the priority and moral value assigned to death versus life in a vegetative or physically helpless state, or the relative valuation of spiritual salvation versus physical survival. Next in rank is the "good of the patient-as-person," which compels physicians' beneficence and respect for patients' autonomy. This is the driving principle behind the rule and practice of informed consent (recognition of the patient's right to information bearing upon consent, including granting access to complete information; enhancement of competence in decision making by, e.g., providing translators when needed, suspending the use of drugs adversely affecting mental clarity, etc.). In the ranking also is the *prima facie* "biomedical good" (what ought ideally to be done medically), which is outweighed by the aforementioned higher-order considerations in cases when they and the "biomedical good" conflict (Pellegrino and Thomasma 1981; see also Loewy 1989:54–55).

It is an inescapable irony that the very construction of bioethics and its ground rules encodes the values of particular cultural traditions. Indeed, it could not be otherwise, for ethical first principles are cultural products, shaped by culturally provided moral codes, definitions of a multiplicity of desirable "goods," and rules for rank-ordering conflicting "goods" in various kinds of situations. The central principles of bioethics as we now know it in the United States are derived from Western cultural backgrounds, formal intellectual traditions, and a largely Judeo-Christian moral framework (Kunstadter 1980; Flack and Pellegrino 1992). These principles include autonomy of patients, beneficence of physicians, and the principle of parentalism (to use the gender-neutral form) by which in certain circumstances a physician may override a patient's wishes to act in what s/he judges to be the patient's best interest. Customary practices and professional mandates that derive from these foundational principles include abiding as much as possible by the patient's wishes in matters of treatment, maintenance of a patient's confidentiality, disclosure of diagnosis and prognosis (truth-telling), seeking of informed consent for treatment (includes disclosure), and efforts to determine what constitutes the patient's best interest—generally in circumstances in which the patient's decisional capacity is in question.

Medical problems have emotional, psychological, aesthetic, religious, interpersonal, and practical dimensions that differ across cultures and belief systems and that impel certain kinds of action and constrain others. Ethical principles are not cultural universals (see Kunstadter 1980; Lieban 1991). Moral mandates and ethical convictions differ cross-culturally, as do the specific goals and ends that are cherished. There is cultural variability in the recognition of who may have the authority or the mandate to protect the patient's best interest, and to define in what that best interest consists. In some cultures the concept of individual autonomy does not exist or is not meaningful; the individual's rights and obligations are constituted in the framework of kinship or community networks (de Craemer 1983). This was illustrated in the case of Mr. L. in Chapter 3, and affected, among other things, the consent procedure: "decisional capacity" in Hmong culture resides in the clan and even in community adjudicators, but not properly in individual persons, especially in circumstances of serious consequence (see also Kisken and Kisken 1990). A similar situation holds for many Native American cultures (Barre Toelken, personal communication).

Both the nature of truth and the circumstances for its telling are culturally variable. A number of cultures deem it proper that the disclosure of any diagnosis or prognosis be made to a person other than the patient, for the patient is to be shielded from distress and cared for by others. In these cultural frameworks, such conduct is both customary and considerate, as well as morally correct. In the case of bad news especially, it may be the family's moral duty to protect the patient from negative or frightening information (Long and Long 1982; Meleis and Jonsen 1983; Beyene 1992; Klessig 1992; Muller and Desmond 1992), or to break the news themselves in the appropriate manner and setting (Beyene 1992). Physicians who pursue their professional obligation to disclose information (either toward the end of truth-telling or as a means to obtaining informed consent), especially in the instance of a grave or terminal illness, may be seen to be doing direct harm to the patient or acting in a manner damaging to the patient's best interest (Brotzman and Butler 1992; Beyene 1992), and thereby violating their mandate of beneficence.[10] In situations judged to be medically futile, simply raising the issue of termination of life-sustaining treatment may, from certain cultural perspectives, likewise be seen as contributing to the patient's decline. Such an action would, by those cultures' definitions, constitute a breach of the patient's best interest and a violation of beneficence (Klessig 1992). Ironically, such an action may even violate what bioethics itself would define as the patient's autonomy or right to self-determination, since that autonomy may in some value systems involve the patient's sovereign right to be protected from disclosures that remove hope. Death may be a matter for the determination of God, not mortals, and miraculous intervention may be considered to be possible at any stage—but only in the presence of active faith and hope; to destroy hope is therefore to hasten or contribute to the death of the patient (Beyene 1992).

Giving genuinely equal weight to all patients' belief systems will pose epistemological and ontological challenges for bioethics. May we grant as serious considerations assertions that persons have (one or more) souls? That souls have obligations and destinies? That the health of souls may be as important or more important than the health of bodies? That souls and spirits, if improperly treated, may afflict or endanger the living? That spiritual salvation may take precedence over physical survival (even in apparently remediable situations)? That God or other supernatural agents may intervene to heal (even in apparently hopeless or futile situations)? That there are instrumental relationships between the living and the dead? That such relationships should be taken into account in deliberations at the beginning and at the end of life? That knowledge may be gained by direct apprehension, through dreams, or by supernatural agency? That such knowledge is a sound and reasonable basis for decision and action? That individual autonomy is meaningless or undesirable, or that familial or community good inherently takes precedence over individual benefit? These are not rhetorical questions. Not only are these concerns well represented in a growing body of ethnographic and ethics literature, but all of these are convictions that are held by people whom I myself have interviewed, and with whom I have worked. They are, in other words, real convictions that are deeply held by members of patient populations in the United States today. To deny them in medical settings is to deny the patient's very reality, risking serious psychological and emotional impact on patient and family alike and raising genuine ethical concerns.

What weight is to be given to these considerations in ethical deliberation? What justification could be used for failure to give them due attention? When a "reasonable person" standard is applied in instances of substituted judgment, whose cultural construction of what the "reasonable person" would want or believe will shape it? Medical ethics presupposes coming to a choice of action from among a number of possible "right" courses. It enshrines individual autonomy, recognizes differences in point of view, and abjures the use of force, including mental, psychological, and ideological coercion. Does exclusive application of a hegemonic ontology and epistemology in defining the field of acceptable considerations constitute in some cases a use of ideological force, and therefore a coercive action inimical to the very heart of the ethical endeavor? How are these difficult boundaries to be drawn so that "realities are neither rigidly fixed nor entirely subject to *ad hoc* interpretation" (Loewy 1989:24)? Bioethics by its very nature is a discipline of questions and of competing claims and mandates. It is critical to the moral inquiry which is its business that the process be open and fair. Due consideration of patients' values and beliefs cannot be guided alone by their degree of familiarity, strangeness, or propriety in the estimation of the ethicist or clinician: these are not inherent qualities of propositions, but consequences of exposure and knowledge, products of judgment by culturally supplied and personally honed sets of standards. In the future it will be difficult, but essential, to "prevent [the] preemptory and premature rejection" (Flack and Pellegrino 1992:viii) of ideas and values which have not heretofore formed a part of the essential framework upon which bioethics is founded.[11]

Education and Training of Health Professionals

Promotion of changes in practice, if it is to have any far-reaching or long-lasting effect, must be underwritten by parallel changes in the education and training of health professionals. One of the critical shifts required is that of fundamental orientation to professional and patient roles and knowledge: to bring about a genuine recognition that the health professional's goals, values, and professional belief and knowledge system is but *one* of the significant viewpoints that will be brought to bear in any encounter with patients. This orientation is already one of the cornerstones of the field of transcultural nursing and should be incorporated into the education of all health professionals. All of us are aware that even within our own epistemological frameworks there are multiple ways in which to interpret a problem or a set of observations, and therefore a variety of reasonable ways to respond. This basic recognition can be broadened to include the patient's belief system as another of the recognized ways in which reasonable people respond to a given set of health circumstances, and this can happen irrespective of professional agreement with particular patients' reasons or conclusions. Heretofore the customary professional presumption has been that the layperson's perspective is necessarily problematic to the extent that it differs from the professional point of view. Training in a more accommodating professional mindset will permit the patient's perspective to be treated as a resource, a source of information to be engaged, rather than as a set of "complications" or obstacles to be overcome (see Delbanco 1992; Gerteis et al. 1993; Hufford 1993a).

The best outcome of an interaction cannot be gained without an effort to understand what motivates *all* parties. An understanding of one's own conceptual framework is thus as necessary as an understanding of others' worldviews to the promotion of fairness in judgment and productivity in efforts at conflict resolution. A productive model is furnished by contemporary ethnography, the descriptive study of culture. A primary research method of the social sciences,[12] ethnography provides a very useful tool for developing both greater self-awareness (reflexivity) and the capacity to better understand patients' belief systems. The method itself can be adapted to some facets of provider education and skills training (see Stein 1982b). The inclusion in a patient history of a few open-ended questions about health beliefs, goals for treatment, and other important personal values adapts it in brief to the clinical setting. Full-scale use may be made in needs assessment projects preliminary to the establishment of community-based practices (Snider and Stein 1987), to the design and delivery of specialized services, or to public health efforts (e.g., Weidman 1978). Most germane to all of provider education, however, is not necessarily the method itself but the ethnographic perspective, particularly its recognition of the expertise and knowledge of the cultural *insider*.[13] This is a stance which differs from and moves beyond empathy. It aims to grasp how individuals and communities *themselves* understand their lives, define their needs, and set their priorities (in this case, with respect to health).

Ideally, the ethnographic perspective assumes a relationship between the "observer" and the "observed" (e.g., the health professional and the patient or patient population) which recognizes that each is privy to certain important orders of knowledge and information. "Observers" aim to learn *from*—not just about—the "observed." This approach has clinical applicability to both diagnosis and treatment, in addition to its obvious relevance for provider-patient relations. For example: patients define what is and is not considered a "symptom" for them, and assign meaning to symptoms in ways that influence when they turn to someone for care, what kinds of care they choose and from whom, and what they say about their problem. They also weigh in the balance their goals for treatment against what treatments are obtainable from various sources, and what their desirable and undesirable aspects are. If making the best of a condition or its symptoms is more important to a person than achieving a remission with considerable loss of function, or if retaining the ability to engage in certain activities is more important than relieving or preventing exacerbation of associated pain, these preferences will guide patients' choices of and responses to treatment.

Health professionals need to balance these important personal goals with medical goals in formulating treatment recommendations. Both viewpoints must be engaged:

[O]nly the patient *knows* the effects of [an illness and of] prior treatment decisions upon *his or her* quality of life, while only the provider has a full understanding of the pathophysiological consequences of those same decisions. . . . It is not that the physician should generally try to see things *entirely* from the patient's perspective. . . . It is rather that *only* the patient can truly occupy that perspective, and the patient therefore has access to essential information for which he or she is the only valid source. (Hufford 1993a:169)

An ethnographic perspective requires self-awareness in order to avoid projection of one's own values, categories, and other assumptions onto others thereby obscuring from view their frame of reference. At the same time, it contributes to the achievement and refinement of self-awareness through the illumination of areas of congruence and incongruence between two parties' sets of expectations and values.

New information will have to be incorporated into the professional knowledge base. Curricula should address cultural issues and uses of vernacular healing systems in all teaching areas to which any psychosocial aspects of health, illness, and care are relevant. Members of local patient populations, and clients and practitioners of vernacular healing systems prominent in the locality, make informative guest lecturers and discussants. Inclusion of general overviews of cultural repertoires and of vernacular healing systems, together with specific examples drawn from the immediate practice area, will give health professionals both specific background information and theoretical models: ways of thinking about the multiplicity of points of view that are held by reasonable people for sound and comprehensible reasons. All manner of assumptive stereotyping should be foregrounded, including those encounters in which "culture" or significant difference in worldview between patients and care providers are *not* anticipated as factors. This may be the case when patients do not fit prevailing expectations, or when their differences in worldview are of relatively low profile to others (though not necessarily of minor significance). An example of the former case is the extensive use of alternative health care resources by middle-class, well-educated, and thoroughly acculturated patients (including extremely high rates for some classes of illness; see Kronenfeld and Wasner 1982). An example of the latter is any instance in which care providers incorrectly assume shared belief systems with patients on the basis of shared ethnicity, race, educational background, or social class (see Branch and Paxton 1976; Weidman 1982; Dowling 1987). Inclusion of such material will, if presented fairly, focus attention on making individual patients more visible, complete, and understandable as people, and keep both preventive and curative health care efforts in the context of persons and their lives:

Ideally physicians should define their diagnostic and therapeutic goals in terms of the everyday life and function of individual patients. Unfortunately that ideal is seldom met . . . because doctors seem to be trained to focus on diseases almost to the exclusion of how sick persons actually live their lives in families and communities. In part the problem arises because physicians are trained from the first days of medical school to disregard the knowledge they bring with them of everyday life and human function as irrelevant to medicine. (Cassell 1984:16)

Educational changes must also provide for the acquisition of relevant new skills and competencies. It has become almost a commonplace in recent years to exhort health professionals to develop cultural sensitivity, and more recently, to acquire cultural *competence*.[14] "Sensitivity" denotes awareness and implies responsiveness, but has the ring of being ancillary to the job: a respectful and generous attitude, politically correct, but not actually required for effectiveness. "Competence," on the other hand, is critical. It is the essential quality of being "fit, qualified or capable," and of "having the requisite ability" to do the job effectively. Cultural competence is pertinent to many health care-related endeavors: administration, education, planning, analysis, policy making, and provision of services and care. Cultural competence does not require the health professional to be a social scientist, nor to memorize reams of facts about numerous cultural groups and "how they think" about health and illness. In fact, to undertake the latter is to invite stereotyping.[15] What it does require is the capacity to assess one's own work, as well as to assess patients, in cultural terms (Hufford 1990). It entails recognition of patients as possessors of authoritative points of view, and elicitation and engagement of patients' values and preferences. This step will come more easily to some health professions than to others because of existing and historical orientations to clients, for example, nursing's philosophical stance of engagement with patients as contrasted with medicine's general stance of detachment (Anspach 1987; Hoffmaster 1992).

Presently "culture" is thought of in health care as being pertinent to certain patients, as "part of what makes *some* patients 'different'— especially makes them different from care providers and from the system in general" (Hufford 1990:35). But it cannot be overstressed that *all ideas and values are the products of culture.* Ideas about health, illness, and care are cultural, regardless of whether they are learned throughout life within a specific cultural heritage group; acquired through new affiliations or changes in lifestyle; learned in the library; gleaned from talking with members of a social network formed around a particular interest, illness experience, or health threat; or acquired in formal professional training. Cultural factors shape all people, providers and patients alike. Cultural competence applies to interactions with *all* patients, irrespective of heritage, *and* to providers' self-understanding as well. The culturally competent provider will routinely "consider . . . cultural perspectives as part of total client assessment" (Henkle and Kennerly 1990:146) and see "acceptance of individual differences as important components of client care" (ibid.:147). Just as it is now standard procedure for clinicians to observe universal precautions with respect to body fluids, it should become standard procedure to observe "universal considerations" with respect to elicitation of and responsiveness to patients' health-related beliefs and values, goals and desires.

Adding Sociocultural Context to the Health Care Encounter

Elicitation of the patient's perspective should be included in history-taking and should cover certain basic categories at a minimum: explanatory models of illness, goals and preferences for treatment, and measures of care undertaken outside the conventional health care system. Patients' explanatory models of illness (Kleinman 1975, 1980) contain information that is pertinent, and at times even critical, to clinical success, including patients' views of "(1) etiology; (2) time and mode of onset; (3) pathophysiology; (4) course, including . . . degree of sickness . . . ; and (5) [recommended] treatment" (Blumhagen 1982:301; see also Nations, Camino, and Walker 1985). A few well-put questions and a receptive attitude are simple and effective elicitation tools (Kleinman, Eisenberg, and Good 1978). Different individuals and cultural groups value symptoms differently, some causing greater distress and implying much more serious risk or significant loss than others. Patients' and providers' interpretations of the presenting symptoms may well be at variance (Cassell 1984). Failure to discover these meanings may result in misunderstandings that can affect both the success of a particular clinical encounter and long-term therapeutic success as well as the patient-provider relationship. Goals for treatment may vary radically between patients with the same disease, or between any given patient and clinicians. These differences too can compromise the success of therapeutic efforts and may also lead to quite different assessments of what actually constitutes therapeutic success (see Delbanco 1992; Hufford 1993). Since beliefs and explanations pertaining to health are responsive to experience and new input and are thus changeable over time, explanatory models and goals for treatment ought to be elicited in the history-taking at each illness episode (Blumhagen 1982; Hufford, 1984, 1985b, 1993b) in extended relationships with the same patients. Inquiries about uses of nonbiomedical healing modalities should be a routine part of the patient history (Eisenberg et al. 1993).

In any given practice locality, familiarity with common health practices, as well as with vernacular terms for body parts and functions, for diseases and dysfunctions, and of course for "folk illnesses" is of considerable utility. Since folk illnesses have been shown to have a measurable impact on morbidity and mortality (Rubel, O'Nell, and Collado-Ardón 1984), a knowledge of folk illness categories and a capacity to respond to them seriously are valuable clinical assets. Health professionals taking into account patients' health belief systems will need to be able to assess (independently or through consultation) which vernacular health care practices they feel need changing in particular circumstances and which do not. Such case-based assessment substitutes informed judgment for reflex rejection of the unfamiliar. Since "folk beliefs can support a wide range of effective behavior, without being modified," (Egeland 1978:192), providers need not relentlessly "educate" patients to agree with professional perceptions of all matters. With respect for patients' epistemologies, health professionals can build common ground with patients to work toward mutually important goals, even when their specific rationales and constructions of the situation differ.

More than simply learning how to elicit and integrate new orders of information from patients, clinicians and other health professionals must also become able to exchange information, including why they believe their own preferences and recommendations to be important. Much of this is to say that physicians and other health professionals will need to be able to engage in genuine dialogue with patients, to negotiate—sometimes across widely divergent belief systems—and to promote accommodative rather than authoritarian strategies in patient-provider interactions. An understanding of the biases produced by ethnocentrism and its counterpart, medicocentrism, will contribute to flexibility. Patients have as much to contribute to biomedicine as to gain from it (Reiser 1993). The introduction of nonbiomedical values as *equally important* determinants of action holds the potential to help dissolve an impasse, to foster mutual trust between patients and clinicians, and to improve the quality and responsiveness of health care. Note that none of this is to suggest that providers ought to abandon or downplay the significance of their professional beliefs and values or of their clinical knowledge and expertise. Far from it. It is rather to say that along with this vital information should be included in consideration additional critical information: that which in the end governs how people respond both to their health concerns and to medical advice.

Recapitulation

The spectrum of health care resources in United States today is characterized by a broad plurality of systems of health beliefs and practices.
Conventional professional Western medicine, though it is the officially
sanctioned system of care, is only one of the healing resources to which
innumerable people in this country routinely have recourse. The remainder I have called vernacular health belief systems: the extensive
variety of folk and popular healing modalities undertaken outside the
domain of conventional medicine. By examining, both in general and
in depth, a sampling of vernacular health beliefs and practices readily
discoverable in the United States in the current decade, this study has
attempted to illuminate some of the ways in which people's experiences, needs, beliefs, and values influence their health care choices,
and to address the implications of those choices for health professions
education and health care design and delivery.

The long-standing prediction of modernization—that as science and
medicine progressed and education became more widely accessible,
folk and popular healing systems would decline and be replaced—has
not been borne out in actuality. Vernacular health care systems have
persisted alongside medical advancement, and they remain quite vital
at present. Indeed, many such systems have recently experienced an
upsurge in patronage and popularity, both in the United States and in
other complex, modern societies. Vernacular healing systems have
adherents among every ethnicity and social class, and at all levels of
educational attainment. They address all aspects of health: preventive
behaviors, optimal health maintenance routines, nutritional concerns,
therapeutic actions and substances, rehabilitation, management of
acute and chronic illness, handling of birth and death, coping with
suffering, overall attitudes and lifestyles. New variants develop continually.

The familiar stereotypes of marginality, ignorance, and desperation
that have attached to use of nonconventional healing strategies are
inadequate to a genuine understanding of vernacular health belief
systems and the people who use them. These misleading images seriously distort the picture, both in clinical encounters and in the literature. They misrepresent the majority of both the systems and their
adherents, and they entirely overlook very large numbers of users of
these pervasive health care resources. The equally prominent misconception that people using vernacular healing resources typically do so
to the exclusion of conventional medical care generates a good deal of
distress among health professionals on the basis of a false premise.
Though this is sometimes the case, it is in fact much more common that

both types of health care are used, either serially or simultaneously. A form of self-triage operates in the selection of treatment combinations that, in an individual's own opinion, best address particular health concerns. The individual himself or herself manages the integration of the selected therapeutic systems.

Clearly, this active and complex sphere of vernacular health belief and practice has significant implications for the health professions, both in education and training, and in clinical activities. These implications are likely to become more salient in the foreseeable future, given the pressures for change being brought to bear on the official health care system: from structural changes in the ownership, management, and delivery of care; to the altered constellation of health care needs of an aging and increasingly ethnically and culturally diverse population; to the expense, distresses, and ethical dilemmas of burgeoning medical technologies; to a steadily mounting public disaffection with the procedures, values, and interaction styles of conventional medical care. In this climate, it is predictable that the parallel streams of unofficial healing traditions and the alternatives that they offer will continue to flourish and to expand their constituencies.

It is important therefore for vernacular healing systems to be well studied, thoroughly described, and well understood in all of their aspects. This will require interdisciplinary efforts, pursued with rigor of scholarship and avoidance of polemic. Such study must incorporate (and continue to verify) the recognition that vernacular health beliefs and practices, like conventional medical care, are systematic bodies of thought that are fundamentally rational, and which are bolstered by lengthy histories of ideas, considerable social support, and reputations for efficacy sustained by experience, observation, and evaluative processes. It must take into account patients' own authority and agency, and be descriptive, rather than prescriptive in nature. Attention needs to be directed both to illuminating and obviating the risks some vernacular healing actions pose, and to understanding and encouraging the ways in which these systems function as significant and effective therapeutic resources.

Patients will continue to make (and have the right to make) treatment choices in keeping with their own values and preferences. Health professionals need to be equipped to understand the basis of those choices, as well as to be explicitly aware of their own values so that they can better understand their responses to patients. Such an understanding must encompass an appreciation of the relationship of culture and worldview to values and to definitions of and responses to health, illness, and care—for all people, regardless of heritage or professional training. The biopsychosocial model of illness is gaining recognition in many areas of medicine and is well accepted in nursing, if not yet very thoroughly integrated into the routine clinical practices of either. Vernacular healing resources, and the myriad factors that sustain their use, are part of a thorough application of that model.

The conception of the patient-provider relationship as a therapeutic alliance, common in the professional literature, remains more theoretical than actual. A reconfiguration of responsibility and authority, a recognition of the ideal patient role as one of full participant, will be necessary to realization of the model. This will require the capacity of health professionals to accept the patient as an active co-shaper of the relationship and of health care choices and actions, rather than as a limited partner to whom various duties are merely delegated. It is time to put recognition into standard practice, to translate theories, ideas, and intentions into action toward the end of creating more humane and responsive health care through facilitation of understanding and communication, and promotion of mutual respect, between care providers and patients. This humanitarian concern addresses as well such very practical issues as improving the quality of care and increasing the satisfaction of patients and providers alike.

Notes

1. To the health professional frustrated by patients who apparently will not take action on their own behalf, this will seem an ironic statement. Two considerations apply: (1) that different individuals take up authoritative roles to differing degrees, and any given person will take them up differently depending on particular circumstances at the time of "patienthood"; and (2) that the decision to relinquish all responsibility to health professionals is a form of exercise of patients' authoritative agency. That is, they make firm choices about health care—including the entire continuum between choices to turn it over entirely to others, and choices to run the show themselves.

2. The creation in the summer of 1992 of the Office of Alternative Medicine, under the auspices of the National Institutes of Health, may change this situation, although their initial two-year budget of $2 million, to include both staffing/administration and research grants, permits only a handful of projects funded at $30,000 each—very small potatoes by usual NIH research grant standards. Nevertheless, it is the first such sizeable effort with government sponsorship, and is also noteworthy for its requirement that all projects must be collaborative efforts between investigators with conventional research experience and representatives of the alternative therapy or system under investigation (see National Institutes of Health 1993).

3. The example cited refers to interviewees whose cultural backgrounds did not include familiarity with traditional Chinese medicine (TCM) or acupuncture; they had all learned about TCM through their own research or by word of mouth. Patients to whose cultural backgrounds TCM is indigenous are likely to prefer the traditional practitioner to the physician-acupuncturist, too: not

because they are specifically seeking a new paradigm or a different view of their illnesses, but because they know through life experience and cultural teaching that the traditional practitioner is indicated by the situation and that s/he has a greater depth of knowledge and experience. In addition, such a practitioner is likely to share both linguistic and conceptual interpretive and communicative frameworks with the patient.

4. These are matters of both federal and state regulation. The FDA ruling on importation for personal use of limited quantities of foreign pharmaceuticals, mentioned in Chapter 4, is an example of an area which is federally regulated; the legal statuses of lay midwives and licensed acupuncturists are examples of state regulatory jurisdiction.

5. Even the growing practice of seeking second and third opinions *within* the conventional medical system may signal a disinclination (on the part of both patients and health professionals) to believe there is a single solution for any health problem of even minor complexity.

6. It is incorrect to think of some people or groups as "ethnic" and others not. All people can also be defined, or can define themselves, in terms of ethnicity (see Stern and Cicala 1991).

7. Mr L. was criticizing his physicians' ethnocentrism, although that was not his name for either their cognitive position or their lack of conscious awareness of its presumptions.

8. This simplistic view also overlooks the obvious fact that if proper knowledge were all that were required to induce health-promoting behavioral change, health professionals would themselves be its very models: "slim, agile, nonsmoking, temperate eaters of complementary protein, low fat and cholesterol," and so on (Milio 1976, quoted in Egeland 1978:191).

9. These statements are obviously generalizations that oversimplify the unpredictability of the contexts in which much bioethical debate occurs. General principles sometimes conflict with one another, and situations arise in which action must be taken but the patient's views cannot be known or obtained. The purpose of this section is to identify briefly some of the issues relevant to full consideration of the patient's point of view.

10. In some cultural frameworks, speaking openly of ills is considered to *cause* or *create* those ills. A colleague who acts as a cross-cultural mediator recounted the following example: A Tohono O'odham (Papago) man complained to the Traditional Indian Alliance in Tucson, Arizona (a health care organization), that his doctor was killing him. In reply to questioning, the doctor said that he had simply told the man that if he didn't take his medication for diabetes, he would die. The mediator suggested restating the medical message in positive terms, such as "If you *do* take your medicine, you will feel better" (Barre Toelken, personal communication).

11. Cross-cultural, or transcultural, considerations in biomedical ethics are beginning to become an increasingly salient topic in the literature, and may be expected to be the focus of symposia, conferences, debates, and much publication in the next decade.

12. See, for example, James Spradley, *The Ethnographic Interview* (New York: Holt, Rinehart, and Winston 1979) and *Participant Observation* (New York: Holt, Rinehart, and Winston 1980); Grant McCracken, "The Long Interview" (Qualitative Research Methods Series, no. 13, Newbury Park, CA: Sage Publications 1988); Charles Briggs, *Learning How to Ask: A Sociolinguistic Appraisal of the Role of the Interview in Social Science Research* (Cambridge: Cambridge Uni-

versity Press 1986); and Martyn Hammersley and Paul Atkinson, *Ethnography: Principles in Practice* (London: Routledge 1992).

13. I refer here specifically to contemporary ethnography and the epistemological, philosophical, and ethical stances that inform it. Ethnography, like other methodologies, has a long history of parentalism and of biases that have belittled the subjects of study or failed to accredit the viewpoint of cultural insiders. Like other methods and bodies of knowledge, it can of course also be used unethically or used to promote the interests of more powerful groups (to whom the ethnographers usually belong) over those of less powerful groups (to whom the subjects of study most often belong).

14. This term is in use already in both grass-roots and "official" settings, e.g., U.S. Department of Health and Human Services, Office for Substance Abuse Prevention publishes *Cultural Competence for Evaluators* (DHHS publication ADM 92–1884, 1992), one title in an OSAP Cultural Competence Series.

15. It is practical and useful, however, to be acquainted with the demographics of one's practice area, and to bear in mind the health belief systems and self-care practices that are frequently associated with the populations represented there (see, e.g., Stein 1982a; Snider and Stein 1987). Such information alerts the health professional to some of the common possibilities, just as epidemiological information keeps certain diagnostic possibilities in the consciousness.

Appendix: Practical Tools

The materials that follow are practical tools for thinking, research, teaching, and practice. They can be used as curriculum materials and guidelines for students, both for content mastery and skills training; as slides and handouts for topical presentations to students and colleagues; as guides to research and fact-finding; as concept maps for clinical practice and service design; as stimuli to critical thinking; and no doubt in other applications.

Basic Questions About Health Systems provides a list of questions to guide research into any specific health belief system, and should lead to a fairly complete description of the system. The more complete the description, the greater the possibility of genuine understanding of the system and its rationales. In clinical practice, the better the understanding, the greater the likelihood of successful intersystem negotiation. And of course, the more successful the negotiation, the greater the odds of satisfactory outcomes for all parties involved (providers and patients alike).

Discovering and Working with Patients' Nonconventional Health Beliefs and Practices can be used as a teaching tool for students in the health professions, and as a practice guideline for established care givers and service providers. It is a good companion piece to the *Clinical Decision Tree* that immediately follows it, which outlines in graphic form a suggested general course of decision making regarding patients' uses of nonconventional healing resources.

Eliciting the Patient's Explanatory Model provides some basic questions that can be included in clinical history taking to facilitate patients' descriptions of their own understandings of and preferences regarding their illness and treatment; explanatory notes and cautions alert students and health professionals to corollary considerations. This piece can be used as both a teaching tool and a practice guideline.

The immediately following exercise, *Taking a Health Beliefs History,* was developed as a practice exercise for health professions students and incorporates the explanatory model elicitation, but does not refer to a specific illness episode. It contains both explanatory text and a description of the health beliefs history that can be used as an assignment outline for a focused interview and write-up. At the Medical College of Pennsylvania, this exercise is assigned in conjunction with the annual Culture, Communication, and Health Day that is a part of the required second-year course in Community and Preventive Medicine (see Rubenstein et al. 1992). Anyone is an appropriate subject for the interview, since all persons have health beliefs and practices; it is not necessary to find an interviewee whose health beliefs diverge from the medical model (although it is also not difficult to find one).

The guide entitled *Resources* alerts students, researchers, and other interested parties to a substantial but by no means exhaustive number and variety of informational resources helpful for research and fact-finding. Specific parenthetical illustrations given are from Philadelphia but others could quickly be substituted for any locality or region.

Finally, *Importing an Ethnographic Perspective to Health Care* suggests some ways in which the perspective of modern ethnography—that of discovering, seeking to understand, and responding respectfully to the worldviews and lifeworlds of others—might be applied in and by the health professions. It is applicable to enhancement of students' and providers' awareness, sensitivity, and cultural competence; to design and delivery of more patient-responsive health care and related services; and to improvement and enrichment of provider-patient relationships.

Basic Questions About Health Systems

For the predominant health belief systems in your locality or represented in your patient population (wherever you ultimately find yourself in practice), gathering information in response to these questions should give you a fairly thorough sense of the systems' workings, and so facilitate understanding and negotiation. Think of these as research questions. That is, they are not necessarily usable as direct questions to patients, but they identify categories of information it would be helpful to have about any health belief system in order to produce an accurate and fairly complete description.

What are the primary goals of the system? (E.g., prevention of disease; pain control; enhancement of wellness; treatment of chronic disease; spiritual growth; spiritual salvation; preservation of internal and/or external balance or harmony; avoidance of synthetic substances; minimal intervention.)

Who uses the system, or to whom is it primarily accessible? (E.g., members of a particular ethnic or cultural heritage group; people with specific diseases/dysfunctions; members of specific religious denominations; members of specific interest or identity groups.)

How extensive, varied, or specialized are its applications? (E.g., pediatric; general healing; women's health; geriatric; veterinary; certain conditions only [burns, warts, bleeding, bonesetting, pregnancy and childbirth].)

Adapted from David J. Hufford, "American Healing Systems: An Introduction and Exploration." Hershey, PA: Milton S. Hershey Medical Center, Pennsylvania State University Medical School, 1984. Used by permission.

What is the system's referral network? (E.g., family members; community members; physicians; practitioners from other nonconventional systems; testimony of the healed; print media; health food stores.)

What classes of health and disease does the system recognize and address? (E.g., physical, emotional, mental, spiritual; folk illness categories such as *susto*, high blood, or livergrown; asymptomatic disease or prodromal sequences; diseases of imbalance, disharmony, energy blockage, or impurity.)

How are symptoms interpreted within the system?
   Generally? (E.g., dangerous, and to be eliminated; expressions of the body's needs, and not to be interfered with unless absolutely necessary; indicators of specific energy blockage.)
   Specifically? (E.g., rashes as infections or impurities "coming out"; fevers as signs of excessive "heat" in the body or as mechanisms promoting "sweating out" of toxins or impurities in the blood; musculoskeletal pain as a sign of "cold" lodged in the body; respiratory or other symptoms as particularly dangerous.)

What causes for illness does the system recognize? (E.g., energy blockages, deficits, or excesses; spinal subluxations; exposure to cold or to harsh weather; improper nutrition; constitutional predisposition; environmental influences; "nerves"; fright; emotional or mental distress; malign human agency such as witchcraft, hexes, or the evil eye; spiritual deficiency; sin; supernatural influences.)

How important is it to identify and address ultimate, as opposed to proximate, causes for illness? (E.g., germs may be the proximate cause of a disease, but other causes are implied in the fact that they make a particular person sick at a particular time while others who may have been exposed are spared.)

How are common health/illness terms distinctively defined by the system? (E.g., *asma* or *fatiga*; terms such as "anemia" used as euphemisms for feared or stigmatized diseases such as TB or cancer, or "headache" as a euphemism for conditions causing embarrassment, such as menstruation. Does "healed" mean physically well, or does it have other meanings? Does "healthy" mean entirely symptom-free, disease-free by other measures, or optimally functioning given certain unavoidable limitations?)

Can therapeutic measures be undertaken at home or elsewhere, on one's own or with the aid of family members? What are these? (E.g., preparation of herbal teas or special diets; avoidance of specific foods or other substances; massages; vitamin/mineral supplementation; prayer.)

Are there specialist practitioners? If so, how are they selected and trained? (E.g., birth order [seventh son]; divine calling; family tradition; appointment by a religious or secular authority; formal schooling; apprenticeship; use of standardized printed text materials; oral tradition; supernatural selection.)

What kinds of specialists are there? (E.g., lay midwives; bonesetters; massagers; injectionists; diviners/diagnosticians [as distinct from curers]; bloodstoppers; herbalists; priests; mediums; "straight" vs. "mixing" chiropractors; shamans; singers.)

What do practitioners do? (E.g., diagnosis; recommendations or prescriptions; massages; spinal manipulation; needling; ritual cleansing; injection; guided imagery; soul restoration.)

What is the relationship of these therapeutic actions to the illness and its melioration? (E.g., spinal manipulation corrects subluxations to improve the flow of vital energy; homeopathic remedies stimulate the body's healing energy; some herbs are prescribed according to the doctrine of signatures, some for a pharmacological effect, and others because they produce a specific action—carminative, diaphoretic, purgative.)

What are the responsibilities of practitioners? (E.g., provide information; teach self-care techniques; give specific treatments; supply medications; evaluate progress; help patient to cope with illness.)

What are the responsibilities of patients/clients? (E.g., follow suggested treatment regimens; make lifestyle changes; keep records of own self-care activities and observed responses; show sufficient faith; avoid sin; think positively.) Are patients/clients held responsible or accountable for their own illness or health?

What are the risks and costs of the system (from both the insider's and the outsider's perspectives)? (E.g., travel to distant treatment sites; expensive foods or medicaments; potential toxicities and side effects; debilitating treatment regimens; physical or spiritual danger; dietary insufficiencies; willingness of third-party payors to cover expenses.)

How are the successes and failures of treatments and practitioners evaluated? (E.g., mobilization of body's own healing capacity; superior healing capacity of natural vs. synthetic medicaments; divine providence; shared blame for failure because of patient error or inability to follow recommended therapies; insufficient faith on the part of the patient; some practitioners are skilled or good and others are not; inevitability of a certain percentage of failures in any system.)

How does the system view suffering and death? (E.g., suffering is always bad and may indicate that the sufferer is not in a state of grace; coping with suffering can be spiritually or morally uplifting; suffering can be "offered up" for specific religious intentions to the benefit of self and others; death is only a stage in a spiritual continuum; people die when it is their time or when it is God's will.)

What does this system provide for healing and for coping with illness that conventional medicine does not provide? (E.g., a holistic approach; more natural therapeutics; spiritual guidance; methods for dealing with supernatural causes and afflictions; recognition of the importance of proper diet and nutrition to health and healing; extensive personal contact with healer; extensive participatory rights for patients; family or community involvement in therapeutic regimen; explanations for illness and suffering, and for selection of particular individuals to fall ill at particular times.)

How does this system view interaction with conventional medicine? (E.g., medicine is excellent for mechanical problems, required surgeries, and trauma, while this system is better at controlling symptoms and promoting overall healing; medicine addresses proximate causes and this system addresses ultimate causes; sufficient faith and expiation of sin obviates the need for medical intervention altogether; medicine is excellent for monitoring the progress which is principally achieved through the therapeutic regimen of this system; medicine is aggressive and seeks rapid results while this system is gentler and views proper healing as a gradual process; medicine is good for some aspects of the illness and this system is good for others.)

Discovering and Working with Patients' Nonconventional Health Beliefs and Practices

1. Become familiar with the region in which you practice.
Some nonconventional health belief systems are closely connected with particular ethnic, religious, or other specific identity groups. Some, such as the numerous New Age healing systems, are associated largely with "mainstream" populations and are widely and unpredictably distributed among them. What is the profile of your area or patient population? What healing resources are represented?

2. Be familiar with circumstances that encourage use of alternative or complementary therapies.
For example, chronic or recurrent illness (even if medically minor), very serious illness, or poor medical prognosis often prompt a broadening of healing resources to include nonconventional healing practices, even among those not previously familiar with or receptive to such systems or practices.

3. Become familiar with specific nonconventional therapies closely associated with particular health conditions seen often in your practice or specialty.
Remember that these will include both health maintenance or "wellness" practices, and therapeutic or remedial practices.

4. Check during initial history for:

- patient explanatory model for the presenting complaint
- lifestyle cues, religious or spiritual considerations

Adapted from David J. Hufford, "What Every Health Professional Should Know About Folklore." In Michael Owen Jones, ed., *Putting Folklore to Use*. Lexington: University Press of Kentucky, 1993. Used by permission.

- patient preferences for therapeutic approaches
- patient treatment goals

Any of these topics may give cues to beliefs and values indicating that use of nonconventional therapies is likely.

5. Give "permission" for your patients to raise issues of nonconventional therapies or health beliefs.
Present yourself as open to patient beliefs, and respond without judgment. Be frank about what *you* do not know (e.g., if you have no familiarity with herbalism or the hot/cold classification of a particular medication, etc.), and ask for further information. Ask directly what the patient is doing/has done to treat the illness and how that seems to be working. Make it clear that you intend to work together with the patient. Ask for specific information from the patient about alternative therapies, for your own information and for the medical record.

6. Listen for "non-disclosing" cues.
Sometimes, passing references may be made to nonconventional beliefs and practices, in a manner that is deliberately ambiguous. This allows the patient to test for reactions before committing him or herself to fuller disclosure. If unnoticed or unresponded to, such "testing" may not be repeated, and further information may not be forthcoming. If responded to nonjudgmentally with requests for further explanation, these cues may prove to be openers for a more detailed description of health beliefs and practices.

7. Whenever a patient encounters *personally* serious health problems, renew "permission" and check again for nonconventional health beliefs/practices as at initial history.
Beliefs change over time and in response to many kinds of circumstances, including confronting a serious or personally threatening or frightening illness. Remember that an illness does not have to be grave from a medical point of view in order to present a serious threat from the patient's point of view.

8. Negotiate the best possible mutually agreeable treatment program.
Explain the important points of concern you have, and point out any differences in interpretation that may be significant. Discuss possible changes in the patient's therapeutic preferences for medical reasons, and where possible show how these can be consistent with the patient's belief system. Also discuss therapeutic preferences of yours which you feel are negotiable, or which can be undertaken in steps.

9. Consider consultation with a nonmedical specialist.
Spokespersons for or practitioners within particular belief systems or nonconventional healing systems can provide additional information and explain the system's rationales. Social scientists (folklorists, anthropologists, sociologists), clergy, social service professionals, for example, may be able to provide additional information, serve as mediators, or help to construct persuasive arguments that are consistent with patient belief systems.

Decision Tree for Detecting and Dealing with Clinically Important Patient Involvement in Non-Conventional Health Practices and Beliefs

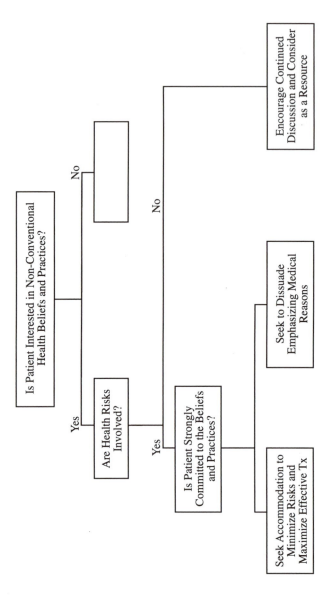

From David J. Hufford, "American Healing Systems: An Introduction and Exploration." Hershey, PA: Milton S. Hershey Medical Center, Pennsylvania State University Medical School, 1984. Used by permission.

Eliciting the Patient's Explanatory Model

The wording of questions will vary with the characteristics of *the patient*, *the problem*, and *the setting*, but we suggest the following set of questions to elicit the patient explanatory model. Patients may often hesitate to disclose their models to doctors. Clinicians need to be persistent in order to show patients that their ideas are of genuine interest and importance for clinical management.

Explanatory Model

(1) What do you think caused your problem?
(2) Why do you think it started when it did?
(3) What do you think your sickness does to you?
    How does it work?
(4) How severe is your sickness?
    Will it have a long or a short course?
(5) What kind of treatment do you think you should receive?

Several other questions will elicit the patient's therapeutic goals and the psychosocial and cultural meaning of his illness, if these issues have not already been incorporated into his answers:

Goals

(6) What are the most important results you hope to receive from this treatment?
(7) What are the chief problems your sickness has caused for you?
(8) What do you fear most about your sickness?

Quoted and adapted from Kleinman, Eisenberg, and Good. "Culture, Illness, and Care: Clinical Lessons from Anthropologic and Cross-Cultural Research." *Annals of Internal Medicine* 88:251–258, 1978, p. 256. Used by permission.

Purpose and Adaptability of Questions

These questions should help to illuminate a patient's characterization and explanation of a presenting problem, and will generally elicit some related health beliefs and practices as well as other important values. The questions can be selectively included in any history-taking. The form in which they appear here is a suggested form: they may need to be modified in the particular patient interview in order to be made more understandable, more specific to the situation, and so forth. Not all of the questions will be appropriate to every interview. Any additional questions that seem pertinent at the time or that arise from the conversation should of course be added.

Capabilities That Facilitate Disclosure

- The ability to question, listen, and repeat patients' descriptions *without the necessity to agree* with them
- An open, non-judgmental attitude
- The capacity not to require agreement with all points of your own explanatory model
- Tolerance for ambiguity, if the explanatory model is confusing to you
- The capacity to admit what you don't know, both within your own system, and about other systems
- Awareness that when your explanation and your patient's are incongruent, *understanding* is more important than agreement (and agreement may not be possible)

Cautions and Reminders

1. Whatever information you get in response to your questions should be considered carefully, even if, to your way of thinking, it seems not to pertain to the problem. If this happens, ask the question again later in a slightly different way, or go back to the same question. If the response is the same, you are probably hearing an important part of the patient's explanatory model. (For example, mention of a serious family fight prior to onset of a disease may imply that some physical violence was involved, that distress can make you sick, that sickness may be a punishment for disruption of social relations and obligations, or that an injured or angered party may be able to cause the perceived offender to become sick in retaliation.) Considerations such as these may have an effect on responses to medical advice, recourse to nonbiomedical therapies, patient outlook or emotional state, therapeutic outcome, etc.

2. Any response of yours that appears judgmental, impatient, or dismissive will discourage further disclosure. No one is willing to expose him-/herself to ridicule or rejection, and patients generally feel no particular need to acquaint clinicians with their nonconventional health beliefs and practices: they are accustomed to managing the interaction of the conventional medical system with whatever other approaches to health care they use. It is up to the clinician to create the climate that encourages this exchange of information.

3. In any given interview (and even over the longer term relationship), you will elicit only a portion of the information that is pertinent. Some may not seem pertinent to the patient; some may be considered private; some may not be considered safe or proper to report (e.g., things that might be sacred, whose legal status is unknown or illegal, or that are felt to be likely to provoke negative reactions, retaliation, etc.). Be encouraging, even persistent, but avoid being or appearing coercive. Continue to inquire over the course of your relationship with the patient.

4. Be frank about the things that you don't understand or with which you are unfamiliar (e.g., parts of patients' explanatory models, or treatment modalities with which you are not acquainted). If you *have* heard any of it before, use observations to that effect to encourage continued conversation (e.g., "Oh yes, I've heard that from other people, too").

5. If there are significant conflicts between the patient's explanatory model and yours, state your own views, preferences, and concerns clearly and honestly and explain your *reasons*. Rely on persuasion and well-supported explanation, not appeals to authority. Focus your persuasive efforts on significant points only: you may have to be prepared to compromise, as will the patient. Where conflicting explanations do *not* appear to interfere with a patient's acceptance of medical advice or to threaten the desired therapeutic outcome, there is no need to address them or to try to "educate" patients to agree with you. Remember, it is more important for you and the patient to *understand* each other's views than it is for you to agree with each other. The importance of agreement comes in the treatment negotiation, which should be much facilitated by a caring and open-minded approach on the part of the provider.

Exercise: Taking a Health Beliefs History

Many patients use preventive, health maintenance, and treatment measures that fall outside of the conventional health care system. Many hold models of health, illness, and care that are not congruent with the conventional medical model. Patients' health belief systems may derive from their culture of ancestry or group identity, or they may have been discovered and adopted from a variety of other sources. The reasons that people have for holding quite different notions of health, illness, and treatment from those represented in the medical model vary widely. They include (to cite only a few examples):

- acceptance as part of an ethnic or religious cultural heritage (e.g., Pennsylvania German powwowing or "sympathy healing," or the mandates of *any* religion);
- lifestyle factors adopted to harmonize with a consciously selected philosophical stance (e.g., a macrobiotic or natural foods diet or a preference for naturally derived medicines);
- efforts to multiply therapeutic options in the face of a particular illness (e.g., cancer, HIV/AIDS, chronic fatigue, MS, chronic pain syndromes, common colds, migraine);
- dissatisfaction with results or treatments obtained from the conventional biomedical system (e.g., drugs with undesirable side effects, treatments that are invasive or extremely unpleasant, treatments that do not appreciably ameliorate the illness or improve quality of life).

A review of even this brief list should make it apparent that health beliefs and values that differ significantly from those of conventional biomedicine are *by no means* confined to particular ethnic or denominational groups. In fact, they are not necessarily even more common in such groups, in spite of long-standing stereotypical impressions to the contrary.

It is important for health professionals to gain some understanding of patients' health beliefs and practices, as well as of related cultural values, because they can have many clinically significant implications: for communication and understanding (in both directions); for accuracy of diagnosis; for appropriateness of treatment recommendations; for potential interactions between nonconventional and conventional therapeutic modalities; for the ways in which patients respond to medical advice and integrate medical treatment recommendations into their lives; and for outcomes. The more complete and accurate information you have about your patient's explanations of health and illness, and about treatments used in addition to (or sometimes instead of) those you recommend, the more likely you are to be successful in negotiating a treatment program that both you and your patient can understand and find agreeable.

Within any group, there is always a wide range of awareness and adoption of a particular system of values, beliefs, and practices. This means that while knowledge of a pattern of health beliefs common to a given identity-group gives you a very useful frame of reference when working with patients from that group, it is *not predictive* from individual to individual. Different individuals also have differing degrees of commitment to particular beliefs and associated practices. This variation in commitment has important implications for successful negotiation with the patient's belief system (Hufford 1977a, 1984, 1988a). (For example, especially profound levels of commitment are associated with less willingness to change in response to medical preferences or pressures, just as health professionals' strength of commitment to their medical beliefs and values is associated with reduced willingness to compromise.)

To find out what is important for a given patient, what explanatory model of illness s/he holds, what goals and expectations s/he has for treatment, and what personal beliefs and values might have an effect on his or her responses to the clinical encounter and to treatment recommendations, you need to ask on a case by case basis. It is useful to include such a health beliefs history in your information-gathering from patients.

It is important to bear in mind that most people view health professionals as persons in positions of authority, and often as persons with very fixed ideas about what is right or important. This makes patients very cautious about revealing anything they feel might result in their jeopardizing access to medical services, having their deeply felt concerns dismissed as trivial, or being made to feel foolish by provoking a derisory or irritable reaction. Patients manage their degrees of disclosure in the clinical encounter according to their own assessments of the situation, and *they* are the ones who in the end make the decisions about how they will respond to medical recommendations. It is important, for all of these reasons, to elicit from patients in a compassionate and nonjudgmental way their important concerns, beliefs, and values that may have implications for health and health care. You can usually learn several relevant pieces of information with just a few well-put questions and an accepting manner.

As this becomes more familiar to you through practice, you will be able to assess these issues with relative ease and to incorporate a few key questions in the basic history-and-physical assessment. Findings can be used in negotiating a treatment plan that, though it will often involve compromises on *both* sides, is acceptable to both you and your patient and therefore more likely to succeed. Over the course of longer-term relationships with individual patients, the health beliefs history can be fleshed out and updated.

Elements in the Health Beliefs History

You should focus on three basic elements in the health beliefs history:

- specific values, beliefs and practices relevant to the current state of health or illness (or to health and illness generally);
- source of and depth of commitment to those beliefs, values, and practices;
- likelihood of compromise, including areas in which compromise is most likely to be successful.

Some examples are given below.
1. *Specific values, beliefs and practices that might be relevant to health and health care*:

- understandings of how particular illnesses are acquired and progress, what preventive and treatment measures are considered important, what treatment measures have been taken to date, what things ought to be avoided;
- religious or philosophical concepts about life and death, the nature and meaning of suffering, what constitutes a good life, what constitutes a good death, what it is to be a good person, moral imperatives;
- dietary laws, preferences, and proscriptions (general and situational, e.g., special dietary considerations for holy times, for cyclical purifications, or for certain health conditions);

- any beliefs and practices specifically identified with current states of health and illness, e.g., home remedies, first-aid and preventive measures, lifestyle modifications;
- participation in any nonbiomedical healing systems or recourse to alternative practitioners or self-care measures.

2. *Assessment of source of, and depth of commitment to, particular beliefs, values, and practices*:

- strength of identification with a particular system or identity-group culture;
- religious grounds, and level of involvement with and commitment to religious identity;
- relation of particular beliefs/practices to broader moral mandates;
- relation of particular beliefs/practices to other strongly held philosophical positions;
- length of time involved with given beliefs/practices;
- prevalence of same or similar beliefs/practices in community of peers, close social network, family (i.e., breadth and depth of social support for beliefs/practices);
- personal experience (or personal experience of close others) of efficacy or ascribed efficacy of practices;
- presence of serious or personally troubling health conditions, especially if conventional medical responses are limited or unsuccessful;
- personal goals for treatment.

3. *Factors that support successful negotiation*:

- provider's attitude of openness and cooperation (includes its expression through minimal communicative cues such as subtleties of tone of voice, facial expressions, body language, eye contact, posture);
- provider's ability to explain, in plain language, reasons supporting medical preferences;
- provider's ability to explain, in plain language but without implied personal criticism, grounds for disagreement or concern with patients' preferences or practices;
- provider's capacity to tolerate divergences from the medical model;
- provider's ability to share decision making, and to make concessions on some points;
- patient beliefs/practices that are not closely associated with or derived from religious or moral mandates or other strong convictions;
- relatively short duration of patient familiarity with beliefs/practices;

- patient beliefs/practices not strongly identified with or supported by person's cultural heritage or other identity-group;
- availability of another member of patient's identity-group who can provide other interpretations for beliefs/practices, within the same or very similar framework of values (e.g., in the case of a religious belief with a scriptural basis, someone who could provide a counter argument also based in scripture);
- high level of patient (and significant others) satisfaction with and trust of conventional medical care and care givers.

Responding to the Health Beliefs History

In responding to the findings of the health beliefs history, mention any significant implications of particular aspects of the patient's belief system for conventional clinical care. Identify opportunities as well as challenges. Consider any misgivings you may have about any health-related practices or actions in which your patient is involved and assess why you feel as you do. Suggest possible points of compromise, and note particular factors that might support successful negotiation between yourself as care provider and this particular person as patient.

Resources

Once you are established in a practice area, it will behoove you to gain some depth of understanding of the demographics and cultural diversity of your general area, and of your particular patient population. To find out more about specific populations or groups of people and their commonly represented values, cultural preferences and practices—and specifically, health beliefs and practices—you *do* have to make a search. This is a partial list of some of the resources you could use in your region of practice to pursue such information. (Examples listed in parentheses are located in Philadelphia, PA.)

Resource People

Colleges and universities, social service agencies, religious and chaplaincy organizations, grass-roots community organizations, and ethnic group or other identity-group associations are good sources of people who might be able to provide information or consultation as well as guide your further searches. At universities, call the folklore, anthropology, and sociology program or department offices, or any department that conducts ethnographic studies—sometimes education, or regional or urban planning, for instance. If there is a local college of pharmacy, see if they have a pharmacognosist on staff: this is a good resource person for information about pharmacological properties of herbal medicaments; toxicologists may be able to inform you about plant toxicities. If there are botanical gardens or arboreta in your area, consult with their botanists about medicinal plants. If there is a school of nursing, find out if they have specialists in transcultural nursing. If there are refugee resettlement agencies, find out what groups they work with, and what background information they can provide. Ethnic associations and some social service organizations can also provide information and referrals, or help locate translators, if needed. Don't overlook healers and purveyors of self-care supplies (herbs, religious articles, vitamin and mineral supplements, etc.) in your community.

Libraries

Public libraries, university libraries, medical and nursing libraries, specialty libraries. Use their indices to find articles in the medical and nursing literature, the social sciences literature (including anthropology, folklore, and sociology—all of which address health beliefs and behavior), the literatures of psychology, public health, and religious studies (all religions have something to say about health and healing), and the popular and special-interest press. In the literature of health care, nursing (their computerized index is called CINAHL) and public health are richly supplied with articles that deal with cultural and psychosocial aspects of health and illness, and they do so more often and in more depth then the medical journals tend to do. The Modern Language Association (MLA) indexes several folklore and anthropology journals. *Dissertation Abstracts* will turn up titles in this subject area from a number of disciplinary perspectives. These are original studies based on research or fieldwork, and many are not published elsewhere.

Journals that frequently address cultural and belief issues in health care include *Social Science and Medicine*, *Culture, Medicine and Psychiatry*, *Medical Anthropology Quarterly*, *Journal of Health and Social Behavior*, *Holistic Nursing Practice*, *Western Journal of Medicine*, *Journal of Transcultural Nursing*, and a number of others in the behavioral and social sciences.

Literature that addresses many of the same kinds of issues and practical problems found in health care negotiations includes the literature on international business negotiations, material on cross-cultural counseling, and material on cross-cultural conflict resolution (or conflict resolution generally). Literature dealing with medicine in nonindustrialized countries and in combat conditions may include useful examples of workable solutions achieved by modifying usual medical expectations and procedures.

Special Databases

These can be searched at many libraries, or the libraries can help you find out how to hook up to their networks. Examples are CAIN, the computerized AIDS information network; HOMEONET, the homeopathic information network; and NAPRALERT, a database of scientific information on medicinal plants and natural substances.

City, County, State, and U.S. Government Offices

Try health departments, of course; the census office has demographic information for the area; city and county planning offices publish demographic maps of various sorts, based on most recent analyzed census data. In Philadelphia, the mayor's office has special commissions (e.g., on Neighborhoods, on Puerto Rican-Latino Affairs, on Sexual Minorities, on Women). The Pennsylvania governor's office has a Heritage Affairs Commission that deals with ethnic and nationality groups, among other things; under the auspices of this commission is the state folklorist's office, which commissions and carries out ethnographic work throughout the state. These offices also have empaneled at different times specialized task forces that may be pertinent.

Consulates

The consular offices for specific nationalities can help you locate other information about nationality groups in your area.

The Telephone Book

Use it to find special offices and associations that can give you further information about the group or topic you're pursuing. Use all of its sections, because things are listed according to all manner of classification systems, and have all sorts of unpredictable names. For example:

In the **Blue Pages** (government offices), look up HUMAN SERVICES listings. There try subheadings that may be pertinent, such as:

- HEALTH/COMMUNITY SERVICES—To find groups specific to a particular disease or disorder (e.g. Lupus, HIV/AIDS), ethnic associations (Chinese Benevolent Association, Korean Association of Greater Philadelphia), social service organizations dealing with specific populations (Nationalities Service Center; Council of Neighborhood Organizations)
- COUNSELING/INFORMATION GIVERS and REFERRAL SERVICES—(Mayor's Office of Community Services)
- MENTAL HEALTH/SPECIALIZED AGENCIES—(Asociación Puertorriqueños en Marcha; Hispanic Mental Health Institute; Southeast Asian Mental Health Program)
- NEIGHBORHOOD ORGANIZATIONS AND PROGRAMS—(Council of Spanish Speaking Organizations)

In the **White Pages**, look up identity-group listings by the descriptive name of the group. This won't turn up all of the relevant organizations and associations, because some have other kinds of names (Taller Puertorriqueño), some are not listed (Hmong Association), and some groups don't have identity-specific associations (middle-class Anglos). But you will find many for specific ethnic/nationality/identity groups (examples include African-American, American Indian, Cambodian, Gay and Lesbian, Greek Orthodox, Irish, Islamic, Lithuanian, Ukranian among many, many others.) Also look under ASSOCIATION, COALITION, COUNCIL, ORGANIZATION, SOCIETY, UNION, and other related terms, since many specialized organizations have names which begin with these words.

In the **Yellow Pages,** look for general headings that may lead to specific groups or populations, for example:

- ASSOCIATIONS—Read through the listings, as names may not be what you're expecting. This will yield organizations specific to purposes (refugee resettlement), populations, and also diseases/disorders. The latter may have information about what sorts of alternative or complementary therapies are used for the specific disorder.
- CHURCHES and other places of worship—Good places to pursue information about religious beliefs and their relationship to conventional medical care. Several have education or public relations offices; otherwise, speak to the clergy member in charge.
- CLINICS—Includes many conventional medical care facilities, and clinics serving particular populations or offering specialized therapies.
- CONSULATES
- COUNSELORS
- HUMAN SERVICES ORGANIZATIONS
- MUSEUMS—You may find some that focus on a particular group (African-American Historical and Cultural Museum) and others that have exhibits, collections, or other information of use to you (Balch Institute for Ethnic Studies, University of Pennsylvania Museum of Anthropology), including occasional special exhibits dealing with historical, regional, or ethnic health care practices. They may also sponsor an occasional forum or conference on a pertinent topic. Get on their mailing lists.
- NEWSPAPERS—Gives names of local papers, including many for specific ethnic, nationality, or identity groups. These give a sense of the community and its interests, carry advertisements for health

care products and physicians or other providers serving the particular group. (Philadelphia area examples include *Au Courant*; *The Irish Edition*; *Korean Guardian*; *Main Line Times*; *South Philadelphia Review-Chronicle*; *Germantown Courier*; *Philadelphia Gay News*; *Ukranian Daily Paper*, and many others.)

- PHARMACIES—Scan the listings; some may have specialties such as homeopathic pharmaceuticals (Palmer Apothecary; a few on the Main Line) or others (e.g., Hausmann's specializes in "foreign and unusual prescriptions").
- SOCIAL SERVICE ORGANIZATIONS—In Philadelphia, this heading includes the Asian American Council of Greater Philadelphia, BEBASHI (Blacks Educating Blacks About Sexual Health Issues), the Center for Advancement in Cancer Education (an information center for both conventional and nonconventional cancer therapies), the Migrant Education Program, PRANA (New Age counseling services), and the Philadelphia Refugee Service Center, among many others. It also has listings for many organizations focused on a specific disease or disorder—again, a possible source for information about support networks and their particular views of a health problem; and about alternative therapies that arise for almost all serious illnesses.

In addition, try specific headings for the system or practice you are interested in researching. The Philadelphia book has headings, for example, for ACUPUNCTURE, CHIROPRACTORS, CHRISTIAN SCIENCE PRACTITIONERS, HEALTH FOOD and DIET PRODUCTS, HERBS, HOLISTIC PRACTITIONERS, HOMEOPATHS, HYPNOTISTS, MEDITATION INSTRUCTION, NATUROPATHS, NUTRITIONISTS, PARAPSYCHOLOGISTS, REFLEXOLOGISTS, and YOGA INSTRUCTION (among others). These headings are useful in pursuing the health belief systems of many patients who do not identify themselves with a particular ethnic or nationality group and whose interest group affiliations cannot as readily be looked up as ethnic and nationality group associations can. ETHNIC RESTAURANTS may sometimes provide leads or an entry into an ethnic community whose other public resources are difficult for outsiders to find or that do not have listings in the book.

In addition, try the group-specific resources in nearby large cities. For example, Gay Men's Health Crisis (New York) has a wealth of information, and an excellent archive, about HIV alternative therapies; the International Hospital Liaison Committee of the Jehovah's Witnesses has its offices in New York; and so on.

Local General Circulation Newspaper(s)

Contact the one with the largest circulation. Find out who covers human interest stories about health care, alternative health care, culture-specific health practices, and talk to them. Find out if they have a health care "beat." See if you can use their archive of, or index to, such stories they have previously printed.

Herb Stores

Almost all have information on the properties and uses of most of their herbs and may have books and other printed material as well. These are the same books that members of the system use for references and thus are wonderful resources for understanding what members of the community are using and reading. (Penn Herb Company, in Philadelphia, is one of the largest suppliers nationwide.)

Religious Goods Stores

May have information about particular religious/spiritual items used in connection with healing—from saints' medals to *elekes* to special candles and incenses, to amulets and charms—and the belief contexts of their use. A visit will acquaint you with many of the common items, some of which you may then recognize in the course of your practice.

Health Food Stores

Such stores typically have informational pamphlets relating to particular foods or supplements, and may also have related magazines or books that give insight into the philosophy, approach to health, and so forth. They frequently distribute the local "alternative network" news publications, which contain articles explaining various practices or philosophies, and which also contain advertisements for products, services and service providers, and informational seminars on scores of health-related topics. These are good resources for obtaining further information (or names of contacts for further information) about any systems represented in their pages. (In Philadelphia, these alternative network publications include *Prana*, *Connexions*, and *New Frontier*; all are distributed free of charge.)

Book Stores

Both general and specialty. Browse through their Health, Fitness, Diet, and Self-Improvement sections to find information on health-related philosophies and practices of many "mainstream" patients. Also check their Religion/Spirituality and Occult sections. Make sure to check out your local New Age bookstore for health and healing literature in abundance.

In-House Resources

If you are affiliated with a hospital, find out if it has a patient relations department, a patient advocacy service, a language bank, a department of social work or social services. Get to know the range of services that each of these provides, and how to get in touch with them efficiently. Consider helping to add needed services, as well.

Importing an Ethnographic Perspective to Health Care

Modern ethnography (the decription of culture) strives to understand how a culture or group understands itself, and to accurately represent the point of view of group members, or cultural insiders. This effort entails recognition that worldviews that differ from that of the ethnographer (usually a professional or scholar) are not necessarily less valid, and are equally deserving of respect. Application of this attitude to health care can facilitate the development of more patient-centered and patient-responsive services and providers. The questions that follow offer guidelines for importing an ethnographic perspective to health care settings.

- **What can I learn**
from this patient or from members of this group of people about the way individuals and the group define the world, order their concerns, understand right behavior, assess circumstances, define health and illness, establish goals for life and for treatment of illness, etc.?

- **How can I incorporate**
the concerns and perspectives of this patient or patient population into the ways in which I structure and deliver health care: shaping of procedures and protocols, office hours, scheduling, waiting room arrangement, furnishings, uses of space, forms of address and conversation, uses of time, inclusion of ethnically significant or valued foods in dietary plans, treatment planning and decisions, etc.?

- **What can I modify**
in my own thinking and behavior to facilitate establishment of relationships of trust and mutual respect (e.g., understanding provider education and patient education as two sides of the same coin; understand-

ing that two views of a health problem and its appropriate solutions may have to be taken into account; understanding that patients' goals are at least as important as providers' goals in formulating a plan for care)?

• **How can I negotiate**
treatment and prevention plans that are acceptable both to me and to my patients, even if we have different beliefs about why things are important or how they work (remembering that negotiation means *both* sides will probably have to compromise)?

• **How can I establish a working partnership**
in which *both* points of view contribute to outcomes at all levels (including, e.g., design as well as delivery of health care services, design and operation of health care facilities, institutional and broader health policy change and implementation)?

Glossary

Acculturation. The process of adaptation to a culture other than one's culture of origin or first learned culture; borrowing or assimilation of traits from one cultural repertoire to another.

Adherent. (n.) Proponent, participant, or follower; (adj.) showing commitment to a proposition or course of action; current synonym or substitute term for "compliant," used in reference to patients' actions with respect to medical advice or prescription; thought by many to be more respectful of patients than "compliant," because of its differences in connotation regarding authority relations and personal integrity.

Agency. The capacity, condition, or state of acting or exerting power; means by which an end is achieved or a purpose accomplished.

Agent. A person responsible for his acts; a person capable of deliberate action; one who acts or exerts power. In medical usage, any substance capable of producing an effect; an immediate cause (e.g., an infectious *agent*).

Ascites. Accumulation of serous fluid in the abdominal cavity.

Authority. Grounds, warrant, or convincing force; power to influence or compel opinion or behavior; "a status, quality, or claim that compels trust or obedience" (Starr 1987:9). Social authority allows for shaping or control of action through the issuing of commands or orders (civil and military authorities; parents; teachers; health professionals) and may be explicitly or implicitly underwritten by the capacity to use force. Cultural authority entails consensual recognition of the capacity to make trustworthy judgments about the nature of reality "through definitions of fact and value" (Starr 1987:13). Acceptance of others' authority substitutes for derivation of principles or conclusions by exercise of private judgment (Starr 1987).

Autonomy. The right of self-governance or self-regulation; the right of freedom from dominion by the will of others. Patient autonomy is the ethical principle that recognizes patients' rights to self-determination in acceptance or refusal of specific aspects of care.

Axiom. A proposition accepted as true on its intrinsic merit; an established rule or principle; a self-evident truth. A "fundamental statement, that cannot be deduced from other statements" (Angeles 1981: 22) but which may serve as a basis or starting point for other inferences.

AZT. Azidothymidine, zidovudine; antiretroviral drug of the nucleoside analogue class which was the first FDA-approved treatment to combat HIV. It was approved in 1987 for general availability (seven years after recognition of HIV disease and its epidemic character), and was the only approved anti-HIV agent until late 1991.

Belief. A conviction that something is true or accurate, or acceptance of a proposition as true; "the quality of being held to be certain" (Hufford, "Belief Glossary," unpublished; used by permission). As used in this work, "local knowledge" (where "local" refers to any group or individual possessing such knowledge). Belief and knowledge both involve mental or intellectual acceptance of something as true, actual, or real on the basis of some form of authoritative support for the conclusion.

Beneficence. The principle in medical ethics that obligates physicians and other health professionals to act in kindness and for the purpose of doing good.

Bioethics. Application of ethical principles to medical decision making, and to the conduct of health professionals with respect to patients and to research subjects; also called medical ethics and biomedical ethics.

CD-4 cells. A type of lymphocyte or white blood cell involved in the immune system's infection-fighting capabilities; also called T-helper cells, or in the common parlance, "T-cells." HIV penetrates and destroys these cells. In everyday speech, "CD-4 cells" and "T-cells" are interchangeable usages.

CMV retinitis. Infection of the retina of the eye caused by cytomegalovirus (CMV). CMV infections of various kinds are common to people with HIV disease; CMV retinitis causes blindness if not aggressively treated.

Compliance. The act or quality of submission or obedience to the desires or demands of others. In medical usage, the act or process of carrying out "doctors' orders" or closely following medical advice, which is considered very desirable if not requisite in patient behavior. Reflects the professional point of view and the assumption that the physician should have authoritative status in directing patient behavior.

Compliant. Submissive or disposed to yield to the will of others. In medical usage, refers to patients who are obedient to medical advice or "doctors' orders," and who take medications and follow regimens according to prescription and instructions. Considered at minimum a desirable quality of patients, sometimes a duty or responsibility of patienthood. Reflects the professional point of view and the assumption that the physician should have authoritative status in directing patient behavior.

Conventional. Usual and customary, normative; requires contextualization to be a meaningful descriptor (i.e., conventional where, or under what circumstances, or by whose consensus, or with respect to what).

Conventional medicine. Used here to indicate the officially sanctioned medical system of the United States; also called Western, academic, or scientific medicine, or biomedicine.

Cultural evolutionism. The theory that cultures pass through developmental stages analogous to those of species or individuals, presumed to be a continuous and unidirectional process moving from simpler and "lower" (more "primitive") forms to more complex and "higher" (more "civilized") forms. The cultures of the scholars were considered examples of more civilized stages, while those of many of their subjects of study were considered examples of more primitive or "less evolved" stages.

ddC. Dideoxycytidine, an antiretroviral drug in the class known as nucleoside analogues; approved in June 1992 for use in HIV disease as a combination therapeutic agent.

ddI. Dideoxyinosine (or didanosine), an antiretroviral drug in the class known as nucleoside analogues; approved in October 1991 for use in HIV disease.

Doctrine of signatures. The theory that the essential properties or "virtues," and thus the medicinal indications, of plants and other substances are revealed or mirrored in aspects of their outer appearance; e.g. bloodroot, because of its copious bright red sap, is indicated for strengthening the blood, walnuts for problems with the head or brain, liverleaf for liver ailments. This theory might have either a religious or a secular interpretation: either that God has marked remedies with a "signature" (Crellin and Philpott 1990), or that it is natural that like substances treat like organs or conditions, and Nature has so constituted beneficial plants that humans can learn them by the "signatures" that suggest their uses.

Emic. Of the categories or viewpoint of insiders to a given culture or belief system.

Enculturation. The process of learning or acquiring one's culture of origin.

Endoscopy. Direct visual inspection of interior areas or cavities of the body, performed by insertion of an optical instrument.

Epistemology. The theory or study of the nature and origins of knowledge.

Ethnicity. Shared cultural identity or cultural heritage, which forms a part of the lifestyle and shared sense of identity of the members of a group. Ethnicity is a cultural, not a biological, characteristic and is mutable. It is incorrect (though common) to assume that some people can be defined in terms of ethnicity and others cannot.

Ethnobotany. The study of plants and their classifications, names, and uses in relation to specific cultures.

Ethnocentrism. The belief that one's own cultural mores are superior or more "correct" than those of others; the conscious or unconscious practice of interpreting other cultures or the actions of their members in terms of the values and norms of one's own culture.

Ethnography. The practice of describing or writing about culture. Current ethnography emphasizes cultural representation from the insider's or member's point of view.

Etic. Of the categories or viewpoint of outsiders to a given culture or belief system, specifically, of scientists or academics interpreting systems or cultures other than their own.

Evidence. Material, narrative, or experiential support for the veracity, credibility, or reliability of an idea or proposition. Definitions of what constitutes evidence under what conditions, and of the requirements of evidential weight to establish a given contention, are established within, and vary among, specific epistemological frameworks.

Folk belief. Unofficial belief that has a shared social dimension (i.e., as distinguished from "an idiosyncratic belief in the delusional system of a psychotic" person [Hufford, "Belief Glossary," unpublished; used by permission]). Note that the designation "folk belief" tells some things about the social status of the belief, but *does not* tell or imply anything about its accuracy.

Fraud. Knowing, intentional deception or misrepresentation. Health fraud definitely exists but, properly defined, does not include practitioners or purveyors who are sincere in their belief in the benefits of the substances, methods, or practices they represent.

Free radicals. Groups of atoms that carry an unpaired electron and are therefore unstable and very reactive (Dorland's Illustrated Medical Dictionary). For some members of the holistic healing and health foods movements, free radicals are a matter of concern. They are understood as byproducts of oxidation in cells and are thought to initiate "chain reaction[s] of molecular and chemical changes within cells and tissues" (Monte 1989). In this context, free radicals are implicated in the genesis of cancers and (other) immune disorders.

Functionalism. Theoretical stance that explains the existence and persistence of cultural traits either as a function of a given set of social circumstances or constraints or in terms of the social function(s) of the traits themselves, or both.

Gesunkenes kulturgut. Literally, "sunken cultural materials"; the theory that knowledge and innovation are produced in the elite strata of society and gradually filter down to ordinary people, or the "masses." Also known as the "trickle-down" theory.

Given. (adj.) Assumed as actual or hypothetical; (n.) something taken for granted, a basic assumption; a principle taken to be axiomatic.

Health behavior. For my purposes, all actions taken with respect to good or ill health—including any purposive health maintenance activities, and all actions intended to be preventive, diagnostic, palliative, meliorative, curative, or rehabilitative—irrespective of their outcomes, or of the social sphere in which they are undertaken (home, hospital, house of worship, healer's premises, health clinic, etc.).

Hematemesis. Vomiting blood.

HIV. Human immunodeficiency virus, identified as the infectious agent of the acquired immunodeficiency syndrome (AIDS) and of the spectrum of illnesses and symptomatologies that make up the broad category of HIV disease.

Iatrogenic. Adverse effects or conditions caused by the interventions of or occurring as a result of treatment by a physician or other health professional.

Intersubjective. Interrelating two consciousnesses; sharing of subjective experience and understanding among two or more subjects, in such a way as to create mutual validation and verification of events or experiences which may not be accessible to objective verification; consensual, where consensus is achieved through such validation processes.

Knowledge. As used here, and as broadly construed, "justified belief"; that which is held to be certain or true. Belief and knowledge both involve mental or intellectual acceptance of something as true, actual, or real on the basis of some form of authoritative support for the conclusion.

KS/Kaposi's sarcoma. Cancerous condition of the blood vessel walls, usually characterized by reddish or purple spots on the skin (though it can also occur internally); it is a frequent manifestation of HIV disease.

Lymphocytes. White blood cells central to immune system functions of creating antibodies to foreign substances, destroying invading organisms, and stimulating or modulating the overall immune response.

Macrophage. Cells that both engulf foreign substances in the body and interact with lymphocytes to facilitate production of antibodies.

Märchen. Folktale, sometimes referred to in popular parlance as a "fairy tale"; characterized by formulaic openings and closings ("once upon a time . . . ," "and they lived happily ever after").

Medicocentrism. The conscious or unconscious practice of interpreting the actions and beliefs of patients (or anyone else) in terms of the values and norms of medicine; the belief that medical views, values, and explanations are the standard against which other views are to be tested for correctness.

Memorate. A first-person narrative, usually of a supernatural experience or encounter.

Motif. The smallest meaningful image in a story; motifs "travel" and are found in many story settings. Examples include witches riding people, black dogs as incarnations of the Devil, identification through the fitting of a shoe, and so forth.

Natural. Occurring in nature; not synthesized or manufactured.

Neng. English phonetic rendering of the Hmong name for a helping spirit which a shaman calls upon for assistance in acquiring information pertinent to diagnosis and to treatment recommendations and other actions required to restore a patient to health.

Nonconventional. Not in the realm of the conventional; not the same as that which is recognized as conventional. Use of the formulation "non-" implies that the term is not a member of the same class as its root adjective, and may not necessarily be judged by the same standards and expectations (e.g., natural/nonnatural; American/non-American).

Nosology. The branch of medical science that deals with the classification of diseases; a disease classification system.

Official. Authorized, authoritative; proceeding from an office or post of authority; prescribed, sanctioned, or recognized as authoritative. "This definition implies social structures (the office from which the authorization comes) possessing a certain amount of political power" (Hufford, "Belief Glossary," unpublished; used by permission). The definition is necessarily relative or context-bound: all religious healing is unofficial with respect to biomedicine in the United States, but within its own context may be further analyzed into official theological principles, interpretations, and actions as compared to unofficial or grassroots beliefs and practices.

Ontology. The theory or study of Being or of the reality status of things.

PCP. The common abbreviation for *Pneumocystis carinii* pneumonia. This type of pneumonia is extremely rare, except as a result of immunocompromise; it is one of the very serious opportunistic infections of AIDS, and a frequent cause of death in PWAs.

Pharmacognosy. The branch of pharmacology that deals with the features of natural drugs, their constituents, chemistry, and effects.

Phenomenology. For the purposes of this book, the study of accounts of experience and the study of phenomena *through* experience; subjects' reports of their conscious experiences, taken as primary data (Havens 1960). (Does not refer here to formal phenomenological theories of philosophy.)

Philology. The study of comparative historical linguistics; the study of human speech in or through literature (written and oral), as a means of understanding cultural history.

Pluralism. "A state of society in which members of diverse ethnic, racial, religious, or social groups maintain an autonomous participation in and development of their traditional culture or special interest within the confines of a common civilization" (Merriam-Webster's Collegiate Dictionary, Tenth Edition).

Positivism. A theory that positive knowledge can only be based on "natural phenomena and their properties and relations as verified by the empirical sciences" (Merriam-Webster's Collegiate Dictionary, Tenth Edition); embodies the belief that religious and metaphysical thought are (1) developmentally antecedent to scientific thought and (2) noncognitive and inherently incapable of producing knowledge. Implicit or explicit assertion that scientific knowledge is certain, objective, and represents reality accurately and is the only knowledge that can *be* certain to represent reality accurately.

PWA. Person (or people) with AIDS; in general usage, refers to the full spectrum of HIV-positive persons, irrespective of presence or absence of symptoms or of specific "AIDS-defining" illnesses. Coined in the HIV community, the term reflects a deliberate social and political message that those who are HIV+ are *persons*, not patients, not victims; reflects a conscious demedicalization of the image of PWAs, and rejects the connotations of vulnerability and powerlessness implied by the term "victim."

Quack. (n.) Properly defined, the term is restricted in referent to one who pretends to have medical skill or misrepresents him-/herself as a physician or a person having medical knowledge; (adj.) falsely represented as medical. Entails charlatanism or fraud. In medical usage especially, this term is often overextended to cover any nonbiomedical practitioner, healing substance, or healing action irrespective of presence or absence of fraud; in such usages, the term it is meant to be condemnatory and dismissive.

Reflexivity. The state or stance of directing attention onto oneself. In scholarship, the principle of subjecting oneself and one's methods to the same scrutiny as is turned upon one's subject, of including one's approaches and biases and their effects upon the subject, in the account of the research results. Self-awareness.

Reification. Objectification or "thing-ification"; treating an abstract notion as an actual or concrete thing. "The fallacy of taking abstractions and regarding them as actually existing entities that are causally efficacious and ontologically prior and superior to their referents" (Angeles 1981:243).

Reify. To objectify an abstraction (see reification).

Role. The set of behaviors and expectations culturally defined as appropriate to or required of a particular status or position (e.g., teacher, healer, parent).

Scientific. Relating to, characterized by, or derived by application of, the methods and principles of science.

Scientistic. Characterized by the conviction that the methods and requirements of the natural sciences are the only genuine means to reliable knowledge, and that these methods should be employed for all areas of investigation; by extension, characterized by the conviction that all findings not obtained or verifiable by scientific methods are necessarily of questionable validity.

Sclerotherapy. Treatment by the injection of hardening solutions.

Shaman. A ritual intermediary between other persons and the spirit world, generally dealing with illness or other misfortune; a specialist healer, found in many cultures around the world, who deals directly with supernatural entities in obtaining information necessary to diagnosis and treatment, or in carrying out treatment procedures. The shaman is thought to leave his or her body and enter the spirit realm, where s/he engages in various kinds of activities. Unlike a medium (whose spirit is also thought to leave the body), the shaman does not become a vessel for other entities to use or speak through, and is able to remember all that happened while s/he was out of the body.

Shunt. In medical usage, an artificially created passage between two naturally occurring channels, especially blood vessels.

Sick role. In sociological theory, a set of expectations provided for sick persons by society; the sick role is understood both to enable sick persons to remove themselves from everyday obligations without reprisal, and to obligate them to adopt meliorative attitudes and actions with respect to their sickness. The theory is both controversial, and pervasive and influential in the thinking of academics and health professionals.

Supernatural. In common usage, "referring to an order that is objectively real, qualitatively different from the everyday material world, that interacts with this world in certain ways, and that includes persons" and other beings or noncorporeal entities (Hufford, "Belief Glossary," unpublished; used by permission).

T-cells. Common name for T-helper cells; used interchangeably in common speech with the name CD-4 cells (q.v.).

Traditional. Customary and of long-standing acceptance and definition; exhibiting continuity over time and space; passed down generationally. The precise referent of the term is often situational, and its understood meaning may derive from the context of its use. For example, "traditional medicine" usually connotes biomedicine to a physician or other health professional but connotes folk medicine or ethnomedicine to an anthropologist, folklorist, ethnobotanist, or New Age healing proponent.

"Trickle-down" theory. See *gesunkenes Kulturgut.*

Unconventional. Not conventional, in the sense of: opposite of or contrary to conventional; not bound by or in accordance with convention. Implies negation of the root adjective "conventional," and so connotes something strange or out of the ordinary. Use of the formulation "un-" implies that the term and its obverse are members of the same class, and may be judged by the same set of standards and expectations (e.g., natural/unnatural; American/un-American).

Varices. Enlarged and distended veins.

Vernacular. The mode of expression of a group or class, as contrasted with an official sanctioned, formal, or idealized mode of expression. In the usage "vernacular health belief system," a system native to or firmly held by the people who use it; what people *actually* do when they are sick, when they wish to prevent sickness, or when they are responsible for others who are ailing, as compared to what they "ought" to do according to an official set of standards. The analogy is to vernacular language: that is, how people *actually* speak, as opposed to how a textbook of grammar dictates that they should properly speak.

Worldview. A comprehensive perceptual and conceptual schema of the nature of life and of reality; intricate, systematic "ways of seeing," of apprehending and defining reality, which are patterned and encoded at all levels of expression and interpretation. Worldviews determine the character of what is real or true, and how it is reliably to be known.

Bibliography

Abrams, Donald I.
   1990   "Alternative Therapies in HIV Infection." *AIDS* 4:1179–1187.
Ackerknecht, Erwin H.
   1971   *Medicine and Ethnology: Selected Essays*. Baltimore: Johns Hopkins
          University Press.
Ackerman, Terrence F.
   1989   "Conceptualizing the Role of the Ethics Consultant: Some Theoret-
          ical Issues." In J. C. Fletcher, N. Quist, and A. R. Jonsen, eds., *Ethics
          Consultation in Health Care*. Ann Arbor: Health Administration
          Press, 1989, pp. 37–52.
Adams, Laura M., and Merritt E. Knox
   1988   "Traditional Health Practices: Significance for Modern Health
          Care." In W. A. Van Horne and T. V. Tonnesen, eds. *Ethnicity and
          Health*. Madison, WI: The University of Wisconsin System Institute
          on Race and Ethnicity, pp. 134–156.
AIDS Treatment News
          Edited and published by John S. James. P.O. Box 411256, San
          Francisco, CA 94141.
Aiken, Linda, and David Mechanic, eds.
   1987   *Applications of Social Science to Clinical Medicine and Health Policy*. New
          Brunswick, NJ: Rutgers University Press.
Alive and Kicking
          Newsletter printed and distributed by We the People: People Living
          with AIDS/HIV of the Delaware Valley, Inc., 425 South Broad
          Street, Philadelphia, PA, 19147.
Allister, D. S.
   1981   *Sickness and Healing in the Church*. Oxford: Latimer House.
Altman, Dennis
   1986   *AIDS in the Mind of America*. Garden City, NY: Anchor Press/Double-
          day.
Alver, Bente Gullveig
   1982   "Folk Medicine as an Open Medical System." In T. Vaskilampi and
          C. MacCormack, eds., *Folk Medicine and Health Culture: Role of Folk
          Medicine in Modern Health Care*. (Proceedings of the Nordic Research
          Symposium, 27–28 August, 1981, Kuopio, Finland.) Kuopio: The
          University of Kuopio, pp. 124–139.

Alver, Bente Gullveig, and Torunn Selberg
    1984   "Alternative Medicine in Today's Society." *Temenos* 20:7–25.
    1987a   "Folk Medicine as Part of a Larger Concept Complex." *Arv* 43:21–
          44.
    1987b   "Trends in Research on Folk Medicine in the Nordic Countries."
          Ethnologia Scandinavica (1987):59–70.
American Foundation for AIDS Research (AmFAR)
          AIDS/HIV Experimental Treatment Directory (Updated and Published
          Quarterly), 733 3rd Avenue, 12th Floor, New York, NY 10017.
Anderson, Barbara G., J. R. Toledo, and Nancy Hazam
    1982   "An Approach to the Resolution of Mexican-American Resistance to
          Diagnostic and Remedial Pediatric Heart Care." In N. J. Chrisman
          and T. W. Maretzki, eds., *Clinically Applied Anthropology*. Dordrecht,
          The Netherlands: D. Reidel Publishing Company, pp. 325–350.
Anderson, Gwen, and Bridget Tighe
    1976   "Gypsy Culture and Health Care." In P. Brink, ed., *Transcultural
          Nursing: A Book of Readings*. Englewood Cliffs, NJ: Prentice-Hall, pp.
          256–262.
Anderson, John Q.
    1968   "Magical Transference of Disease in Texas Folk Medicine." *Western
          Folklore* 27(2):191–199.
Anderson, W. H., B. B. O'Connor, R. R. MacGregor, and J. S. Schwartz
    1991   "Recourse to Complementary Therapies of HIV-Positive Patients
          Continuing to Seek Conventional Treatment." VII International
          Conference on AIDS: Abstracts, Volume 2 (Abstract and poster
          WD4197).
    1993   "Patient Use and Assessment of Conventional and Alternative
          Therapies for HIV Infection and AIDS." *AIDS* 7(4):561–566.
Andrews, Theodora
    1982   (With the Assistance of William A. Corya and Donald A. Stickel, Jr.)
          *A Bibliography on Herbs, Herbal Medicine, "Natural" Foods, and Uncon-
          ventional Medical Treatment*. Littleton, CO: Libraries Unlimited.
Angeles, Peter A.
    1981   *Dictionary of Philosophy*. New York: Barnes and Noble Books.
Anspach, Renée R.
    1987   "Prognostic Conflict in Life-and-Death Decisions: The Organiza-
          tion as an Ecology of Knowledge." *Journal of Health and Social Be-
          havior* 28:215–231.
    1990   "The Language of Case Presentation." In P. Conrad and R. Kern,
          eds. *The Sociology of Health and Illness: Critical Perspectives*. 3d ed. New
          York: St. Martin's Press, pp. 319–338.
Arensberg, Conrad, and Arthur H. Niehoff
    1975   "American Cultural Values." In J. Spradley and M. Rynkiewich, eds.
          The Nacirema: Readings on American Culture. Boston: Little, Brown,
          pp. 363–378.
Arkko, Pertti J., Birgit L. Arkko, Onni Kari-Koskinen, and Penti J. Taskinen
    1980   "A Survey of Unproven Cancer Remedies and Their Users in an
          Outpatient Clinic for Cancer Therapy in Finland." *Social Science and
          Medicine* 14A:511–514.
Arno, Peter, and Karyn Feiden
    1992   *Against the Odds: The Story of AIDS Drug Development, Politics, and
          Profits*. New York: Harper Collins Publishers.

Ashley, Leonard R. N.
  1986   "Folk Remedies for the Common Cold." *New York Folklore* XII(3/4):
          143–146.
Badgley, Laurence
  1987   *Healing AIDS Naturally*, 2d ed. Foster City, CA: Human Energy
          Press.
Baer, Hans A., ed.
  1987   *Encounters With Biomedicine: Case Studies in Medical Anthropology*.
          Montreux, Switzerland: Gordon and Breach Science Publishers.
Baker, David, and Richard Copeland
  1992   "Selecting and Using Alternative Treatments for HIV and AIDS:
          Treatments, Resources, Questions. (Revised 7/92)." Photocopied
          packet distributed at VIII International Conference on AIDS, Am-
          sterdam, The Netherlands.
Bamforth, Nick
  1987   *AIDS and the Healer Within*. New York: Amethyst Books.
Banks, S. A., and E. A. Vastyan
  1973   "Humanistic Studies in Medical Education." *Journal of Medical Edu-
          cation* 48:248–257.
Banks, Samuel A.
  1979   "The Doctor's Dilemma: Social Sciences and Emerging Needs in
          Medical Education." In W. R. Rogers and D. Barnard, eds., *Nourish-
          ing the Humanistic in Medicine: Interactions with the Social Sciences*.
          Pittsburgh: University of Pittsburgh Press, pp. 277–296.
Barker, Judith C.
  1992a   "Cultural Diversity—Changing the Context of Medical Practice." In
          Cross-Cultural Medicine—A Decade Later [Special Issue]. *Western Jour-
          nal of Medicine* 157 (September):248–254.
  1992b   (ed.) *Cross Cultural Medicine—A Decade Later* [Special Issue]. *Western
          Journal of Medicine* 157(3).
Barnes, Barry, and David Bloor
  1982   "Relativism, Rationalism, and the Sociology of Knowledge." In Mar-
          tin Hollis and Steven Lukes, eds., *Rationality and Relativism*. Cam-
          bridge: MIT Press, pp. 21–47.
Barnes, Barry, and David Edge, eds.
  1982   *Science in Context. Readings in the Sociology of Science*. Cambridge, MA:
          MIT Press.
Barrett, Linda K., and Evon Z. Vogt
  1969   "The Urban American Dowser." *Journal of American Folklore* 82(325):
          195–213.
Barrick, Mac E.
  1964   "Folk Medicine in Cumberland County." *Keystone Folklore Quarterly*
          9(3):100–110.
Barton, S. E., D. A. Hawkins, D. M. Jadresic, and B. G. Gazzard
  1989   "Alternative Treatments for HIV Infection" (Letter). *British Medical
          Journal* 298(June 3):1519–1520.
Bascom, William
  1953   "Folklore and Anthropology." *Journal of American Folklore* 66:283–
          290.
Becker, Marshall H.
  1974   (ed.) *The Health Belief Model and Personal Health Behavior*. Thorofare,
          NJ: Charles B. Slack, Inc.

1986   "The Tyranny of Health Promotion." *Public Health Reviews* 14:15–25.

Being Alive
      Monthly HIV/AIDS newsletter. 4222 Santa Monica Boulevard, Los Angeles, CA 90029.

Beiser, Edward N.
1992   "Medical Ethics in an Outpatient Setting: Conflicting Cultural Values." *Rhode Island Medicine* 75(8):413–416.

Beiser, M.
1977   "Ethics in Cross-Cultural Research." In E. F. Foulks, ed., *Current Perspectives in Cultural Psychiatry*. Jamaica, NY: Spectrum, pp. 125–137.

Benedict, Ruth
1946   *Patterns of Culture*. New York: Penguin Books.

Benedict, Susan
1990   "Nursing Research Priorities Related to HIV/AIDS." *Oncology Nursing Forum* 17(4):571–573.

Bennett, Gillian
1984   "Women's Personal Experience Stories of Encounters with the Supernatural: Truth as an Aspect of Storytelling." *Arv* 40:79–88.
1987   *Traditions of Belief*. London: Penguin Books.

Berger, Peter L., and Thomas Luckmann
1967   *The Social Construction of Reality*. New York: Anchor Books.

Berger, Stuart M.
1985   *Dr. Berger's Immune Power Diet*. New York: New American Library.
1986   *Dr. Berger's Immune Power Cookbook*. New York: New American Library.

Bergman, Robert M.
1973   "A School for Medicine Men." *American Journal of Psychiatry* 130(6):663–666.

Berkow, Robert (editor-in-chief)
1982   *The Merck Manual of Diagnosis and Therapy*, 14th ed. Rahway, NJ: Merck Sharpe & Dohme Research Laboratories.

BETA: Bulletin of Experimental Treatments for AIDS
      Published by the San Francisco AIDS Foundation. Box 426182, San Francis co, CA 94142.

Bethell, Tom
1988   "Gays on Parade." *American Spectator* 21(September):9–11.

Beyene, Yewoubdar
1992   "Medical Disclosure and Refugees—Telling Bad News to Ethiopian Patients." *Western Journal of Medicine* 157(3):323–327.

Bihari, Bernard
1992   "Hypericin for the Treatment of HIV Disease: An Update." *BETA: Bulletin of Experimental Treatments for AIDS* (May):33–34.

Biltz, Nan
1989   "Healing with Gemstones." Unpublished manuscript, University of Pennsylvania, Philadelphia.

Birrer, Richard B., ed.
1987   *Urban Family Medicine*. New York: Springer-Verlag.

Black, William George
1883   *Folk-Medicine: A Chapter in the History of Culture*. London: The Folk-Lore Society.

Bleich, J. David
  1989   "The Obligation to Heal in the Judaic Tradition." In R. M. Veatch, ed., *Cross Cultural Perspectives in Medical Ethics: Readings*. Boston: Jones and Bartlett Publishers, pp. 44–57.
Bletzer, Keith V.
  1980   *Selected References in Medical Anthropology*. Monticello, IL: Vance Bibliographies.
Bliatout, Bruce Thowpaou (Thojpov Npliajtub)
  1982a   *Hmong Sudden Unexpected Nocturnal Death Syndrome: A Cultural Study*. Portland, OR: Sparkle Publishing Enterprises.
  1982b   "Understanding the Differences Between Asian and Western Concepts of Mental Health and Illness." Paper presented to the Department of Health and Human Services—Region VII, Kansas City, Missouri, May 20–22. Portland, OR: Southeast Asian Refugee Federation Orientation Center.
  1986   "Guidelines for Mental Health Professionals to Help Hmong Clients Seek Traditional Healing Treatment." In Glenn L. Hendricks, Bruce T. Downing, and Amos Deinard, eds., *The Hmong in Transition*. New York: Center for Migration Studies of New York, and Southeast Asian Refugee Studies Project of the University of Minnesota, pp. 349–364.
Blumhagen, Dan
  1980   "Hyper-Tension: A Folk Illness With a Medical Name." *Culture, Medicine and Psychiatry* 4:197–227.
  1982   "The Meaning of Hypertension." In N. J. Chrisman and T. W. Maretzki, eds., *Clinically Applied Anthropology*. Dordrecht, The Netherlands: D. Reidel Publishing Company, pp. 297–324.
Bø, Olav
  1963   "Rational Folk-Medicine." *Arv* 18/19 (Symposium on Folk Medicine, ed. by Carl Herman Tillhagen):301–311.
Boas, Franz
  1901   "The Mind of Primitive Man." *Journal of American Folklore* 14(52):1–11.
  1904   "Some Traits of Primitive Culture." *Journal of American Folklore* 17(67):243–254.
Body Positive
    Monthly newsletter for HIV+ people. 2095 Broadway, Suite 306, New York, NY 10023.
Booth, William
  1988   "An Underground Drug for AIDS." *Science* 241(September 9): 1279–1281.
Bosk, Charles L.
  1985   "The Fieldworker as Watcher and Witness." Hastings Center Report (June):10–14.
  1987   "Professional Responsibility and Medical Error." In Linda Aiken and David Mechanic, eds., *Applications of Social Science to Clinical Medicine and Health Policy*. New Brunswick, NJ: Rutgers University Press, pp. 460–477.
Boumbulian, Paul J., W. D. MacGregor, T. L. Delbanco, S. Edgman-Levitan, D. R. Smith, and R. J. Anderson
  1991   "Patient-Centered, Patient Valued Care." *Journal of Health Care for the Poor and Underserved* 2(3):338–346.

Bowser, Benjamin P.
  1992   "African-American Culture and AIDS Prevention." *Western Journal of Medicine* 157(3):286–289.
Boyd, Michael R.
  1989   "Blue-Green Algae Kill HIV in Culture." *Science News* 136(August 26):141.
Branch, Marie F., and Phyllis Perry Paxton, eds.
  1976   *Providing Safe Nursing Care for Ethnic People of Color.* New York: Appleton-Century-Crofts.
Brendle, Thomas R., and Claude W. Unger
  1935   *Folk Medicine of the Pennsylvania Germans: The Non-Occult Cures.* Norristown, PA: Pennsylvania German Society.
Brigden, Malcolm L.
  1987   "Unorthodox Therapy and Your Cancer Patient." *Postgraduate Medicine* 81(1):271–280.
Brink, Pamela J.
  1976   (ed.) *Transcultural Nursing: A Book of Readings.* Englewood Cliffs, NJ: Prentice-Hall.
  1989   "Editorial: Ethics Across Cultures." *Western Journal of Nursing Research* 11(5):518–519.
Brody, Garry S.
  1980   "Holistic Medicine and Unscientific Cults." *Western Journal of Medicine* 133(2):172–173.
Brody, Howard, and David Sobel
  1979   "A Systems View of Health and Disease." In David Sobel, ed., *Ways of Health: Holistic Approaches to Ancient and Contemporary Medicine.* New York: Harcourt Brace Jovanovich, pp. 87–103.
Brotzman, G. L., and Butler D. J.
  1992   "Cross-Cultural Issues in the Disclosure of a Terminal Diagnosis: A Case Report." *The Journal of Family Practice* 32(4):426–427.
Brown, Ray, Mario Ramirez, and E. Fuller Torrey
  1972   "Could the Hangup be Medical Folklore?" *Patient Care* (September 30):61–75.
Brown, Waln K.
  1973   "Greek Traditional Medical Practices as Revealed in a Manuscript from the Island of Levkas." *Keystone Folklore Quarterly* 18(3):103–126.
Browne, Ray B.
  1958   *Popular Beliefs and Practices from Alabama.* (University of California Folklore Studies, No. 9.) Los Angeles: University of California Press.
Brush, Stephen G.
  1974   "The Prayer Test." *American Scientist* 62:561–563.
Buchwald D., Panwala S., and Hooton, T. M.
  1992   "Use of Traditional Health Practices by Southeast Asian Refugees in a Primary Care Clinic." *Western Journal of Medicine* 156(5):507–511.
Buonanno, Michael
  1984   "Becoming White: Notes on an Italian-American Explanation of the Evil Eye." *New York Folklore* 10(1/2):39–53.
Byington, Robert H.
  1964a   "Popular Beliefs and Superstitions from Pennsylvania." *Keystone Folklore Quarterly* 9(1):3–12.
  1964b   "Powwowing in Pennsylvania." *Keystone Folklore* 9(3):111–117.

Cabrera, Lydia
  1986a *El Monte* (Notas sobre las religiones, la magia, las supersticiones, y el folklore de los negros criollos y el pueblo de Cuba). Miami: Ediciones Universal.
  1986b *Reglas de Congo: Palo Monte/Mayombe*. Miami: Ediciones Universal.
Cannon, Walter B.
  1942 " 'Voodoo' Death." *American Anthropologist* 44(2):169–181.
Cartwright, Christine A.
  1982 " 'To the Saints Which Are at Ephesus . . .': A Case Study in the Analysis of Religious Memorates." *Western Folklore* 41(Winter):57–70.
Casdorph, H. Richard
  1976 *The Miracles*. Plainfield, NJ: Logos International.
Cassell, Eric
  1975 "Preliminary Explorations of Thinking in Medicine." *Ethics in Science and Medicine* 2(1):1–13.
  1976 "Moral Thought in Clinical Practice: Applying the Abstract to the Usual." In H. T. Engelhardt and D. Callahan, eds., *Science, Ethics and Medicine* (Volume I, The Foundations of Ethics and Its Relationship to Science). Hastings-on-Hudson, NY: Hastings Center Institute of Society, Ethics, and Life Sciences, pp. 147–160.
  1982 "The Nature of Suffering and the Goals of Medicine." *New England Journal of Medicine* 306:639–645.
  1984 *The Place of the Humanities in Medicine*. Hastings-on-Hudson, NY: Hastings Center Institute of Society, Ethics, and Life Sciences.
Cassileth, Barrie
  1986 "Unorthodox Cancer Medicine." *Cancer Investigation* 4(6):591–598.
  1989 "The Social Implications of Questionable Cancer Therapies." *Cancer* 63(7):1247–1250.
Cassileth, Barrie, and Helene Brown
  1988 "Unorthodox Cancer Medicine." *Cancer* 38(3):176–186.
Cassileth, Barrie, Edward Lusk, Thomas Strouse, and Brenda Bodenheimer
  1984 "Contemporary Unorthodox Treatments in Cancer Medicine: A Study of Patients, Treatments, and Practitioners." *Annals of Internal Medicine* 101:105–112.
Cate, Pat
  1986 "An ABC of Alternative Medicine: Bach Flower Remedies." *Health Visitor* 59(September):276–277.
Caudill, William
  1953 "Applied Anthropology in Medicine." In A. Kroeber, ed., *Anthropology Today*. Chicago: University of Chicago Press, pp. 771–806.
Centers for Disease Control and Prevention
  1993 *HIV/AIDS Surveillance Report* 5(1).
Chambers, Erve
  1989 *Applied Anthropology: A Practical Guide*, 2d ed. Prospect Heights, IL: Waveland Press.
Charmaz, Kathy
  1991 *Good Days, Bad Days: The Self in Chronic Illness and Time*. New Brunswick, NJ: Rutgers University Press.
Chesney, Alan P., Barbara L. Thompson, Alfredo Guevera, Angela Vela, and Mary Frances Schottstaedt
  1980 "Mexican-American Folk Medicine: Implications for the Family Physician." *Journal of Family Practice* 11:567–574.

Chindarsi, Nusit
  1976   *The Religion of the Hmong Njua*. Bangkok, Thailand: Siam Society.
Chocron, Daya Sarai
  1986   *Healing with Crystals and Gemstones*. York Beach, ME: Samuel Weiser.
            (Originally published in German by Heinrich Hugendubel Verlag,
            Munich, 1983.)
Chomsky, Noam
  1957   *Syntactic Structures*. The Hague: Mouton.
Chow, Effie
  1976   "Cultural Health Traditions: Asian Perspectives." In M. F. Branch
            and P. P. Paxton, eds., *Providing Safe Nursing Care for Ethnic People of
            Color*. New York: Appleton-Century-Crofts, pp. 99–114.
Chowchuvech, Supatra
  1983   "The West Philadelphia H'mong Community." Master's Thesis,
            University of Pennsylvania, Philadelphia.
Chrisman, Noel J.
  1977   "The Health Seeking Process: An Approach to the Natural History
            of Illness." *Culture, Medicine and Psychiatry* 1(4):351–378.
  1982   "Anthropology in Nursing: An Exploration of Adaptation." In N. J.
            Chrisman and T. W. Maretzki, eds., *Clinically Applied Anthropology*.
            Dordrecht, The Netherlands: D. Reidel Publishing Company, pp.
            117–140.
Chrisman, Noel, and Arthur Kleinman
  1983   "Popular Health Care and Lay Referral Networks." In David Me-
            chanic, ed., *Handbook of Health, Health Care, and Health Professions*.
            New York: Free Press, pp. 569–591.
Chrisman, Noel, and Thomas J. Maretzki
  1982a   *Clinically Applied Anthropology: Anthropologists in Health Science
            Settings*. Dordrecht, The Netherlands: D. Reidel Publishing Com-
            pany.
  1982b   "Anthropology in Health Science Settings." In N. J. Chrisman and
            T. W. Maretzki, eds. *Clinically Applied Anthropology*. Dordrecht, The
            Netherlands: D. Reidel Publishing Company, pp. 1–34.
Christakis, Nicholas A.
  1992   "Ethics are Local: Engaging Cross-Cultural Variation in the Ethics
            for Clinical Research." *Social Science and Medicine* 35(9):1079–1091.
Clark, Margaret M. (special guest editor)
  1983   *Cross-Cultural Medicine* [Special Issue]. *The Western Journal of Medicine*
            139(6).
Clark, Matt
  1985   "AIDS Exiles in Paris." *Newsweek* 106(August 5):71.
Clarke, John R.
  1987   "What Do Physicians Know? Thoughts About Clinical Knowledge."
            In David J. Newell and Ira W. Gabrielson, eds., *Medicine Looks at the
            Humanities*. Lanham, MD: University Press of America, pp. 27–34.
Clarke, Loren K., and Malcolm Potts, eds.
  1988   *The AIDS Reader*. Boston: Branden Publishing Company.
Clouser, K. Danner, and David J. Hufford, eds.
  1993   "Nonorthodox Medical Systems: Their Epistemological Claims"
            [Special Issue]. *Journal of Medicine and Philosophy* 18(2).
Cobb, Beatrix
  1954   "Why Do People Detour to Quacks?" In E. Gartley Jaco, ed., *Pa-
            tients, Physicians, and Illness*. New York: The Free Press, pp. 283–287.

Colbruno, Michael
   1990   "The Black AIDS Dilemma." *San Francisco Sentinel* (February 9):10.
Colson, Anthony C.
   1971   The Differential Use of Medical Resources in Developing Coun-
           tries." *Journal of Health and Social Behavior* 12: 226–237.
Comas-Diaz, Lillian
   1981   "Ethnicity and Treatment: Puerto Rican Espiritismo and Psycho-
           therapy." *American Journal of Orthopsychiatry* 51(4):636–645.
Conrad, Peter
   1985   "The Meaning of Medications: Another Look at Compliance." *So-
           cial Science and Medicine* 20(1):29–37.
Conrad, Peter, and Rochelle Kern, eds.
   1986   *The Sociology of Health and Illness: Critical Perspectives*, 2d ed. New
           York: St. Martin's Press.
   1990   *The Sociology of Health and Illness: Critical Perspectives*, 3d ed. New
           York: St. Martin's Press.
Coodley, Gregg
   1991   "Nutritional Problems in HIV-infected Patients." *AIDS Medical Re-
           port* 4(9):93–99.
Cortese, Anthony
   1990   *Ethnic Ethics: The Restructuring of Moral Theory*. Albany: State Univer-
           sity of New York Press.
Coulter, Harris L.
   1975   *Homeopathic Medicine*. St. Louis: Formur.
Crellin, John K., and Jane Philpott
   1990   *Herbal Medicine Past and Present* (2 volumes). Volume 1: *Trying to Give
           Ease*. Volume 2: *A Reference Guide to Medicinal Plants*. Durham, NC:
           Duke University Press.
Crepeau, Pierre, ed.
   1985   *Medecine et Religion Populaires/Folk Medicine and Religion* (National
           Museum of Man, Mercury Series, Paper No. 53). Ottawa: Canadian
           Centre for Folk Culture Studies.
Critical Path
           Edited by Kiyoshi Kuromiya. Newsletter of the Critical Path AIDS
           Project, 2062 Lombard Street, Philadelphia, PA 19146.
Croom, Edward M., Jr.
   1983   "Documenting and Evaluating Herbal Remedies." *Economic Botany*
           37:13–27.
Cross, Alan W., and Larry R. Churchill
   1982   "Ethical and Cultural Dimensions of Informed Consent." *Annals of
           Internal Medicine* 96:110–113.
Curry, F. J.
   1968   "Neighborhood Clinics for More Effective Outpatient Treatment of
           Tuberculosis." *New England Journal of Medicine* 279:1262–1267.
Curt, Gregory A., Gale Katterhagen, and Francis X. Mahaney
   1986   "Immunoaugmentative Therapy: A Primer on the Perils of Unproved
           Treatments." *Journal of the American Medical Association* 255(4):505–507.
Daniel, E. Valentine, and Judy F. Pugh, eds.
   1984   *South Asian Systems of Healing* (*Contributions to Asian Studies*, Vol. 18).
           Leiden, The Netherlands: E. J. Brill.
Danielson, Kimberly J., Donna E. Stewart, and Gerald P. Lippert
   1988   "Unconventional Cancer Remedies." *Canadian Medical Association
           Journal* 138(11):1005–1011.

Dao, Yang
　1982　"Why Did the Hmong Leave Laos?" In Bruce T. Downing and
　　　　Douglas P. Olney, eds., *The Hmong in the West*. Papers of the 1981
　　　　Hmong Research Conference, University of Minnesota. Minneapo-
　　　　lis: Southeast Asian Refugee Studies Project, Center for Urban and
　　　　Regional Affairs, University of Minnesota, pp. 3–18.
D'Arcy, P. F.
　1991　"Adverse Reactions and Interactions with Herbal Medicines. Part 1:
　　　　Adverse Reactions." *Adverse Drug Reactions and Toxicological Reviews*
　　　　10(4):189–208.
Davis, E. Wade
　1988　*Passage of Darkness. The Ethnobiology of the Haitian Zombie*. Chapel
　　　　Hill: University of North Carolina Press.
Davis, Fred
　1991　*Passage Through Crisis: Polio Victims and Their Families*. New Bruns-
　　　　wick, NJ: Transaction Press. (Originally published in 1958.)
Davis, Kenneth W.
　1969　"Weather Signs in Central Texas." *Western Folklore* 28(3):169–174.
de Craemer, Willy
　1983　"A Cross-Cultural Perspective on Personhood." *Milbank Memorial
　　　　Fund Quarterly/Health and Society* 61(1):19–34.
de Groot A. C., and Weyland, J. W.
　1992　"Systemic Contact Dermatitis from Tea Tree Oil." *Contact Dermatitis*
　　　　27(4):279–280.
de Vries, Manfred F. R. K.
　1982　"Abominable Snowman or Bigfoot: A Psychoanalytic Search for the
　　　　Origin of Yeti and Sasquatch Tales." *Fabula* 23(3/4):246–261.
de Wert, Elly
　1984　"Folk Healers as Part of Local Health Care System. A Case Study in
　　　　Northern Norway." *Temenos* 20:101–121.
Dean, Kathryn
　1981　"Self-Care Responses to Illness: A Selected Review." *Social Science
　　　　and Medicine* 15A:673–687.
　1989a　"Conceptual, Theoretical, and Methodological Issues in Self-Care
　　　　Research." *Social Science and Medicine* 29(2):117–124.
　1989b　"Self-Care Components of Lifestyles: The Importance of Gender,
　　　　Attitudes, and the Social Situation." *Social Science and Medicine* 29(2):
　　　　137–152.
　1989c　(ed.) *Social Science and Medicine* 29(2). [Special Issue on Health Self-
　　　　Care]
DeFriese, Gordon, A. Woomert, P. A. Guild, A. B. Stickler, and T. R. Konrad
　1989　"From Activated Patient to Pacified Activist: A Study of the Self-
　　　　Care Movement in the United States" [Special Issue on Health Self-
　　　　Care] *Social Science and Medicine* 29(2):195–204.
Deinard, Amos S.
　1986　"Introduction, Part 4: Health Care Issues." In Glenn L. Hendricks,
　　　　Bruce T. Downing, and Amos Deinard, eds., *The Hmong in Transi-
　　　　tion*. New York: Center for Migration Studies of New York and
　　　　Southeast Asian Refugee Studies Project of the University of Min-
　　　　nesota, pp. 333–336.
Delbanco, Thomas
　1992　"Enriching the Doctor-Patient Relationship by Inviting the Patient's
　　　　Perspective." *Annals of Internal Medicine* 116(5):414–418.

Derr, Celeste, Y. Serrano, J. Cruz, and S. Faruque
 1992 "HIV and Drug Use Prevention in Hispanic Communities Through Botánicas." VIII International Conference on AIDS: Abstracts, Volume 2 (Abstract and Poster PoB3392).
Devereux, George
 1961 "Shamans as Neurotics." *American Anthropologist* 63(5):1088–1090.
 1978 *Ethnopsychoanalysis—Psychoanalysis and Anthropology as Complementary Frames of Reference.* Berkeley: University of California Press.
DiGiacomo, Susan M.
 1987 "Biomedicine as a Cultural System: An Anthropologist in the Kingdom of the Sick." In H. A. Baer, ed., *Encounters with Biomedicine: Case Studies in Medical Anthropology.* Montreux, Switzerland: Gordon and Breach Science Publishers, pp. 315–346.
Dillner, Elisabet
 1963 "Lisa of Finshult and Her 'Smöträ.'" *Arv* 18/19 (Symposium on Folk Medicine, ed. by Carl Herman Tillhagen):275–289.
DiPalma, Michael
 1984 "A Natural Way to Health." *New Frontier* (May):7, 30.
Dobkin de Rios, Marlene
 1969 "Fortune's Malice: Divination, Psychotherapy, and Folk Medicine in Peru." *Journal of American Folklore* 82(324):132–141.
Donovan, J. L., and D. R. Blake
 1992 "Patient Non-Compliance: Deviance or Reasoned Decision-Making?" *Social Science and Medicine* 34(5):507–513.
Donovan, J. L., D. R. Blake, and W. G. Fleming
 1989 "The Patient Is Not a Blank Sheet: Lay Beliefs and Their Relevance to Patient Education." *British Journal of Rheumatology* 28:58–61.
Dowling, Patrick T.
 1987 "Cross-Cultural Medicine: Overview." In R. Birrer, ed., *Urban Family Medicine.* New York: Springer-Verlag, pp. 220–221.
Downing, Bruce T., and Douglas P. Olney, eds.
 1982 *The Hmong in the West.* Papers of the 1981 Hmong Research Conference, University of Minnesota. Minneapolis: Southeast Asian Refugee Studies Project. Center for Urban and Regional Affairs, University of Minnesota.
Drake, Donald C.
 1988 "AIDS Now Centering on Urban Poor." *Philadelphia Inquirer*, June 20, 1988.
Dunbabin, D. W., G. A. Tallis, P. Y. Popplewell, and R. A. Lee
 1992 "Lead Poisoning from an Indian Herbal Medicine." *Medical Journal of Australia* 157(11/12):835–836.
Dundes, Alan
 1961 "Brown County Superstitions." *Midwest Folklore* 11(1):25–56.
 1965 (ed.) *The Study of Folklore.* Englewood Cliffs, NJ: Prentice-Hall.
 1971 "Folk Ideas as Units of Worldview." *Journal of American Folklore* 84(331):93–103.
 1981 (ed.) *The Evil Eye: A Folklore Casebook.* New York: Garland Publishing.
Dunnigan, Timothy
 1986 "Processes of Identity Maintenance in Hmong Society." In Glenn L. Hendricks, Bruce T. Downing, and Amos Deinard, eds., *The Hmong in Transition.* New York: Center for Migration Studies of New York

and Southeast Asian Refugee Studies Project of the University of Minnesota, pp. 41–54.

Durbin, Paul T.
1984   *A Guide to the Culture of Science, Technology, and Medicine*. New York: Free Press.

Dwyer, J., R. Bye, P. Holt, and S. Lauze
1988   "Unproven Nutritional Therapies: What Is the Evidence?" *Nutrition Today* 23(2) 25–33.

Easlea, Brian
1980   *Witch-Hunting, Magic and the New Philosophy: An Introduction to Debates of the Scientific Revolution, 1450–1750*. Sussex, UK: Harvester Press.

Edwards, J. Guy, and David Gill
1981   "Psychiatry and the Occult." *The Practitioner* 225 (January):83–88.

Egawa, Janey, and Nathaniel Tashima
1982   "Indigenous Healers in Southeast Asian Refugee Communities." San Francisco: Pacific Asian Mental Health Research Project.

Egeland, Janice A.
1978   "Ethnic Value Orientation Analysis." *Miami Health Ecology Project Report, Volume II*. Miami: University of Miami.

Eisenberg, D. M., R. C. Kessler, C. Foster, F. E. Norlock, D. R. Calkins, and T. L. Delbanco
1993   "Unconventional Medicine in the United States." *New England Journal of Medicine* 328 (January 28):246–252.

Eisenberg, Leon
1977   "Disease and Illness: Distinctions Between Professional and Popular Ideas of Sickness." *Culture, Medicine, and Psychiatry*, 1:9–23.

Eisenberg, Leon, and Arthur Kleinman
1981   *The Relevance of Social Science for Medicine*. Dordrecht, The Netherlands: D. Reidel Publishing Company.

Eliade, Mircea
1964   *Shamanism: Archaic Techniques of Ecstasy* (Translated from the French by Willard R. Trask). Bollingen Series LXXVI. Princeton, NJ: Princeton University Press. (Originally published in French as *Le chaminisme at les techniques archaiques de l'extase*, Librairie Payot, Paris, 1951.)

Ellerman, Daniel
1988   "Report on the Survey of Persons with AIDS/ARC" (Prepared for the Philadelphia Commission on AIDS). Philadelphia: Leonard Davis Institute of Health Economics, University of Pennsylvania.

Elesh, David, and Paul T. Schollaert
1972   "Race and Urban Medicine: Factors Affecting the Distribution of Physicians in Chicago." *Journal of Health and Social Behavior* 13:236–249.

Elliot-Binns, C.P.
1973   "An Analysis of Lay Medicine." *Journal of the Royal College of General Practitioners* 23:255–264.

Engel, George L.
1977   "The Need for a New Medical Model: A Challenge for Biomedicine." *Science* 196:129–136.

1985   "Commentary on Schwartz and Wiggins: Science, Humanism, and the Nature of Medical Practice." *Perspectives in Biology and Medicine* 28:362–366, 1985.

Engelhardt, H. Tristram, Jr.
1982   "Bioethics in Pluralist Societies." *Perspectives in Biology and Medicine*
        26:64–78.
1989   "Ethics and the Resolution of Controversies: A Closer Look at the
        Brink." In R. M. Veatch, ed., *Cross Cultural Perspectives in Medical
        Ethics: Readings*. Boston: Jones and Bartlett Publishers, pp. 187–
        192.
Erich, Oswald A., and Richard Beitl, eds.
1955   *Wörterbuch der deutschen Volkskunde*, 2d ed. Stuttgart: A. Kroner.
Ewing, A. C.
1951   *The Fundamental Questions of Philosophy*. London: Routledge and
        Kegan Paul.
Fabrega, Horacio, Jr.
1974   "Ladino Theories of Disease: A Case Study." In H. Fabrega, Jr., ed., *Disease and Social Behavior*. Cambridge, MA: MIT Press, pp. 223–256.
Fabrega, Horacio, and Daniel B. Silver
1970   "Some Social and Psychological Properties of Zinacanteco Shamans." *Behavioral Science* 15(6):471–486.
Falk, L. A., B. Page, and W. Vesper
1973   "Human Values and Medical Education from the Perspectives of
        Health Care Delivery." *Journal of Medical Education* 48:152–157.
Farley, Eugene S.
1988a   "Cultural Diversity in Health Care: The Education of Future Practitioners." In W. A. Van Horne and T. V. Tonnesen, eds., *Ethnicity and
        Health*. Madison: University of Wisconsin System Institute on Race
        and Ethnicity, pp. 36–57.
1988b   "Preface." In W. A.Van Horne and T. V. Tonnesen, eds., *Ethnicity
        and Health*. Madison: University of Wisconsin System Institute on
        Race and Ethnicity, pp. 1–11.
Faw, Cathy, Ron Ballentine, Lois Ballentine, and Jan van Eys
1977   "Unproved Cancer Remedies: A Survey of Use in Pediatric Outpatients." *Journal of the American Medical Association* 238:1536–1538.
Feyerabend, Paul
1988   *Against Method*, rev. ed. London: Verso. (First published in 1975 by
        New Left Books.)
Finkler, Kaja
1985   *Spiritualist Healers in Mexico: Successes and Failures of Alternative Therapeutics*. South Hadley, MA: Bergin and Garvey.
Firestone, Melvin M.
1962   "Sephardic Folk-Curing in Seattle." *Journal of American Folklore*
        75(298):301–310.
Fisher, Sue
1986   *In the Patient's Best Interest: Women and the Politics of Medical Decisions*.
        New Brunswick, NJ: Rutgers University Press.
Fisher, Sue, and Alexandra D. Todd
1983   *The Social Organization of Doctor-Patient Communication*. Washington,
        DC: Center for Applied Linguistics.
Flack, Harley E., and Edmund D. Pellegrino, eds.
1992   *African-American Perspectives on Biomedical Ethics*. Washington, DC:
        Georgetown University Press.
Flaskerud, Jacquelyn H., and Evelyn Ruiz Calvillo
1991   "Beliefs About AIDS, Health, and Illness Among Low-Income Latina Women." *Research in Nursing and Health* 14:431–438.

Flaskerud, Jacquelyn H., and Cecilia E. Rush
   1989   "AIDS and Traditional Health Beliefs and Practices of Black Women." *Nursing Research* 38(4):210–215.

Flaskerud, Jacquelyn H., and Joyce Thompson
   1991   "Beliefs About AIDS, Health and Illness in Low-Income White Women." *Nursing Research* 40(5):266–271.

Fletcher, John C., Norman Quist, and Albert R. Jonsen, eds.
   1989   *Ethics Consultation in Health Care*. Ann Arbor, MI: Health Administration Press.

Forssén, Anja
   1982   "Illness in a Traditional East African Tribe." In T. Vaskilampi and C. MacCormack, eds., *Folk Medicine and Health Culture: Role of Folk Medicine in Modern Health Care*. (Proceedings of the Nordic Research Symposium, 27–28 August 1981, Kuopio, Finland.) Kuopio: University of Kuopio, pp. 235–256.

Foster, George M., and Barbara G. Anderson
   1978   *Medical Anthropology*. New York: Alfred A. Knopf.

Foucault, Michel
   1975   *The Birth of the Clinic: An Archaeology of Medical Perception*. New York: Random House.

Foulks, Edward F.
   1980   "The Concept of Culture in Psychiatric Residency." *American Journal of Psychiatry* 137:811–816.

Foulks, Edward F., Daniel Freeman, Florence Kaslow, and Leo Madow
   1977   "The Italian Evil Eye: Mal Occhio." *Journal of Operational Psychiatry* 8(2):28–34.

Foulks, Edward F., Jacqueline B. Persons, and Lawrence R. Merkel
   1986   "The Effect of Patients' Beliefs About Their Illnesses on Compliance in Psychotherapy." *American Journal of Psychiatry* 143(3):340–344.

Frank, Jerome
   1974   *Persuasion and Healing: A Comparative Study of Psychotherapy*, rev. ed. New York: Schocken Books.
   1975   "The Faith That Heals." *Johns Hopkins Medical Journal* 137:127–131.

Freidson, Eliot
   1961   *Patients' Views of Medical Practice*. New York: Russell Sage Foundation.
   1973   *Profession of Medicine*. New York: Dodd, Mead and Company.
   1987   "The Medical Profession in Transition." In Linda Aiken and David Mechanic, eds., *Applications of Social Science to Clinical Medicine and Health Policy*. New Brunswick, NJ: Rutgers University Press, pp. 63–79.

Friedl, John
   1982   "Explanatory Models of Black Lung: Understanding the Health-Related Behavior of Appalachian Coal Miners." *Culture, Medicine and Psychiatry* 6:3–10.

Fulder, S., and R. Munro
   1982   *The Status of Complementary Medicine in the United Kingdom*. London: Threshold Foundation.

Galanti, Geri-Ann
   1991   *Caring for Patients from Different Cultures*. Philadelphia: University of Pennsylvania Press.

Gamson, Josh
  1989   "Silence, Death, and the Invisible Enemy: AIDS Activism and Social
          Movement 'Newness.'" *Social Problems* 36(4):351–367.
Gardner, Rex
  1983   "Miracles of Healing in Anglo-Celtic Northumbria as Recorded by
          the Venerable Bede and His Contemporaries: A Reappraisal in the
          Light of Twentieth Century Experience." *British Medical Journal*
          287:1927–1933.
Garrison, Vivian
  1982   "Folk Healing Systems as Elements in the Community Support
          Systems of Psychiatric Patients." In U. Reuveni, R. Speck, and J.
          Speck, eds., *Innovative Interventions: Healing Human Systems*. New
          York: Human Sciences Press, pp. 58–95.
Garrity, Thomas F.
  1981   "Medical Compliance and the Clinician-Patient Relationship: A Re-
          view." *Social Science and Medicine* 15E:215–222.
Geddes, William Robert
  1976   *Migrants of the Mountains: The Cultural Ecology of the Blue Miao (Hmong
          Njua) of Thailand*. Oxford: Clarendon Press/Oxford University Press.
Gerson, Elihu
  1976   "The Social Character of Illness: Deviance or Politics?" *Social Science
          and Medicine* 10:219–224.
Gerteis, Margaret, Susan Edgman-Levitan, Jennifer Daley, and Thomas L.
  Delbanco, eds.
  1993   *Through the Patient's Eyes: Understanding and Promoting Patient-
          Centered Care*. San Francisco: Jossey-Bass Publishers.
Gevisser, Mark
  1988   "Battling the FDA: AIDS Movement Seizes Control." *The Nation*
          (December 19):677–678, 680.
Gevitz, Norman, ed.
  1988   *Other Healers: Unorthodox Medicine in America*. Baltimore: Johns
          Hopkins University Press.
Gillin, John
  1948   "Magical Fright." *Psychiatry* 11(4):387–400.
Glaser, Barney, and Anselm Strauss
  1967   *The Discovery of Grounded Theory: Strategies for Qualitative Research*.
          New York: Aldine Publishing Company.
Glassbrenner, Kimberly
  1985   "Seeking 'Indian-Acceptable' Ways to Fight Hypertension." *Journal
          of the American Medical Association* 254(14):1877–1878.
Glazier, D. M., and Glazier R., Jr.
  1990   "Understanding Alternative Therapies Often Used to Fight HIV
          Infection." *AIDS Medical Report* (July):77–86.
Glymour, Clark, and Douglas Stalker
  1983   "Engineers, Cranks, Physicians, and Magicians." *New England Jour-
          nal of Medicine* 308:960–965.
Goldstein, Diane E.
  1983   "The Language of Religious Experience and Its Implications for
          Fieldwork." *Western Folklore* 42(2):105–113.
  1987   "Sharing in the One: An Ethnography of Speaking in a Mystical
          Religious Community." PhD Dissertation, University of Pennsylva-
          nia, Philadelphia.

1991   (ed.) *Talking AIDS: Interdisciplinary Perspectives on Acquired Immune Deficiency Syndrome*. ISER Research and Policy Papers No. 12. St. Johns, Newfoundland: Institute of Social and Economic Research.

Goldstein, Kenneth S.
1964   "The Collecting of Superstitious Beliefs." *Keystone Folklore Quarterly* 9(1):13–22.

Gong, Victor, ed.
1986   *Understanding AIDS*. New Brunswick, NJ: Rutgers University Press.

González-Wippler, Migene
1973   *Santería: African Magic in Latin America*. New York: Julian Press.
1982   *The Santería Experience*. Englewood Cliffs, NJ: Prentice-Hall, Inc.
1989   *Santería: The Religion*. New York: Harmony Books.

Good, Byron
1977   "The Heart of What's the Matter: The Semantics of Illness in Iran." *Culture, Medicine and Psychiatry* 1:25–58.

Good, Mary-Jo Del Vecchio, and Byron Good
1982   "Patient Requests in Primary Care Clinics." In N. J. Chrisman and T. W. Maretzki, eds., *Clinically Applied Anthropology*. Dordrecht, the Netherlands: D. Reidel Publishing Company, pp. 275–296.

Gordon, James S.
1984   "Holistic Health Centers in the United States." In J. Warren Salmon, ed., *Alternative Medicines—Popular and Policy Perspectives* (Contemporary Issues in Health, Medicine, and Social Policy). New York: Tavistock Publications, pp. 229–251.

Gould, Stephen Jay
1981   *The Mismeasure of Man*. New York: W. W. Norton & Company.

Graham, Joe S.
1985   "Folk Medicine and Intracultural Diversity Among West Texas Mexican Americans." *Western Folklore* 44(3):168–193.

Greenblatt, R. M., H. Hollander, J. R. McMaster, and C. J. Henke
1991   "Polypharmacy Among Patients Attending an AIDS Clinic: Utilization of Prescribed, Unorthodox, and Investigational Treatments." *Journal of Acquired Immune Deficiency Syndromes* 4:136–143.

Greene, L. W.
1970   "Should Health Education Abandon Attitude Change Strategies?" *Health Education Monographs* 30.

Grieve, Mrs. M.
1982   *A Modern Herbal*, Revised (with an Index of Scientific Names). New York: Dover Publications. (Originally published in 1931 by Harcourt Brace and Company.)

Gross, Jane
1987   "AIDS Victims Grasp at Home Remedies and Rumors of Cures." *New York Times*, May 15. Reprinted in Loren Clarke and Malcolm Potts, eds., *The AIDS Reader*. Boston: Branden Publishing Company, 1988, pp. 178–183.

Grossinger, Richard
1982   *Planet Medicine: From Stone Age Shamanism to Post-Industrial Healing*, rev. ed. Boston: Shambala Publications.

Gunda, Béla
1962   "Gypsy Medical Folklore in Hungary." *Journal of American Folklore* 75(296):131–146.

Gustafson, Kirk R., et al.
1989   "AIDS-Antiviral Sulfolipids from Cyanobacteria (Blue-Green Algae)." *Journal of the National Cancer Institute* 81:1254–1258.
Guzley, Gregory
1992   "Alternative Cancer Treatments: Impact of Unorthodox Therapy on the Patient with Cancer." *Southern Journal of Medicine* 85(May): 519–523.
Hahn, Robert A., and Atwood D. Gaines
1985   *Physicians of Western Medicine. Anthropological Approaches to Theory and Practice.* Dordrecht, The Netherlands: D. Reidel Publishing Company.
Hamilton, Joan
1989   "From China, a Drug That Takes Aim at AIDS." *Business Week* (April 29):29.
Hammer, Joshua
1988   "Inside the Illegal AIDS Drug Trade (Dextran Sulfate Smuggled into U.S. from Japan)." *Newsweek* 112(August 15):41–42.
Hand, Roger
1989   "Alternative Therapies Used by Patients With AIDS" (Letter to the Editor). *New England Journal of Medicine* 320(10):672–673.
Hand, Wayland D.
1958   "Popular Beliefs and Superstitions from Pennsylvania, Part I." *Keystone Folklore Quarterly* 3(3):61–74.
1961   *The Frank C. Brown Collection of North Carolina Folklore* (Volume 6, Popular Beliefs and Superstitions from North Carolina). Durham, NC: Duke University Press.
1964   *The Frank C. Brown Collection of North Carolina Folklore* (Volume 7, Popular Beliefs and Superstitions from North Carolina). Durham, NC: Duke University Press.
1976   (ed.) *American Folk Medicine: A Symposium.* Berkeley: University of California Press.
1980   *Magical Medicine: The Folkloric Component of Medicine in the Folk Belief, Custom, and Ritual of the Peoples of Europe and America* (Selected Essays of Wayland D. Hand). Berkeley: University of California Press.
Hänninen, Osmo
1982   "On the Physiology of the Healing Methods in Folk Medicine." In T. Vaskilampi and C. MacCormack, eds., *Folk Medicine and Health Culture: Role of Folk Medicine in Modern Health Care.* (Proceedings of the Nordic Research Symposium, 27–28 August 1981, Kuopio, Finland.) Kuopio: University of Kuopio, pp. 53–69.
Hansen, Ann
1959   "Folk Medicine from Clarkston, Utah." *Western Folklore* 18(2):107–111.
Hanson, Norwood Russell
1972   *Observation and Explanation: A Guide to the Philosophy of Science.* London: George Allen and Unwin.
Harrell, David E., Jr.
1975   *All Things Are Possible: The Healing and Charismatic Revivals in Modern America.* Bloomington: Indiana University Press.
Harwood, Alan
1971   "The Hot-Cold Theory of Disease: Implications for the Treatment

of Puerto Rican Patients." *Journal of the American Medical Association* 216:1153–1158.

1977a   "Puerto Rican Spiritism: An Institution with Preventive and Therapeutic Functions in Community Psychiatry." *Culture, Medicine and Psychiatry* 1(2):135–153.

1977b   *Rx: Spiritist as Needed.* New York: John Wiley and Sons.

1981a   (ed.) *Ethnicity and Medical Care.* Cambridge, MA: Harvard University Press.

1981b   "Mainland Puerto Ricans." In Alan Harwood, ed., *Ethnicity and Medical Care.* Cambridge, MA: Harvard University Press. pp. 397–481.

Hasan, K. A.
1986   "Medical Anthropology: An Overview." In Roger Pearson, ed., *Essays in Medical Anthropology.* Washington, DC: Mankind Quarterly (Monograph no. 2), pp. 2–22.

Hastings, Arthur C., James Fadiman, and James Gordon, eds.
1981   *Health for the Whole Person: The Complete Guide to Holistic Medicine.* Boulder, CO: Westview Press.

Hatch, E. LeRoy
1969   "Home Remedies Mexican Style." *Western Folklore* 28(3):163–168.

Hautman, Mary Ann, and Janet Kreider Harrison
1982   "Health Beliefs and Practices in a Middle-Income Anglo-American Neighborhood." *Advances in Nursing Science* (April):49–64.

Havens, Joseph
1960   "The Participant's vs. the Observer's Frame of Reference in the Psychological Study of Religion." *Journal for the Scientific Study of Religion* 1:79–87.

Helman, Cecil G.
1978   "Feed a Cold, Starve a Fever—Folk Models of Infection in an English Suburban Community, and Their Relationship to Medical Treatment." *Culture, Medicine and Psychiatry* 2:107–137.

1982   "Prevailing Beliefs and Attitudes of British Patients in General Practice: Some Examples and Their Clinical Implications." In T. Vaskilampi and C. MacCormack, eds., *Folk Medicine and Health Culture: Role of Folk Medicine in Modern Health Care.* (Proceedings of the Nordic Research Symposium, 27–28 August 1981, Kuopio, Finland.) Kuopio: University of Kuopio, pp. 143–163.

1984   *Culture, Health and Illness. An Introduction for Health Professionals.* Bristol, UK: John Wright and Sons. (2d ed. with additions, 1990.)

Hendricks, Glenn L., Bruce T. Downing, and Amos Deinard, eds.
1986   *The Hmong in Transition.* New York: Center for Migration Studies of New York and Southeast Asian Refugee Studies Project of the University of Minnesota.

Henkle, Joan O., and Susan M. Kennerly
1990   "Cultural Diversity: A Resource in Planning and Implementing Nursing Care." *Public Health Nursing* 7(3):145–149.

Henry, Keith
1988   "Alternative Therapies for AIDS: A Physician's Guide." *Minnesota Medicine* 71(5):297–299.

Herbert, Victor
1986   "Unproven (Questionable) Dietary and Nutritional Methods in

Cancer Prevention and Treatment." *Cancer* 58(8, Supplement): 1930–1941.

Hill, C. E., and H. Matthews
1981　"Traditional Health Beliefs and Practices Among Southern Rural Blacks: A Complement to Biomedicine." In M. Black and J. S. Reed, eds., *Perspectives on the American South*. New York: Gordon and Breach Science Publishers, pp. 307–322.

Hill, Carole E., ed.
1991　*Training Manual in Applied Medical Anthropology*. Washington, DC: American Anthropological Association.

Hoang, Giao N., and Roy V. Erickson
1982　"Guidelines for Providing Medical Care to Southeast Asian Refugees." *Journal of the American Medical Association* 248(6):710–714.

Hoffmaster, Barry
1991　"Morality and the Social Sciences." In G. Weisz, ed., *Social Science Perspectives on Medical Ethics*. Philadelphia: University of Pennsylvania Press, 1991, pp. 241–260.
1992　"Can Ethnography Save the Life of Medical Ethics?" *Social Science and Medicine* 35(12):1421–1431, 1992.

Holbek, Bengkt
1977　"Nordic Folk Belief." (Review of *Nordisk Folktro: Studier Tillägnade Carl-Herman Tillhagen*. Festschrift for Carl-Herman Tillhagen. Stockholm: Nordiska Museet, 1976.) *Ethnologia Scandinavica* (1977): 141–143.

Hollis, Martin, and Steven Lukes, eds.
1982　*Rationality and Relativism*. Cambridge, MA: MIT Press, pp. 21–47.

Honko, Lauri
1963　"On the Effectivity of Folk-Medicine." *Arv* 18/19 (Symposium on Folk Medicine):290–300.
1964　"Memorates and the Study of Belief." *Journal of the Folklore Institute* 1(1):5–20.
1982　"Folk Medicine and Health Care Systems." *Arv* 38:57–85.

Hopkins, Donald R.
1987　"AIDS in Minority Populations in the United States." *Public Health Reports* 102(6):677–681.

Hostetler, John
1976　"Folk Medicine and Sympathy Healing Among the Amish." In Wayland D, Hand, ed., *American Folk Medicine: A Symposium*. Berkeley: University of California Press, pp. 249–258.

Howard, Jan, and Anselm Strauss, eds.
1975　*Humanizing Health Care*. New York: John Wiley and Sons.

Hufford, David J.
1971　"Organic Food People: Nutrition, Health, and World View." *Keystone Folklore Quarterly* (Winter):179–184.
1974　*Folklore Studies and Health: An Approach to Applied Folklore*. PhD Dissertation, University of Pennsylvania, Philadelphia.
1976a　"Ambiguity and the Rhetoric of Belief." *Keystone Folklore* 21(1):11–24.
1976b　"A New Approach to the 'Old Hag': The Nightmare Tradition Reexamined." In Wayland D. Hand, ed., *American Folk Medicine, A Symposium*. Berkeley: University of California Press, pp. 73–86.

1977a   "Christian Religious Healing." *Journal of Operational Psychiatry* 8(2): 22–27.
1977b   "Humanoids and Anomalous Lights." *Fabula* 18(3/4):234–241.
1982a   *The Terror That Comes in the Night: An Experience-Centered Study of Supernatural Assault Traditions.* Philadelphia: University of Pennsylvania Press.
1982b   "Traditions of Disbelief." *New York Folklore Quarterly* 8(3/4):47–55. (Issued in December, 1983.)
1983a   "Folk Healers." In Richard Dorson, ed., *Handbook of American Folklore.* Bloomington: Indiana University Press, pp. 306–313.
1983b   "The Supernatural and the Sociology of Knowledge: Explaining Academic Belief." *New York Folklore* 9(1/2):21–30.
1984   "American Healing Systems: An Introduction and Exploration." (Medical Ethnography Collection, George T. Harrell Library). Hershey, PA: Milton S. Hershey Medical Center, Pennsylvania State University Medical School.
1985a   "Folklore Studies and Health." *Practicing Anthropology* 7:23–25.
1985b   "Health Decision-Making and Systems of Belief." *Journal of Christian Healing* 7:27–31.
1985c   "Reason, Rhetoric, and Religion: Academic Ideology versus Folk Belief." *New York Folklore* 11(1–4):177–194.
1985d   "Ste. Anne de Beaupre: Roman Catholic Pilgrimage and Healing." *Western Folklore* 44:194–207.
1987   "The Love of God's Mysterious Will: Suffering and the Popular Theology of Healing." *Listening: Journal of Religion and Culture* 22(3):225–239.
1988a   "Contemporary Folk Medicine." In Norman Gevitz, ed., *Other Healers: Unorthodox Medicine in America.* Baltimore: Johns Hopkins University Press, pp. 228–264.
1988b   "Inclusionism vs. Reductionism in the Study of the Culture Bound Syndromes." *Culture, Medicine and Psychiatry* 12(4):503–512.
1988c   Contract Report on Unconventional Cancer Therapies, produced for the Office of Technology Assessment, 1988. Unpublished manuscript.
1988d   "Coherence vs. Contradiction in Supernatural Belief." Unpublished paper, presented at the American Folklore Society annual meeting, October, Cambridge, Massachusetts.
1990   "Culturally Sensitive Delivery of Health Care and Human Services." In Shalom Staub, ed., *Proceedings of the Governor's Conference on Ethnicity* (A Conference to Explore the Impact of Pennsylvania's Cultural Diversity on Public Policy). Harrisburg, PA: Pennsylvania Heritage Affairs Commission, pp. 35–37.
1991   "AIDS, Culture, and Authority." In Diane E. Goldstein, ed., *Talking AIDS: Interdisciplinary Perspectives on Acquired Immune Deficiency Syndrome* (ISER Research and Policy Papers, #12). St. John's, Newfoundland: Institute of Social and Economic Research, pp. 7–22.
1992a   "Folk Medicine in Contemporary America." In J. Kirkland, H. Mathews, C. W. Sullivan III, and K. Baldwin, eds., *Herbal and Magical Medicine: Traditional Healing Today.* Durham, NC: Duke University Press, pp. 14–31.
1992b   "Toward a Synthesis of Folk Religion and Folk Belief." Unpublished

paper, presented at a colloquium in honor of Don Yoder, Philadelphia, 17 February.

1993a   "Bringing Quality of Life to Bear in the Clinic." In S. Streufert and F. M. Gengo, eds., *Effects of Drugs on Human Functioning* (Volume 9 of Series: Progress in Basic Clinical Pharmacology). Basel: Karger, pp. 169–178.

1993b   "What Every Health Care Professional Should Know About Folklore." In M. O. Jones, ed., *Putting Folklore to Use*. Lexington: University Press of Kentucky.

1993c   "Epistemologies in Religious Healing." [Special Issue: *Nonorthodox Medical Systems: Their Epistemological Claims*]. *Journal of Medicine and Philosophy* 18(2):175–194.

Hufford, Mary
1991   *American Folklife: A Commonwealth of Cultures*. Washington, DC: Library of Congress.

Hulka, B. S., L. L. Kupper, and J. C. Cassel
1972   "Determinants of Physician Utilization." *Medical Care* 10:300–309.

Hulke, Malcolm, ed.
1979   *The Encyclopedia of Alternative Medicine and Self-Help*. New York: Schocken Books.

Hume, David
1748   "Can We Ever Have Rational Grounds for Belief in Miracles?" (From Hume: *An Enquiry Concerning Human Understanding*. Section X, Parts I and II). In William P. Alston, ed., *Religious Belief and Philosophical Thought: Readings in the Philosophy of Religion*. New York: Harcourt, Brace, and World, 1963.

Huppert, Don
1993   "Figure Skating" (audited financial report of PWA Health Group for FY 1992). *Notes from the Underground* 19(January/February):3.

Hurlich, Marshall, Neal R. Holtan, and Ronald G. Munger
1986   "Attitudes of Hmong Toward a Medical Research Project." In Glenn L. Hendricks, Bruce T. Downing, and Amos Deinard, eds., *The Hmong in Transition*. New York: Center for Migration Studies of New Yorkand Southeast Asian Refugee Studies Project of the University of Minnesota, pp. 427–445.

Hyatt, Harry M.
1970   *Hoodoo; Conjuration; Witchcraft; Rootwork* (5 Volumes). Hannibal, MO: Western Publishing Company (Vols. 1 and 2, 1970); Cambridge, MD: Western Publishing Company (Vol. 3, 1973; Vol. 4, 1974; Vol. 5, 1978).

Hymes, Dell
1972   "On Communicative Competence." In J. B. Pride and Janet Holmes, eds., *Sociolinguistics*. Middlesex, UK: Penguin Books, pp. 269–293.

1973   "Toward Linguistic Competence." *Texas Working Papers in Sociolinguistics*, Working Paper no. 16. Austin: University of Texas Press.

Irish, Andrew C.
1989   "Maintaining Health in Persons with HIV Infection." *Seminars in Oncology Nursing* 5(4):302–307.

Jackson, Jacquelyne Johnson
1981   "Urban Black Americans." In Alan Harwood, ed., *Ethnicity and Health Care*. Cambridge, MA: Harvard University Press, pp. 37–129.

Jacobs, Susan, and Jason Serinus
   1987   "Living with AIDS." *Yoga Journal* (July/August):30–36, 76–78.
Janz, Nancy K., and Marshall H. Becker
   1984   "The Health Belief Model: A Decade Later." *Health Education Quarterly* 11(1):1–47.
Jilek, W. G.
   1971   "From Crazy Witch Doctor to Auxiliary Psychotherapist—The Changing Image of the Medicine Man." *Psychiatria Clinica* (Switzerland) 4(4):200–220.
Johnson, Thomas M., Barry J. Fenton, and Howard F. Stein
   1986   "Race, Ethnic Group, and Disease" (Letter). *Journal of the American Medical Association* 255(9):1138.
Johnson, Thomas M., and Carolyn E. Sargent, eds.
   1990   *Medical Anthropology: Contemporary Theory and Method.* New York: Praeger Publications.
Johnston, Maxene
   1977   "Folk Beliefs and Ethnocultural Behavior in Pediatrics: Medicine or Magic." *Nursing Clinics of North America* 12(1):77–84.
Jones, W. T.
   1967   *The Sciences and the Humanities—Conflict and Reconciliation.* Berkeley: University of California Press.
   1976   "World Views and Asian Medical Systems: Some Suggestions for Further Study." In Charles Leslie, ed., *Asian Medical Systems: A Comparative Study.* Berkeley: University of California Press, pp. 383–405.
Joyce, C. R. B., and R. M. C. Weldon
   1965   "The Objective Efficacy of Prayer: A Double-Blind Clinical Trial." *Journal of Chronic Diseases* 18:367–377.
Kaptchuk, Ted
   1983   *The Web That Has No Weaver: Understanding Chinese Medicine.* New York: Congdon and Weed.
Kasl, S. V., and S. Cobb
   1966   "Health Behavior, Illness Behavior, and Sick Role Behavior." *Archives of Environmental Health* 12(February):246–266, and 12(April):531–541.
Kaslof, Leslie J., editor and compiler
   1978   *Wholistic Dimensions in Healing: A Resource Guide.* Garden City, NY: Doubleday.
Kassler W. J., P. Blanc, and R. Greenblatt
   1991   "The Use of Medicinal Herbs by Human Immunodeficiency Virus-Infected Patients." *Archives of Internal Medicine* 151(November):2281–2288.
Kaufman, Martin
   1988   "Homeopathy in America: The Rise and Fall and Persistence of a Medical Heresy." In Norman Gevitz, ed., *Other Healers: Unorthodox Medicine in America.* Baltimore: Johns Hopkins University Press.
Kay, Margarita
   1973   "Disease Concepts in the Barrio Today." In M. Batey, ed., *Communicating Nursing Research: Collaboration and Competition.* Boulder, CO: Western Interstate Commission for Higher Education, pp. 185–194.

Kelsey, Morton T.
 1973   *Healing and Christianity: In Ancient Thought and Modern Times.* New York: Harper and Row, 1973.
Kenny, Michael G.
 1983   "Paradox Lost: The Latah Problem Revisited." *Journal of Nervous and Mental Disease* 171:159–167.
Kickbusch, Ilona
 1989   "Self-Care in Health Promotion" [Special Issue on Health Self-Care]. *Social Science and Medicine* 29(2):125–130.
Kiecolt-Glaser, Janice, and Ronald Glaser
 1988   "Psychological Influences on Immunity: Implications for AIDS." *American Psychologist* 43(11):892–898.
Kiev, Ari
 1964   (ed.) *Magic, Faith, and Healing: Studies in Primitive Psychiatry Today.* New York: Free Press.
 1968   *Curanderismo: Mexican-American Folk Psychiatry.* New York: Free Press.
Kimball, Charles Patterson
 1970   "A Case of Pseudocyesis Caused by 'Roots.'" *American Journal of Obstetrics and Gynecology* 107(5):801–803.
Kirkland, James, Holly F. Matthews, C. W. Sullivan III, and Karen Baldwin, eds.
 1992   *Herbal and Magical Medicine: Traditional Healing Today.* Durham, NC: Duke University Press.
Kirtley, Bacil F.
 1964   "Unknown Hominids and New World Legends." *Western Folklore* 23(2):77–90.
Kisken, Peter B., and William A. Kisken
 1990   "Consent Problems and the Southeast Asian Refugee." *Wisconsin Medical Journal* 89(11):639–644, 646.
Klein, Norman
 1976   *Health and Community: A Rural American Study.* Dubuque, IA: Kendall/Hunt Publishing Company.
Kleinman, Arthur
 1973   "Toward a Comparative Study of Medical Systems." *Science, Medicine, and Man* 1:55–65.
 1975   "Explanatory Models in Health-Care Relationships." In National Council for International Health, *Health of the Family.* Washington, DC: National Council for International Health, pp. 159–172.
 1977a   "Depression, Somatization and the 'New Cross-Cultural Psychiatry.'" *Social Science and Medicine* 11:3–10.
 1977b   "Cultural Construction of Clinical Reality: Comparisons of Doctor-Patient Interactions in Taiwan." In A. Kleinman, P. Kunstadter, E. Alexander, and J. Gale, eds., *Culture and Healing in Asian Societies: Anthropological and Cross-Cultural Medical Studies.* Cambridge, MA: Schenkman Publishing Company.
 1980   *Patients and Healers in the Context of Culture: An Exploration of the Borderland Between Anthropology, Medicine, and Psychiatry.* Berkeley: University of California Press.
 1982   "Clinically Applied Anthropology on a Psychiatric Consultation-Liaison Service." In N. J. Chrisman and T. W. Maretzki, eds., *Clin-*

ically Applied Anthropology. Dordrecht, The Netherlands: D. Reidel Publishing Company, pp. 83–116.

1983   "The Cultural Meanings and Social Uses of Illness: A Role for Medical Anthropology and Clinically Oriented Social Science in the Development of Primary Care Theory and Research." *Journal of Family Practice* 16(3):539–545.

1984   "Indigenous Systems of Healing: Questions for Professional, Popular and Folk Care." In J. Warren Salmon, ed., *Alternative Medicines— Popular and Policy Perspectives* (Contemporary Issues in Health, Medicine, and Social Policy). New York: Tavistock Publications, pp. 138–164.

Kleinman, Arthur, Leon Eisenberg, and Byron Good
1978   "Culture, Illness, and Care: Clinical Lessons from Anthropologic and Cross-Cultural Research." *Annals of Internal Medicine* 88:251–258.

Kleinman, Arthur, Peter Kunstadter, E. R. Alexander, and James L. Gate, eds.
1978   *Culture and Healing in Asian Societies: Anthropological, Psychiatric, and Public Health Studies.* Cambridge, MA: Schenkman Publishing Company.

Klessig, Jill
1992   "The Effect of Values and Culture on Life-Support Decisions." *Western Journal of Medicine* 157(3):316–322.

Kluckhohn, Florence R.
1953   "Dominant and Variant Value Orientations." In P. Brink, ed., *Transcultural Nursing: A Book of Readings.* Englewood Cliffs, NJ: Prentice-Hall, pp. 63–81. (Reprinted from C. Kluckhohn and H. A. Murray, eds., *Personality in Nature, Society, and Culture.* New York: Alfred A. Knopf, pp. 342–357.)

Knapp, David A., and Deanne E. Knapp
1972   "Decision-Making and Self-Medication: Preliminary Findings." *American Journal of Hospital Pharmacy* 29(12):1004–1012.

Kolata, Gina
1988   "AIDS Patients and Their Above-Ground Underground." *New York Times* (July 10):E32.

Koss, Joan
1975   "Therapeutic Aspects of Puerto Rican Cult Practices." *Psychiatry* 38(2):160–171.

1980   "The Therapist-Spiritist Training Project in Puerto Rico: An Experiment to Relate the Traditional Healing System to the Public Health System." *Social Science and Medicine* 14B:255–266.

Kotarba, Joseph A.
1975   "American Acupuncturists: The New Entrepreneurs of Hope." *Urban Life* 4(2):149–177.

Kreisman, Jerold
1975   "The *Curandero's* Apprentice: A Therapeutic Integration of Folk and Medical Healing." *American Journal of Psychiatry* 132(1):81–83.

Krieger, Dolores
1975   "Therapeutic Touch: The Imprimatur of Nursing." *American Journal of Nursing* 75(5):784–787.

1979a   *The Therapeutic Touch—How to Use Your Hands to Help or Heal.* Englewood Cliffs, NJ: Prentice-Hall.

1979b   "Therapeutic Touch—Searching for Evidence of Physiological Change." *American Journal of Nursing* (April):660–665.

Kroeber, Alfred, ed.
  1953   *Anthropology Today*. Chicago: University of Chicago Press.
Kronenfeld, Jennie J., and Cody Wasner
  1982   "The Use of Unorthodox Therapies and Marginal Practitioners."
          Social Science and Medicine 16:1119–1125.
Kuhn, Thomas
  1970   *The Structure of Scientific Revolutions*, 2d ed., enlarged. (International
          Encyclopedia of Unified Science, Volume 2, Number 2). Chicago:
          University of Chicago Press. (1st ed., University of Chicago,
          1962.)
Kunstadter, Peter
  1980   "Medical Ethics in Cross-Cultural and Multi-Cultural Perspectives."
          Social Science and Medicine 14B:289–296.
Kwitny, Jonathan
  1992   *Acceptable Risks*. New York: Poseidon Press.
Ladd, Holly
  1992   "An AIDS Activist Perspective." *BETA: Bulletin of Experimental Treat-
          ments for AIDS* (May):5.
Laguerre, Michael
  1987   *Afro-Caribbean Folk Medicine*. South Hadley, MA: Bergin & Garvey.
Landy, David, ed.
  1977   *Culture, Disease, and Healing: Studies in Medical Anthropology*. New
          York: Macmillan Publishing Company.
Laney, Sheila
  1993   (Untitled) Address to the 1993 Symposium on Prevention, Medical
          College of Pennsylvania, May 20. Manuscript.
Lathrop, Amy
  1961   "Pioneer Remedies from Western Kansas." *Western Folklore* 20(1):1–
          22.
Lauerman, Connie
  1993   "Alternative Medicine: What Else, Doc?" *Chicago Tribune Magazine*
          (January 24):12–17, 26.
Lebra, W. P., ed.
  1976   *Culture-Bound Syndromes: Ethnopsychiatry and Alternate Therapies*.
          Honolulu: University Press of Hawaii.
Leininger, Madeleine
  1970   *Nursing and Anthropology: Two Worlds to Blend*. New York: John Wiley
          and Sons.
  1977   "Cultural Diversities of Health and Nursing Care." *Nursing Clinics of
          North America* 12(1):5–18.
  1978   *Transcultural Nursing: Concepts, Theories, and Practices*. New York:
          John Wiley and Sons.
  1991   "Transcultural Care Principles, Human Rights, and Ethical Consid-
          erations." *Journal of Transcultural Nursing* 3(1):21–23.
Lemoine, Jacques
  1986   "Shamanism in the Context of Hmong Resettlement." In Glenn L.
          Hendricks, Bruce T. Downing, and Amos Deinard, eds., *The Hmong
          in Transition*. New York: Center for Migration Studies of New York
          and Southeast Asian Refugee Studies Project of the University of
          Minnesota, pp. 337–348.
Leslie, Charles, ed.
  1976   (ed.) *Asian Medical Systems: A Comparative Study*. Berkeley: University
          of California Press.

1980   "Medical Pluralism in World Perspective." *Social Science and Medicine*. 14B:191–195.
Lessa, William A., and Evon Z. Vogt, eds.
1965   *A Reader in Comparative Religion*. New York: Harper and Row.
Lester, Calu, and Larry R. Saxxon
1988   "AIDS in the Black Community: The Plague, the Politics, the People." *Death Studies* 12:563–571.
Levin, Jeffrey S., and Jeannine Coreil
1986   "'New Age' Healing in the U.S." *Social Science and Medicine* 23(9): 889–897.
Levin, Lowell S.
1976   "The Layperson as the Primary Health Care Practitioner." *Public Health Reports* 91(3):206–210.
Levin, Lowell S., and Ellen L. Idler
1981   *The Hidden Health Care System: Mediating Structures and Medicine.* Cambridge, MA: Ballinger Publishing Company.
Levin, Lowell S., Alfred H. Katz, and Erik Holst.
1979   *Self-Care: Lay Initiatives in Health*, 2d ed. New York: Prodist.
Levine, Robert J.
1991   "Informed Consent: Some Challenges to the Universal Validity of the Western Model." *Law, Medicine, and Health Care* 19(3/4):207–213.
Levy, Sandra M.
1989   "Setting the Stage for Infection." *Science News* 136(August 26):141.
Lewin, Ellen, and Virginia Olesen
1985   *Women, Health and Healing: Toward a New Perspective*. New York: Tavistock Publications.
Lewis, Walter L., and Memory Elvin-Lewis
1977   *Medical Botany: Plants Affecting Man's Health*. New York: John Wiley and Sons.
Lieban, Richard W.
1991   "Medical Anthropology and the Comparative Study of Medical Ethics." In G. Weisz, ed., *Social Science Perspectives on Medical Ethics*. Philadelphia: University of Pennsylvania Press, pp. 221–240.
Lister, J.
1983   "Current Controversy on Alternative Medicine." *New England Journal of Medicine* 309:1524–1527.
Lock, Margaret
1987   "Introduction: Health and Medical Care as Cultural and Social Phenomena." In E. Norbeck and M. Lock, eds., *Health, Illness, and Medical Care in Japan: Cultural and Social Dimensions*. Honolulu: University of Hawaii Press, pp. 1–23.
Lock, Margaret, and Deborah Gordon, eds.
1988   *Biomedicine Examined*. Dordrecht, The Netherlands: Kluwer Academic Publishers.
Loewy, Erich H.
1986   "Physicians and Patients: Moral Agency in a Pluralist World." *Journal of Medical Humanities and Bioethics* 7(1):57–68.
1989   *Textbook of Medical Ethics*. New York: Plenum Medical Book Company.
Löfgren, Orvar
1981   "World-Views: A Research Perspective." *Ethnologia Scandinavica* (1981):21–36.

Logan, Michael, and Edward E. Hunt
  1978   *Health and the Human Condition: Perspectives on Medical Anthropology.*
          Belmont, CA: Wadsworth Publishing Company.
Long S. O., and B. D. Long
  1982   "Curable Cancers and Fatal Ulcers—Attitudes Towards Cancer in
          Japan." *Social Science and Medicine* 16:2101–2108.
Lovejoy, N. C., T. A. Moran, and S. Paul
  1988   "Self-Care Behaviors and Informational Needs of Seropositive
          Homosexual/Bisexual Men." *Journal of Acquired Immune Deficiency
          Syndromes* 1(2):155–161.
Lovejoy, Nancy C., and Theresa A. Moran
  1988   "Selected AIDS Beliefs, Behaviors, and Informational Needs of
          Homosexual/Bisexual Men with AIDS or ARC." *International Jour-
          nal of Nursing Studies* 25(3):207–216.
Lovejoy, Nancy C., and Rebecca Sisson
  1989   "Psychoneoruimmunology and AIDS." *Holistic Nursing Practice*
          3(4):1–15.
Lowe, Joan
  1988   "Santería in Philadelphia." Unpublished manuscript, University of
          Pennsylvania, Philadelphia.
Lowenberg, June S.
  1989   *Caring and Responsibility: The Crossroads Between Holistic Practice and
          Traditional Medicine.* Philadelphia: University of Pennsylvania Press.
  1993   "Interpretive Research Methodology: Broadening the Dialogue."
          Advances in Nursing Science 16(2):57–69.
Luft, Harold S.
  1987   "Economic Incentives and Constraints in Clinical Practice." In
          Linda Aiken and David Mechanic, eds., *Applications of Social Science
          to Clinical Medicine and Health Policy.* New Brunswick, NJ: Rutgers
          University Press, pp. 500–518.
Lust, John
  1974   *The Herb Book.* New York: Bantam Books.
Lynd, Robert S.
  1948   *Knowledge for What? The Place of Social Science in American Culture.*
          Princeton, NJ: Princeton University Press. (Sixth Printing. First
          copyrighted 1939.)
MacCormack, Carol
  1982   "Introduction: Traditional Medicine, Folk Medicine, and Alterna-
          tive Medicine." In T. Vaskilampi and C. MacCormack, eds., *Folk Med-
          icine and Health Culture: Role of Folk Medicine in Modern Health Care.*
          (Proceedings of the Nordic Research Symposium, 27–28 August
          1981, Kuopio, Finland.) Kuopio: University of Kuopio, pp. i–xxv.
MacGregor, Frances E.
  1967   "Uncooperative Patients: Some Cultural Interpretations." *American
          Journal of Nursing* 67(1):88–91.
Mackarness, Richard
  1974   "Occultism and Psychiatry." *The Practitioner* 212:363–366.
Malinowski, Bronislaw
  1965   "The Role of Magic and Religion." In W. A. Lessa and E.Z. Vogt,
          eds., *A Reader in Comparative Religion.* New York: Harper and Row,
          pp. 37–46. (Excerpted from "Culture," by Bronislaw Malinowski,
          Encyclopedia of the Social Sciences Volume 4, pp. 634–642, Macmillan
          Publishing Company, 1931.)

Malony, H. Newton, ed.
  1983   *Wholeness and Holiness: Readings in the Psychology/Theology of Mental Health*. Grand Rapids, MI: Baker Book House.
Marcus, George E., and Michael M. Fischer
  1986   *Anthropology as Cultural Critique*. Chicago: The University of Chicago Press.
Marin, B.
  1990   "AIDS Prevention for Non-Puerto Rican Hispanics." In C. G. Leukefeld, R. J. Battjes, and Z. Amsel, eds., *AIDS and Intravenous Drug Use: Future Directions for Community-Based Prevention Research*. (NIDA Research Monograph 93.) Rockville, MD: U. S. Department of Health and Human Services, pp. 35–52.
Marin, B. V., and G. Marin
  1990   "Effects of Acculturation on Knowldege of AIDS and HIV Among Hispanics." *Hispanic Journal of Behavioral Sciences* 12:110–121.
Marin, G.
  1989   "AIDS Prevention Among Hispanics: Needs, Risk Behaviors, and Cultural Values." *Public Health Reports* 104:411–415.
Markle, Gerald E., James C. Petersen, and Morton O. Wagenfield
  1978   "Notes from the Cancer Underground: Participation in the Laetrile Movement." *Social Science and Medicine* 12:31–37.
Marnham, Patrick
  1980   *Lourdes: A Modern Pilgrimage*. New York: Coward, McCann, and Geoghegan.
Martin, Simon
  1988   "Positive AIDS." *Nursing Times* 84(22, June 1):41–43.
Mathisen, Stein
  1988   "Continuity and Change in the Tradition of Folk Medicine." *Arv* 44:169–198.
May, William F.
  1983   *The Physician's Covenant: Images of the Healer in Medical Ethics*. Philadelphia: Westminster Press.
Mayers, Raymond Sanchez
  1989   "Use of Folk Medicine by Elderly Mexican-American Women." *The Journal of Drug Issues* 19(2):283–295.
Mays, Vickie, and Susan D. Cochran
  1987   "Acquired Immunodeficiency Syndrome and Black Americans: Special Psychosocial Issues." *Public Health Reports* 102(2):224–231.
McGinnis, LaMar
  1991   "Alternative Therapies, 1990: An Overview." *Cancer* 67(6, Supplement):1788–1792.
McGuire, Meredith
  1982   *Pentecostal Catholics: Power, Charisma, and Order in a Religious Movement*. Philadelphia: Temple University Press.
  1988   (With the assistance of Debra Kantor). *Ritual Healing in Suburban America*. New Brunswick, NJ: Rutgers University Press.
McGuire, Rick
  1989   "Get Your Alternative Rx Here." *Medical Tribune* (March 30):1, 6, 12.
McIntosh, Karyl
  1978   "Folk Obstetrics, Gynecology, and Pediatrics in Utica, New York." *New York Folklore* 4(1–4):49–59.

Mechanic, David
  1961   "The Concept of Illness Behavior." *Journal of Chronic Disease* 15:
          189–194.
  1972   *Public Expectations and Health Care.* New York: John Wiley & Sons,
          Inc.
  1976a   "Illness, Illness Behavior, and Help-Seeking: Implications for In-
          creasing the Responsiveness of Health Services." In D. Mechanic,
          ed., *The Growth of Beaureaucratic Medicine.* New York: John Wiley
          and Sons, pp. 161–176.
  1976b   (ed.) *The Growth of Beaureaucratic Medicine.* New York: John Wiley
          and Sons.
  1987   "Social Science, Medicine, and Health Policy." In L. Aiken and D.
          Mechanic, eds., *Applications of Social Science to Clinical Medicine and
          Health Policy.* New Brunswick, NJ: Rutgers University Press, pp. 1–
          12.
Meisenhelder, Janice B., and Christopher L. LaCharite, eds.
  1989   *Comfort in Caring: Nursing the Person With HIV Infection.* Glenview, IL:
          Scott, Foresman and Company.
Meleis, A. I., and A. R. Jonsen
  1983   "Ethical Crises and Cultural Differences." *Western Journal of Medicine*
          138(6):889–893.
Meñez, Herminia
  1978   "Encounters with Spirits: Mythology and the Ingkanto Syndrome in
          the Philippines." *Western Folklore* 37(4):249–266.
Meriläinen, Pirkko, Tuula Vaskilampi, and Sirkka Sinkkonen
  1982   "A Pilot Study on the Use of Alternative Treatments in Eastern
          Finland." In T. Vaskilampi and C. MacCormack, eds., *Folk Medicine
          and Health Culture: Role of Folk Medicine in Modern Health Care.* (Pro-
          ceedings of the Nordic Research Symposium, 27–28 August, 1981
          Kuopio, Finland.) Kuopio: University of Kuopio, pp. 190–211.
Mishler, Elliot G.
  1990   "The Struggle Between the Voice of Medicine and the Voice of the
          Lifeworld." In P. Conrad and R. Kern, eds., *The Sociology of Health
          and Illness: Critical Perspectives,* 3d ed. New York: St. Martin's Press,
          pp. 295–307.
Mitchell, G. Duncan, ed.
  1968   *A Dictionary of Sociology.* Chicago: Aldine Publishing Company.
Moffatt, BettyClare, Judith Spiegel, Steve Parrish, and Michael Helquist
  1987   *AIDS: A Self-Care Manual.* Los Angeles: AIDS Project.
Molaghan, Joseph B.
  1991   "Treatment Modalities for Patients with HIV Disease." *Journal of
          Intravenous Nursing* 14(Supplement):525–529.
Monte, Tom
  1989   *The Way of Hope: Michio Kushi's Anti-AIDS Program.* New York:
          Warner Books.
Montgomery, John Warwick, ed.
  1976   *Demon Possession: A Medical, Anthropological, and Theological Sym-
          posium.* Minneapolis: Bethany Fellowship.
Moran, Theresa, N. Lovejoy, C. S. Viele, M. J. Dodd, and D. I. Abrams
  1988   "Informational Needs of Homosexual Men Diagnosed with AIDS
          or AIDS-Related Complex." *Oncology Nursing Forum* 15(3):311–
          314.

Moréchand, Guy
    1968   "Le chaminisme des Hmong." *Bulletin de l'École Française d'Extréme Orient* LIV:54–294.
Morley, Peter, and Roy Wallis
    1978   *Culture and Curing: Anthropological Perspectives on Traditional Medical Beliefs and Practices.* London: P. Owen.
Mottin, Jean
    1980   *The History of the Hmong (Meo).* Bangkok: Odeon Store Ltd. Part. (printed by Rung Ruang Ratana Printing, Bangkok).
    1982   *Allons Faire le Tour du Ciel et de la Terre: Le Chaminisme des Hmong Vu Dans les Textes.* Bangkok: White Lotus.
    1984   "A Hmong Shaman's Séance." *Asian Folklore Studies* 43:99–108.
Muecke, Marjorie
    1983a   "In Search of Healers: Southeast Asian Refugees in the American Health Care System." *Western Journal of Medicine* 139 (December): 835–840.
    1983b   "Caring for Southeast Asian Refugee Patients in the USA." *American Journal of Public Health* 73(4):431–436.
Mullen, Patrick B.
    1969   "The Function of Magic Folk Belief Among Texas Coastal Fishermen." *Journal of American Folklore* 82(325):214–225.
    1971   "The Relationship of Legend and Folk Belief." *Journal of American Folklore* 84:406–413.
Muller, Jessica H., and Brian Desmond
    1992   "Ethical Dilemmas in a Cross-Cultural Context—A Chinese Example." *Western Journal of Medicine* 157(3):323–327.
Murdock, George P.
    1980   *Theories of Illness: A World Survey.* Pittsburgh: University of Pittsburgh Press.
Murphy, Henry B. M.
    1983   "Commentary on 'The Resolution of the Latah Paradox.'" *Journal of Nervous and Mental Disease* 171:176–177.
Murphy, Jane M.
    1976   "Psychiatric Labeling in Cross-Cultural Perspective." *Science* 191: 1019–1028.
Murphy, Joseph M.
    1988   *Santería: An African Religion in America.* Boston: Beacon Press.
Murphy, Murray G.
    1968   "On the Relation Between Science and Religion." *American Quarterly* 20(2):275–295.
Muzzy, Martha
    1986   "Home Remedies." *New York Folklore* 12(3/4):147–152.
National Center for Health Statistics, U.S. Public Health Service
    1978   "Utilization of Selected Medical Practitioners: United States, 1974." (Vital and Health Statistics No. 24.) Bethesda, MD: Public Health Service, Department of Health, Education, and Welfare.
National Institutes of Health
    1993   *NIH Guide for Grants and Contracts* 11(12) March 26; RFA OD-93-002, "Exploratory Grants for Alternative Medicine."
National League for Nursing
    1976   "Ethnicity and Health Care." (Publication no. 14–1625.) New York: National League for Nursing.

Nations, Marilyn K., Linda A. Camino, and Frederic B. Walker
  1985   " 'Hidden' Popular Illness in Primary Care: Residents' Recognition and
          Clinical Implications." *Culture, Medicine and Psychiatry* 9:223–240.
Neighbors, Keith A.
  1969   "Mexican-American Folk Diseases." *Western Folklore* 28(4):249–259.
Ness, Robert C.
  1982   "Medical Anthropology in a Preclinical Curriculum." In N. J. Chris-
          man and T. W. Maretzki, eds., *Clinically Applied Anthropology*. Dor-
          drecht, The Netherlands: D. Reidel Publishing Company, pp. 35–
          60.
Newman, Lucille F.
  1969   "Folklore of Pregnancy: Wives' Tales in Contra Costa County, Cal-
          ifornia." *Western Folklore* 28(2):112–135.
Newshan, Gayle
  1989   "Therapeutic Touch for Symptom Control in Persons with AIDS."
          Holistic Nursing Practice 3(4):45–51.
Nightingale, Stuart L.
  1986   "Immunoaugmentative Therapy." *American Family Physician* 34(6):
          159–160.
  1988   "Immunoaugmentative Therapy: Assessing an Untested Therapy."
          Journal of the American Medical Association 259(23):3457–3458.
  1993   "Public Warning About Herbal Product 'Chaparral.' " *Journal of the
          American Medical Association* 269(3):328.
Noall, Claire
  1959   "Medicine Among the Early Mormons." *Western Folklore* 18(2):157–
          164.
Nolen, William
  1974   *Healing: A Doctor in Search of a Miracle*. Greenwich, CT: Fawcett
          Book Group.
Notes from the Underground
          Newsletter of the PWA Health Group. Published and distributed by
          People With AIDS Working for Health, 150 West 26th Street, Suite
          201, New York, NY 10001.
Nussbaum, Bruce
  1990   *Good Intentions*. New York: Penguin Books.
Nyamathi, Adeline, and Diana M. Shin
  1990   "Designing a Culturally Sensitive AIDS Educational Program for
          Black and Hispanic Women of Childbearing Age." *Clinical Issues in
          Perinatal and Women's Health Nursing* 1(1):86–98.
O'Connor, Bonnie B.
  1985   "The Authority of Experience, and Beliefs About Knowing." Un-
          published paper, presented at American Folklore Society annual
          meeting, Cincinnati, October.
  1986   "Material and Immaterial Essences in Herbal Healing." Unpub-
          lished paper, presented at American Folklore Society annual meet-
          ing, Baltimore, October.
  1989a   "On Choosing Up Sides in the Study of Belief." Unpublished paper,
          presented at American Folklore Society annual meeting, Philadel-
          phia, October.
  1989b   "Educational and Clinical Applications of the Folklorist's Skills."
          Unpublished paper, presented at Society for Health and Human
          Values annual meeting, Washington, DC, October.

1990   "Vernacular Health Belief Systems and Their Implications for Clinical Care." PhD Dissertation, University of Pennsylvania, Philadelphia.

1991a   "Applied Belief Studies and AIDS." In Diane E. Goldstein, ed., *Talking AIDS: Interdisciplinary Perspectives on Acquired Immune Deficiency Syndrome* (ISER Research and Policy Papers, #12). St. John's, Newfoundland: Institute of Social and Economic Research, pp. 83–94.

1991b   "PWA Use and Evaluation of Alternative Therapies for HIV Infection in Philadelphia." VII International Conference on AIDS: Abstracts, Volume 2 (Abstract and poster WD4199).

1993   "The Home Birth Movement in the United States" [Thematic issue: Nonorthodox Medical Systems: Their Epistemological Claims]. *Journal of Medicine and Philosophy* 18(2):147–174.

O'Connor, Bonnie B., J. S. Lazar, and W. H. Anderson.

1992   "Ethnographic Study of HIV Alternative Therapies." VIII International Conference on AIDS: Abstracts, Volume 2 (Abstract and poster PoB3398).

Odegaard, Charles E.

1986   *Dear Doctor: A Personal Letter to a Physician*. Menlo Park, CA: The Henry J. Kaiser Family Foundation.

Orque, Modesta S., Bobbie Bloch, and Lidia S. A. Monrroy

1983   *Ethnic Nursing Care*. St Louis: C. V. Mosby Company.

Paredes, Américo

1977   "On Ethnographic Work Among Minority Groups. A Folklorist's Perspective." *New Scholar* 6:1–32.

Parsons, Talcott

1951   *The Social System*. New York: Free Press.

1975   "The Sick Role and the Role of the Physician Reconsidered." *Milbank Memorial Fund Quarterly* 53:257–278.

Paul, Benjamin

1955   *Health, Culture, and Community: Case Studies of Public Reactions to Health Programs*. New York: Russell Sage Foundation.

Payer, Lynn

1988   *Medicine and Culture: Varieties of Treatment in the United States, England, West Germany, and France*. New York: Penguin Books.

Pedersen, P. J. Draguns, and W. Lonner, eds.

1981   *Counseling Across Cultures*. Honolulu: University of Hawaii Press.

Peel, Robert

1984   *Spiritual Healing in a Scientific Age*. San Francisco: Harper and Row.

Pellegrino, Edmund D.

1974   "Educating the Humanist Physician." *Journal of the American Medical Association* 227:1288–1294.

1979a   *Humanism and the Physician*. Knoxville, TN: University of Tennessee Press.

1979b   "The Sociocultural Impact of Twentieth-Century Therapeutics." In Morris J. Vogel and Charles E. Rosenberg, eds., *The Therapeutic Revolution: Essays in the Social History of American Medicine*. Philadelphia: University of Pennsylvania Press, pp. 245–266.

1979c   "Foreword." In W. R. Rogers and D. Barnard, eds., *Nourishing the Humanistic in Medicine. Interactions with the Social Sciences*. Pittsburgh: University of Pittsburgh Press, pp. ix–xiv.

Pellegrino, Edmund D., and Thomas K. McElhinney
    1982   *Teaching Ethics, the Humanities, and Human Values in Medical Schools: A Ten Year Overview.* Washington, DC: Society for Health and Human Values.
Pellegrino, Edmund D., and David Thomasma
    1981   *A Philosophical Basis for Medical Practice.* New York: Oxford University Press.
Pentikäinen, Juha
    1965   "The Frank C. Brown Collection of North Carolina Folklore. Volumes 6, 7. *Popular Beliefs and Superstitions from North Carolina.*" (Review.) *Temenos* 1:181–185.
Peterson, John L., and Gerardo Marin
    1988   "Issues in the Prevention of AIDS Among Black and Hispanic Men." *American Psychologist* 43(November):871–877.
Philadelphia Inquirer
    1990   "Agency Backs Study of AIDS Drug Tested Underground" (Associated Press). *The Philadelphia Inquirer* (March 10):10A.
Phillips, Jennifer
    1989   "Nurturing the Spirit." In J. B. Meisenhelder and L. LaCharite, eds., *Comfort in Caring: Nursing the Person With HIV Infection.* Glenview, IL: Scott, Foresman and Company, pp. 199–211.
Pocius, Gerald
    1985   "Introductory Bibliography on Folk Medicine." In Pierre Crepeau, ed., *Medecine et Religion Populaires/Folk Medicine and Religion.* (National Museum of Man, Mercury Series, Paper No. 53.) Ottawa: Canadian Centre for Folk Culture Studies, pp. 151–161.
Polanyi, Michael
    1958   *Personal Knowledge.* Chicago: University of Chicago Press.
Polgar, Steven
    1962   "Health and Human Behavior: Areas of Interest Common to the Social and Medical Sciences. *Current Anthropology* 3:159–205.
    1963a   "Health Action in Cross-Cultural Perspectives." In H. E. Freeman, S. Levine, and L. Reeder, eds., *Handbook of Medical Sociology.* Englewood Cliffs, NJ: Prentice-Hall, pp. 397–419.
    1963b   "Health and Human Behavior: Areas of Interest Common to the Social and Medical Sciences." *Current Anthropology* 3:159–205.
Powers, B. A.
    1982   "The Use of Orthodox and Black American Folk Medicine." *Advances in Nursing Science* (April):35–47.
Powles, John
    1979   "On the Limitations of Modern Medicine." In David Sobel, ed., *Ways of Health: Holistic Approaches to Ancient and Contemporary Medicine.* New York: Harcourt Brace Jovanovich, pp. 61–86.
Press, Irwin
    1978   "Urban Folk Medicine: A Functional Overview." *American Anthropologist* 80:71–84.
Primiano, Leonard Norman
    1987   Review of *Household of Faith: Roman Catholic Devotion in Mid-Nineteenth Century America*, by Ann Taves. *Records of the American Catholic Historical Society of Philadelphia* 98:120–122.
    1990   Review of *Living Stones: The History and Structure of Catholic Spiritual*

Life in the United States, by Joseph P. Chinnici, O.F.M. *Records of the American Catholic Historical Society of Philadelphia* 101:64–66.

1993   "Intrinsically Catholic: Vernacular Religion and Philadelphia's 'Dignity.'" PhD Dissertation, University of Pennsylvania, Philadelphia.

Proctor, Robert N.
1991   *Value Free Science? Purity and Power in Modern Knowledge.* Cambridge, MA: Harvard University Press.

Puckett, Newbell Niles
1926   *Folk Beliefs of the Southern Negro.* New York: Dover Publications. (Reprinted 1969.)

Quah, Stella R.
1977   "Self-Medication: A Neglected Dimension of Health Behavior." *Sociological Symposium* No. 19, pp. 20–36.

Rakower, Dena, and Theresa A. Galvin
1989   "Nourishing the HIV-Infected Adult." *Holistic Nursing Practice* 3(4):26–37.

Reichenbach, Hans
1951   *The Rise of Scientific Philosophy.* Berkeley/Los Angeles: University of California Press.

Reimensnyder, Barbara
1982   *Powwowing in Union County.* PhD Dissertation, University of Pennsylvania, Philadelphia.

Reiser, Stanley J.
1992   "Consumer Competence and the Reform of American Health Care." *Journal of the American Medical Association* 267:1511–1515.

1993   "The Era of the Patient. Using the Experience of Illness in Shaping the Missions of Health Care." *Journal of the American Medical Association* 269:1012–1017.

Rempusheski, Veronica
1989   "The Role of Ethnicity in Elder Care." *Nursing Clinics of North America* 24(3):717–725.

Rhodes, Lorna A.
1990   "Studying Biomedicine as a Cultural System." In T. M. Johnson and C. F. Sargent, eds., *Medical Anthropology: Contemporary Theory and Method.* New York: Praeger Publications, pp. 159–173.

Rice, Mitchell F., and Woodrow Jones, Jr.
1987   *Black American Health: An Annotated Bibliography.* New York: Greenwood Press.

Rivera, Elliott
1992   "The Role of the Botánica Spritualist, Folk Healer and the Santero/Santera in the Latino Community Concerning HIV/AIDS, STD's and Substance Abuse." VIII International Conference on AIDS: Abstracts, Volume 2 (Abstract and Poster PoB3399).

Rivera, George, Jr.
1990   "AIDS and Mexican Folk Medicine." *Sociology and Social Research* 75(1):3–7.

Roberson, Mildred H.B.
1987   "Home Remedies: A Cultural Study." *Home Healthcare Nurse* 5(1): 35–40.

1992   "The Meaning of Compliance: Patient Perspectives." *Qualitative Health Research* 2(1):7–26.

Rocereto, LaVerne
1973   "Root Work and the Root Doctor." *Nursing Forum* 12(4):414–426.
Roerderer M, S. W. Ela, F. T. J. Staal, L. A. Hersenberg and L. A. Herzenberg
1992   "N-Acetylcysteine: A New Approach to Anti-HIV Therapy." *AIDS Research and Human Retroviruses* 8(2):209–217.
Rogers, William R., and David Barnard, eds.
1979a   *Nourishing the Humanistic in Medicine: Interactions with the Social Sciences*. Pittsburgh: University of Pittsburgh Press.
1979b   "The Interaction Between Humanistic Social Sciences and Medical Education." In W. R. Rogers and D. Barnard, eds., *Nourishing the Humanistic in Medicine: Interactions with the Social Sciences*. Pittsburgh: University of Pittsburgh Press, pp. 3–24.
1979c   "Some Policy Implications and Recommendations." In W. R. Rogers and D. Barnard, eds., *Nourishing the Humanistic in Medicine: Interactions with the Social Sciences*. Pittsburgh: University of Pittsburgh Press, pp. 297–308.
Romanucci-Ross, Lola
1969   "The Hierarchy of Resort in Curative Practices: The Admiralty Islands, Melanesia." *Journal of Health and Social Behavior* 10:201–209.
Romanucci-Ross, Lola, Daniel E. Moerman, and Lawrence R. Tancredi, eds.
1983   *The Anthropology of Medicine: From Culture to Method*. South Hadley, MA: Bergin and Garvey Publishers.
Rørbye, Birgitte
1982   "Ethnomedicine." *Ethnologia Scandinavica* (1982):53–84.
Rorty, James, and Philip N. Norman
1956   *Bio-Organics: Your Food and Your Health*. New York: Lancer Books.
Rosenberg, Charles
1979   "The Therapeutic Revolution." In Morris J. Vogel and Charles E. Rosenberg, eds., *The Therapeutic Revolution: Essays in the Social History of American Medicine*. Philadelphia: University of Pennsylvania Press, 1979, pp. 3–25.
1987   *The Care of Strangers: The Rise of America's Hospital System*. New York: Basic Books.
Rosenberger, Homer T.
1958   "The Hex Doctor and the Witch of Farrandsville." *Keystone Folklore* 3(2):42–45.
Rowlands, Caroline, and William G. Powderly
1991   "The Use of Alternative Therapies by HIV-Positive Patients Attending the St. Louis AIDS Clinical Trials Unit." *Missouri Medicine* 88(12):807–810.
Rubel, Arthur J.
1964   "The Epidemiology of a Folk Illness: *Susto* in Hispanic America." *Ethnology* 3(3):268–283.
Rubel, Arthur J., Carl O'Nell, and Rolando Collado-Ardón
1984   *Susto: A Folk Illness*. Berkeley: University of California Press.
Rubenstein H. R., B. B. O'Connor, L. Z. Nieman, and E. J. Gracely
1992   "Introducing Students to the Role of Folk and Popular Health Belief-Systems in Patient Care." *Academic Medicine* 67(9):566–568.
Ruby, Jay, ed.
1982   *A Crack in the Mirror: Reflexive Perspectives in Anthropology*. Philadelphia: University of Pennsylvania Press.

Ruiz, Pedro, and John Langrod
1976a "Psychiatrists and Spiritual Healers: Partners in Community Mental Health." In J. Westermeyer, ed., *Anthropology and Mental Health: Setting a New Course*. The Hague: Mouton, pp. 77–81.
1976b "The Role of Folk Healers in Community Mental Health Services." *Community Mental Health Journal* 12(4):392–398.
Salloway, Jeffrey Colman
1973 "Medical Care Utilization Among Urban Gypsies." *Urban Anthropology* 2(1):113–126.
Salmon, J. Warren
1984a (ed.) *Alternative Medicines—Popular and Policy Perspectives* (Contemporary Issues in Health, Medicine, and Social Policy). New York: Tavistock Publications.
1984b "Defining Health and Reorganizing Medicine." In J. Warren Salmon, ed., *Alternative Medicines—Popular and Policy Perspectives* (Contemporary Issues in Health, Medicine, and Social Policy). New York: Tavistock Publications, pp. 252–288.
Salmon, J. Warren, and Howard S. Berliner
1980 "Health Policy Implications of the Holistic Health Movement." *Journal of Health Politics, Policy and Law* 5(3):535–553.
Sanders, Patricia L.
1989 "Acupuncture and Herbal Treatment of HIV Infection." *Holistic Nursing Practice* 3(4):38–44.
Sargant, William
1974 *The Mind Possessed: A Physiology of Possession, Mysticism, and Faith Healing*. Philadelphia: J. B. Lippincott Company.
Saunders, Lyle
1954 *Cultural Difference and Medical Care*. New York: Russell Sage Foundation.
Saunders, Lyle, and Gordon Hewes
1969 "Folk Medicine and Medical Practice." In L. R. Lynch, ed., *The Cross-Cultural Approach to Health Behavior*. Rutherford, NJ: Fairleigh Dickinson University Press.
Scarborough, John, ed.
1987 *Folklore and Folk Medicines*. (Publication No. 10.) Madison, WI: American Institute of the History of Pharmacy.
Schneider, Joseph W., and Peter Conrad
1983 *Having Epilepsy: The Experience and Control of Ilness*. Philadelphia: Temple University Press.
Schreiber, Janet M., and John P. Homiak
1981 "Mexican Americans." In Alan Harwood, ed., *Ethnicity and Health Care*. Cambridge, MA: Harvard University Press. pp. 264–336.
Schwartz, Michael A., and Osborne Wiggins
1985 "Science, Humanism, and the Nature of Medical Practice: A Phenomenological Overview." *Perspectives in Biology and Medicine* 28: 331–61.
Scott, Anne W.
1993 "'Masters of the Ordinary': Integrating Personal Experience and Vernacular Knowledge in Alcoholics Anonymous." PhD Dissertation, University of Pennsylvania, Philadelphia.

Scott, Clarissa S.
1974   "Health and Healing Practices Among Five Ethnic Groups in Miami." *Public Health Reports* 89:524–531.
Segall, Alexander, and Jay Goldstein
1989   "Exploring the Correlates of Self-Provided Health Care Behavior." [Special Issue on Health Self-Care]. *Social Science and Medicine* 29(2):153–162.
Serinus, Jason, ed.
1987   *Psychoimmunity and the Healing Process: A Holistic Approach to Immunity and AIDS*, 2d ed., Revised and Updated. Berkeley: Celestial Arts.
Sheils, W. J., ed.
1982   *The Church and Healing*. Oxford: Published for the Ecclesiastical History Society by Basil Blackwell.
Sherman, Spencer
1988   "The H'mong in America." *National Geographic* 174(October):587–610.
Shilts, Randy
1987   *And the Band Played On: Politics, People and the AIDS Epidemic*. New York: Penguin Books.
Simmons, Ozzie G.
1955   "Popular and Modern Medicine in Mestizo Communities of Coastal Peru and Chile." *Journal of American Folklore* 68(267):57–71.
Simons, Ronald C.
1980   "The Resolution of the Latah Paradox." *Journal of Nervous and Mental Disease* 168:195–206.
1983a   "Latah II—Problems With a Purely Symbolic Interpretation: A Reply to Michael Kenny." *Journal of Nervous and Mental Disease* 171:160–175.
1983b   "Latah III—How Compelling is the Evidence for a Psychoanalytic Interpretation: A Reply to H. B. M. Murphy." *Journal of Nervous and Mental Disease* 171:178–181.
Simons, Ronald C., and Charles Hughes, eds.
1985   *The Culture-Bound Syndromes*. Hingham, MA: Kluwer Academic Publishers.
Simpson, George Eaton
1978   *Black Religions in the New World*. New York: Columbia University Press.
Sinclair, Brett J.
1992   *Alternative Health Care Resources: A Directory and Guide*. West Nyack, NY: Parker Publishing Company.
Singer, Barry, and Victor Benassi
1981   "Occult Beliefs." *American Scientist* 69:49–54.
Skloot, Floyd
1993   "Double Blind: When Healing is a Gamble." *The Sun* 215 (November):4–9.
Smitherman J., and P. Harber P
1991   "A Case of Mistaken Identity: Herbal Medicine as a Cause of Lead Toxicity." *American Journal of Industrial Medicine* 20(6):795–798.
Snider, Gayle F., and H. F. Stein
1987   "An Approach to Community Assessment in Medical Practice." *Family Medicine* 19(3):213–219.

Snow, Loudell
    1973   "'I Was Born Just Exactly With the Gift': An Interview with a
            Voodoo Practitioner." *Journal of American Folklore* 86(341):272–281.
    1974   "Folk Medical Beliefs and Their Implications for Care of Patients: A
            Review Based on Studies Among Black Americans." *Annals of Inter-
            nal Medicine* 81:82–96.
    1983   "Traditional Health Beliefs and Practices Among Lower Class Black
            Americans." *Western Journal of Medicine* 139:820–828.
Snow, Loudell, and Shirley M. Johnson
    1977   "Modern Day Menstrual Folklore." *Journal of the American Medical
            Association* 237:2736–2739.
Sobel, David, ed.
    1979   *Ways of Health: Holistic Approaches to Ancient and Contemporary Medi-
            cine.* New York: Harcourt Brace Jovanovich.
Society for Health and Human Values
    1984   *The Teaching of Humanities and Human Values in Primary Care Resi-
            dency Training: Resource Book.* McLean, VA: Society for Health and
            Human Values.
Soll, Robert W., and Penelope Grenoble
    1984   *Something Can Be Done, and You Can Do It: A New Approach to Under-
            standing and Managing Multiple Sclerosis.* Chicago: Contemporary
            Books.
Sorofman, B., T. Tripp-Reimer, G. M. Lauer, and M. E. Martin
    1990   "Symptom Self-Care." *Holistic Nursing Practice* 4(2):45–55.
Spector, Rachel E.
    1991   *Cultural Diversity in Health and Illness*, 3d ed. Norwalk, CT: Appleton
            and Lange.
Spencer, Norman
    1983   "Medical Anthropology and the AIDS Epidemic: A Case Study in
            San Francisco." *Urban Anthropology* 12(2):141–159.
Spicer, Edward H., ed.
    1977   *Ethnic Medicine in the Southwest.* Tucson: University of Arizona Press.
Spiegel, Allen D.
    1983   *Home Health Care: Home Birthing to Hospice Care.* Owings Mills, MD:
            National Health Publications.
Starr, Paul
    1982   *The Social Transformation of American Medicine.* New York: Basic
            Books.
Stein, Howard F.
    1982a   "The Annual Cycle and the Cultural Nexus of Health Care Be-
            havior Among Oklahoma Wheat Farming Families." *Culture, Medi-
            cine and Psychiatry* 6(1):81–99.
    1982b   "The Ethnographic Mode of Teaching Clinical Behavioral Science."
            In N. Chrisman and T. Maretski, eds., *Clinically Applied Anthropology:
            Anthropologists in Health Science Settings.* Boston: D. Reidel.
    1990a   *American Medicine as Culture.* Boulder, CO: Westview Press.
    1990b   "Psychoanalytic Perspectives." In T. M. Johnson and C. F. Sargent,
            eds., *Medical Anthropology. Contemporary Theory and Method.* New
            York: Praeger Publishers, pp. 73–92.
Steinberg, Charles I.
    1990   "Integrating Traditional Medicine with Other Therapies in the

Treatment of HIV-Infected Individuals." *Maryland Medical Journal* 39(2):183–188.

Stekert, Ellen
1970   "Focus for Conflict: Southern Mountain Medical Beliefs in Detroit." *Journal of American Folklore* 83:115–156.

Stern, S., and J. A. Cicala, eds.
1991   *Creative Ethnicity: Symbols and Strategies of Contemporary Ethnic Life.* Logan: Utah State University Press.

Stevens, Phillips, Jr.
1982   "Some Implications of Urban Witchcraft Beliefs." *New York Folklore* 8(3/4):29–45.

Stimson, Gerry B.
1974   "Obeying Doctor's Orders: A View from the Other Side." *Social Science and Medicine* 8:97–104.

Stoeckle, John D.
1979   "The Tasks of Care: Humanistic Dimensions of Medical Education." In W. R. Rogers and D. Barnard, eds., *Nourishing the Humanistic in Medicine: Interactions with the Social Sciences.* Pittsburgh: University of Pittsburgh Press, pp. 263–276.

Stoller, Paul
1984   "Eye, Mind, and Word in Anthropology." *L'Homme* 24(3/4):91–114.

Strawn, Jill M.
1989   "Complementary Therapies: Maximizing the Mind-Body Connection." In J. B. Meisenhelder and L. LaCharite, eds., *Comfort in Caring: Nursing the Person With HIV Infection.* Glenview, IL: Scott, Foresman and Company, pp. 181–198.

Stuart-Harle, Martin
1984   "Transcultural Medicine: The Average G.P. Isn't Equipped to Deal With It." *The Medical Post* (June 12):56–57.

Studer, Gerald C.
1980   "Powwowing: Folk Medicine or White Magic?" *Pennsylvania Mennonite Heritage* (July):17–23.

Sullivan-Fowler, Micaela, Terry Austin, and Arthur W. Haffner
1988   *Alternative Therapies, Unproven Methods, and Health Fraud: A Selected Annotated Bibliography.* Chicago: American Medical Association, Division of Library and Information Management.

Sumartojo, Esther
1993   "When Tuberculosis Treatment Fails: A Social Behavioral Account of Patient Adherence." *American Review of Respiratory Diseases* 147: 1311–1320.

Svarstad, Bonnie L.
1976   "Physician-Patient Communication and Patient Conformity with Medical Advice." In D. Mechanic, ed., *The Growth of Beaureaucratic Medicine.* New York: John Wiley and Sons, pp. 220–238.

1987   "Patient-Practitioner Relationships and Compliance with Prescribed Medical Regimens." In Linda Aiken and David Mechanic, eds., *Applications of Social Science to Clinical Medicine and Health Policy.* New Brunswick, NJ: Rutgers University Press, pp. 438–459.

Syme, S. Leonard
1984   "Sociocultural Factors and Disease Etiology." In W. Doyle Gentry, ed., *Handbook of Behavioral Medicine.* New York: The Guilford Press, pp. 13–37.

Taylor, Carol
 1973   "The Nurse and Cultural Barriers." In D. Hymnovich and M. Bar-
         nard, eds., *Family Health Care*. New York: McGraw-Hill, pp. 119–
         127.
Taylor, Rosemary R. C.
 1984   "Alternative Medicine and the Medical Encounter in Britain and the
         United States." In J. Warren Salmon, ed., *Alternative Medicines—
         Popular and Policy Perspectives* (Contemporary Issues in Health, Med-
         icine, and Social Policy). New York: Tavistock Publications, pp. 191–
         228.
Thao, Paja
 1986   (Translated in collaboration with Dwight Conquergood.) "I am a
         Shaman." In Brenda Johns and David Strecker, eds., *The Hmong
         World*, Volume 1. New Haven, CT: Yale Council on Southeast Asia
         Studies (Yale Center for International and Area Studies).
Thao, Xoua
 1986   "Hmong Perception of Illness and Traditional Ways of Healing." In
         Glenn L. Hendricks, Bruce T. Downing, and Amos Deinard, eds.,
         The Hmong in Transition. New York: Center for Migration Studies of
         New York and Southeast Asian Refugee Studies Project of the Uni-
         versity of Minnesota, pp. 365–378.
Thompson, Dick
 1989   "Drugs From the Underground (FDA allows wider use of experi-
         mental drugs)." *Time* 134(July 10):49.
Thompson, Stith
 1955   *Motif-Index of Folk-Literature*, rev. ed. Bloomington: Indiana Univer-
         sity Press.
Thompson, William A. R.
 1976   "Herbs That Heal." *Journal of the Royal College of General Practitioners*
         26:365–370.
Tillhagen, Carl Herman, ed.
 1963   *Symposium on Folk Medicine*. Arv 18/19 (1962–63).
Tinling, David C.
 1967   "Voodoo, Rootwork, and Medicine." *Psychosomatic Medicine* 29:483–
         490.
Tobin, Joseph Jay, and Joan Friedman
 1983   "Spirits, Shamans, and Nightmare Death: Survivor Stress in
         H'mong Refugee." *American Journal of Orthopsychiatry* 55(3):439–
         448.
Todd, Alexandra Dundas
 1989   *Intimate Adversaries: Cultural Conflict Between Doctors and Women Pa-
         tients*. Philadelphia: University of Pennsylvania Press.
Todd, Harry F., Jr., and Julio L. Ruffini, eds.
 1979   *Teaching Medical Anthropology: Model Courses for Graduate and Under-
         graduate Instruction*. Washington, DC: Society for Medical Anthro-
         pology.
Toelken, Barre
 1975   "Folklore, Worldview, and Communication." In Dan Ben-Amos and
         Kenneth S. Goldstein, eds., *Folklore: Performance and Communication*.
         The Hague: Mouton.
 1979   *The Dynamics of Folklore*. Boston: Houghton Mifflin Company.

Torrey, E. Fuller
    1969   "The Case for the Indigenous Therapist." *Archives of General Psychiatry* 20(3):365–373.
Treatment Issues
            The Gay Men's Health Crisis Newsletter of Experimental AIDS Therapies. GMHC Medical Information, 129 West 20th Street, New York, NY 10011.
Tripp-Reimer, T.
    1984   "Reconceptualizing the Construct of Health: Integrating Emic and Etic Perspectives." *Research in Nursing and Health* 7(2):101–109.
Tripp-Reimer, T., and L. A. Afifi
    1989   "Cross-Cultural Perspectives on Patient Teaching." *Nursing Clinics of North America* 24(3):613–619.
Tripp-Reimer, T., P. J. Brink, and J. M. Saunders
    1984   "Cultural Assessment: Content and Process." *Nursing Outlook* 32(2): 78–82.
Tripp-Reimer, Toni, and Mary C. Friedl
    1977   "Appalachians: A Neglected Minority." *Nursing Clinics of North America* 12(1):41–54.
Trostle, James A.
    1988   "Medical Compliance as an Ideology." *Social Science and Medicine* 27(12):1299–1308.
Trostle James A., W Allen Hauser, and Ida S. Susser
    1983   "The Logic of Noncompliance: Management of Epilepsy from the Patient's Point of View." *Culture, Medicine and Psychiatry* 7:35–56.
Trotter, Robert T.
    1985   "Folk Medicine in the Southwest: Myths and Medical Facts." *Postgraduate Medicine* 78(8):167–179.
Trotter, Robert T., and Juan Antonio Chavira
    1981   *Curanderismo: Mexican American Folk Healing*. Athens: University of Georgia Press.
Tubesing, Donald A.
    1979   *Wholistic Health—A Whole-Person Approach to Primary Health Care*. New York: Human Sciences Press.
Tung, Tran Minh
    n.d.   "Understanding the Differences Between Asian and Western Concepts of Mental Health and Illness." Typescript.
    1980   *Indochinese Patients: Cultural Aspects of the Medical and Psychiatric Care of Indochinese Refugees*. Falls Church, VA: Action for South East Asians.
Turner, Edith
    1992   *Experiencing Ritual. A New Interpretation of African Healing*. Philadelphia: University of Pennsylvania Press.
Turner, Victor, and Edith Turner
    1978   *Image and Pilgrimage in Christian Culture: Anthropological Perspectives*. Oxford: Basil Blackwell.
Tyler, V. E., E. R. Brady, and J. R. Robbers
    1981   *Pharmacognosy*, 8th ed. Philadelphia: Lea and Febinger.
Ullman, Dana, and Stephen Cummings
    1984   *Everybody's Guide to Homeopathic Medicine*. Los Angeles: J. P. Tarcher.
United States Congress, Office of Technology Assessment
    1990   *Unconventional Cancer Treatments*. (Publication #OTA-H-405.) Washington, DC: U. S. Government Printing Office.

Unschuld, Paul U.
1976   "Western Medicine and Traditional Healing Systems: Competition, Cooperation, or Integration?" *Ethics in Science and Medicine* 3(1): 1–20.
Van Deusen, John, Cynthia Coleman, Le Xuan Khoa, Dung Phan, Hong Hoeung Doeung, Kue Chaw, Liet Tat Nguyen, Phuc Pham, and Thao Bounthinh
1980   "Southeast Asian Social and Cultural Customs: Similarities and Differences, Part I." *Journal of Refugee Resettlement* 1(1):20–39.
Van Horne, Winston A., and Thomas V. Tonnesen, eds.
1988   *Ethnicity and Health*. Madison, WI: University of Wisconsin System Institute on Race and Ethnicity.
Van Ness, Paul N.
1986   "Alternative and Holistic Health Care for AIDS and Its Prevention." Washington, DC: Whitman-Walker Clinic.
1988   *Alternative and Holistic Health Care for AIDS and Its Prevention*: A Sourcebook of Descriptions, Bibliography, and Practitioners in the Washington, DC–Baltimore, Maryland Area, rev. ed. Washington, DC: Whitman-Walker Clinic.
Vaskilampi, Tuula
1982   "Culture and Folk Medicine." In T. Vaskilampi and C. MacCormack, eds., *Folk Medicine and Health Culture: Role of Folk Medicine in Modern Health Care*. (Proceedings of the Nordic Research Symposium, 27–28 August 1981, Kuopio, Finland.) Kuopio: University of Kuopio, pp. 2–16.
Vaskilampi, Tuula, and Carol P. MacCormack, eds.
1982   *Folk Medicine and Health Culture: Role of Folk Medicine in Modern Health Care*. (Proceedings of the Nordic Research Symposium, 27–28 August 1981 Kuopio, Finland.) Kuopio: University of Kuopio.
Veatch, Robert M.
1985   "Lay Medical Ethics." *Journal of Medicine and Philosophy* 10:1–5.
1989   *Cross Cultural Perspectives in Medical Ethics: Readings*. Boston: Jones and Bartlett Publishers.
Vogel, Morris J., and Charles E. Rosenberg, eds.
1979   *The Therapeutic Revolution: Essays in the Social History of American Medicine*. Philadelphia: University of Pennsylvania Press.
Vogel, Virgil J.
1970   *American Indian Medicine*. Norman: University of Oklahoma Press.
1976   "American Indian Foods Used as Medicine." In W. Hand, ed., *American Folk Medicine: A Symposium*. Berkeley: University of California Press, 1976:125–142.
von Sydow, Carl Wilhelm
1948   *Selected Papers on Folklore*. Copenhagen: Rosenkilde and Bagger.
Vuori, Hannu
1982   "WHO and Traditional Medicine." In T. Vaskilampi and C. MacCormack, eds., *Folk Medicine and Health Culture: Role of Folk Medicine in Modern Health Care*. (Proceedings of the Nordic Research Symposium, 27–28 August 1981, Kuopio, Finland.) Kuopio: University of Kuopio, pp. 165–189.
Wagenfield, Morton O., Yvonne M. Vissing, Gerald E. Markle, and James C. Petersen
1979   "Notes from the Cancer Underground: Health Attitudes and Prac-

tices of Participants in the Laetrile Movement." *Social Science and Medicine* 13A:483–485.

Wagner, Roy
    1983   "Visible Ideas: Toward an Anthropology of Perceptive Values." *South Asian Anthropologist* 4(1):1–8.

Wallis, Roy, ed.
    1979   *On the Margins of Science: The Social Construction of Rejected Knowledge.* (Sociological Review Monograph 27.) Stoke-on-Trent, Staffordshire, UK: J. H. Brookes (Printers) Limited.

Wardwell, Walter I.
    1972   "Limited, Marginal, and Quasi-Practitioners." In Howard Freeman, Sol Levine, and Leo G. Reeder, eds., *Handbook of Medical Sociology*, 2d ed. Englewood Cliffs, NJ: Prentice-Hall.
    1988   "Chiropractors: Evolution to Acceptance." In Norman Gevitz, ed., *Other Healers: Unorthodox Medicine in America.* Baltimore: Johns Hopkins University Press, pp. 157–191.

Ware, J. E.
    1987   "The Assessment of Health Status." In Linda Aiken and David Mechanic, eds., *Applications of Social Science to Clinical Medicine and Health Policy.* New Brunswick, NJ: Rutgers University Press, pp. 204–228.

Watson, Wilbur H.
    1984   *Black Folk Medicine: The Therapeutic Significance of Faith and Trust.* New Brunswick, NJ: Transaction Books.

Weidman, Hazel H.
    1978   *Miami Health Ecology Report*, Volume I. Miami: University of Miami.
    1982   "Research Strategies, Structural Alterations, and Clinically Relevant Anthropology." In N. J. Chrisman and T. W. Maretzki, eds., *Clinically Applied Anthropology.* Dordrecht, The Netherlands: D. Reidel Publishing Company, pp. 201–242.

Weil, Andrew
    1983   *Health and Healing.* Boston: Houghton Mifflin Company.

Weisz, George, ed.
    1991   *Social Science Perspectives on Medical Ethics.* Philadelphia: University of Pennsylvania Press. (First published 1990 by Kluwer Academic Publishers, Dordrecht, The Netherlands.)

Wexler, Murray
    1976   "The Behavioral Sciences in Medical Education." *American Psychologist* 31(4):275–283.

White, Emma G.
    1963   "Folk Medicine Among the Pennsylvania Germans." *Journal of American Folklore* 76:95–110.

White, Kerr L., D. Andjelkovic, R. J. C. Pearson, J. H. Mabry, A. Ross, and O. K. Sagen
    1967   "International Comparisons of Medical Care Utilization." *New England Journal of Medicine* 277:516–522.

Williams, Raymond
    1976   *Keywords: A Vocabulary of Culture and Society.* New York: Oxford University Press.

Williams, Rory
    1983   "Concepts of Health: An Analysis of Lay Logic." *Sociology* 17:185–205.

Wilson, Charles Bundy
   1908   "Notes on Folk-Medicine." *Journal of American Folklore* 21(80): 68–73.
Wilson, William A.
   1988   "The Deeper Necessity: Folklore and the Humanities." *Journal of American Folklore* 101(400):156–167.
Wolinsky, Fredric D.
   1980   "Alternative Healers and Popular Medicine." In F. D. Wolinsky, ed., *The Sociology of Health*. Boston: Little, Brown and Company, pp. 291–302.
Wolpe, Paul Root
   1985   "The Maintenance of Professional Authority: Acupuncture and the American Physician." *Social Problems* 32:409–424.
Wright, Anne L., and Wayne J. Morgan
   1990   "On the Creation of 'Problem' Patients." *Social Science and Medicine* 30(9):951–959.
Wright, Peter W. G., and Andrew Treacher, eds.
   1982   *The Problem of Medical Knowledge: Examining the Social Construction of Medicine*. Edinburgh: University of Edinburgh Press.
Wyss, Dennis
   1989   "The Underground Test of Compound Q." *Time* 134(October 9): 18, 21.
Yale Council on Southeast Asia Studies
   1986   *The Hmong World*, Volume 1 (Brenda Johns and David Strecker, eds.). New Haven, CT: Yale Southeast Asia Studies (Yale Center for International and Area Studies).
Yap, P.
   1969   "The Culture-Bound Reactive Syndromes." In W. Caudill and T. Lin, eds., *Mental Health Research in Asia and the Pacific*. Honolulu: East-West Center Press, pp. 35–53.
Yeatman, George W., and Viet Van Dang
   1980   "*Cao Gio* [Coin Rubbing]: Vietnamese Attitudes Toward Health Care." *Journal of the American Medical Association* 244:2748–2749.
Yesalis, Charles E., III, Robert B. Wallace, Wayne P. Fisher, and Rodney Tokheim
   1980   "Does Chiropractic Utilization Substitute for Less Available Medical Services?" *American Journal of Public Health* 70:415–417.
Yoder, Don
   1965   "Official Religion Versus Folk Religion." *Pennsylvania Folklife* 15 (Winter 1965–1966):36–52.
   1966   "Twenty Questions on Powwowing." *Pennsylvania Folklife* 15 (Summer 1966):38–40.
   1972   "Folk Medicine." In Richard Dorson, ed., *Folklore and Folklife: An Introduction*. Chicago: University of Chicago Press, pp. 191–215.
   1974   "Towards a Definition of Folk Religion." *Western Folklore* 33(1):2–15.
   1976   "Hohman and Romanus: Origins and Diffusion of the Pennsylvania German Powwow Manual." In Wayland D. Hand, ed., *American Folk Medicine: A Symposium*. Berkeley: University of California Press, pp. 235–248.
Young, Gordon
   1962   *The Hill Tribes of Northern Thailand*. Bangkok: Siam Society.

Zaretsky, Irving J., and Mark P. Leone
  1974   *Religious Movements in Contemporary America*. Princeton, NJ: Princeton University Press.
Zhang, Qingcai, and Hong-yen Hsu
  1990   *AIDS and Chinese Medicine: Applications of the Oldest Medicine to the Newest Disease*. Long Beach, CA: Oriental Healing Arts Institute.
Zinman, J. M.
  1968   *Public Knowledge: An Essay Concerning the Social Dimension of Science*. Cambridge: Cambridge University Press.
Zola, Irving K.
  1972a   "The Concept of Trouble and Sources of Medical Assistance." *Social Science and Medicine* 6:673–679.
  1972b   "Studying the Decision to See a Doctor." *Advances in Psychosomatic Medicine* 8:216–236.

Index

University of Pennsylvania Press
STUDIES IN HEALTH, ILLNESS, AND CAREGIVING
Joan E. Lynaugh, General Editor

Barbara Bates. *Bargaining for Life: A Social History of Tuberculosis, 1876–1938.* 1992

Michael D. Calabria and Janet Macrae, editors. Suggestions for Thought *by Florence Nightingale: Selections and Commentaries.* 1994

Janet Golden and Charles Rosenberg. *Pictures of Health: A Photographic History of Health Care in Philadelphia.* 1991

Anne Hudson Jones. *Images of Nurses: Perspectives from History, Art, and Literature.* 1987

June S. Lowenberg. *Caring and Responsibility: The Crossroads Between Holistic Practice and Traditional Medicine.* 1989

Peggy McGarrahan. *Transcending AIDS: Nurses and HIV Patients in New York City.* 1994

Elizabeth Norman. *Women at War: The Story of Fifty Military Nurses Who Served in Vietnam.* 1990

Bonnie Blair O'Connor. *Healing Traditions: Alternative Medicine and the Health Professions.* 1995

Anne Opie. *There's Nobody There: Community Care of Confused Older People.* 1992

Elizabeth Brown Pryor. *Clara Barton, Professional Angel.* 1987

Margarete Sandelowski. *With Child in Mind: Studies of the Personal Encounter with Infertility.* 1993

Susan L. Smith. *Sick and Tired of Being Sick and Tired: Black Women's Health Activism in America, 1890–1950.* 1995

Nancy Tomes. *The Art of Asylum-Keeping: Thomas Story Kirkbride and the Origins of American Psychiatry.* 1994

Zane Robinson Wolf. *Nurses' Work, The Sacred and The Profane.* 1988

Jacqueline Zalumas. *Caring in Crisis: An Oral History of Critical Care Nursing.* 1995

This book was set in Baskerville and Eras typefaces. Baskerville was designed by John Baskerville at his private press in Birmingham, England, in the eighteenth century. The first typeface to depart from oldstyle typeface design, Baskerville has more variation between thick and thin strokes. In an effort to insure that the thick and thin strokes of his typeface reproduced well on paper, John Baskerville developed the first wove paper, the surface of which was much smoother than the laid paper of the time. The development of wove paper was partly responsible for the introduction of typefaces classified as modern, which have even more contrast between thick and thick strokes.

Eras was designed in 1969 by Studio Hollenstein in Paris for the Wagner Typefoundry. A contemporary script-like version of a sans-serif typeface, the letters of Eras have a monotone stroke and are slightly inclined.

Printed on acid-free paper.